Comments on **Diabetes at your fingertips** *from readers*

"... in style and substance, this is an excellent book. People with and without diabetes will find it very useful. I recommend every diabetic to own a copy of this interesting book."

Mrs T. M[illegible]ndon

"An excellent book. It is comprehen[illegible] read and understand."

[illegible]von

"**Diabetes at your fingertips** is [illegible] the layman needs."

[illegible]rs P. Pilley, Hornchurch

"I like the form it takes (questions and answers); it makes it much easier to find the specific areas when a problem does arise. Also it makes easier reading for picking up and putting down without having to wade through chapter after chapter of heavy medical jargon which for the lay person can be very difficult to take in and understand."

Mrs Pam Munford, Lincoln

"I have read the book myself from cover to cover and found it to be most informative, up-to-date and presented in a format which is easy to assimilate by the majority of people with diabetes who will undoubtedly relate some question to a particular experience of their own – and find the answer."

Philip Whitmore, Macclesfield

"I think the book is excellent value since it answers all the basic questions of diabetes and has answers to questions I have not seen written down before. (In fact the whole family is interested in reading it.)"

D. Ball, Nottingham

"My family have found the information in your book of great value – it has been a godsend in many ways – we hope that it will help many more in the same situation."

Mrs P. Greasley and family, Stoke-on-Trent

Comments on **Diabetes at your fingertips** *from readers*

"... it will be a very useful reference book for patients and health professionals alike."

Mrs Penny Rodie, Dietitian, BUPA Roding Hospital, Ilford

"My father has very long-standing and brittle insulin-dependent diabetes who thought he knew all there was to know about his condition. However, he was clearly most impressed with your book and has found it informative and useful. He is a man who is extremely difficult to impress and you have achieved it. Well done!"

Mrs Rachel Booker, Cheltenham

"Like a good wine, this book has got better and better over the past 10 years and I will certainly recommend it to my patients, as I have the previous editions. I suppose there must be questions which it does not answer, but it is difficult to think what they are. There is even advice on parachuting and scuba diving which are omitted from many other books.

In summary, I think it is brilliant, exactly what one would have expected from the three authors, all of whom I have known for over 20 years."

Robert Tattersall, Professor of Clinical Diabetes,
Queen's Medical Centre, Nottingham

"When I was diagnosed with type 2 diabetes I read every book I could find on diabetes ... then I came across your book in my doctor's surgery. I sat in the reception area when I went for my diabetes induction course and read your whole book in one day – excellent! So well put together and so informative and easy to understand."

Mrs Clare Mehmet, Stratford

"I have found it extremely helpful and informative, and have learned a lot from it ... your book is so good that I hope more diabetics will get a copy."

Mr E R Carr, North Ferriby

Reviews of **Diabetes at your fingertips**

"What sets this book apart from others is the fact that it answers questions that most books dealing with diabetes cannot. It also surprises the reader with questions one perhaps would not even have thought of.

Overall this is a most interesting and useful book suitable for people with diabetes, their families, health professionals and anyone interested in diabetes. It is a book that once bought will be used over and over again, and works out to be good value."

Balance

"**Diabetes at your fingertips** is an extensively revised and updated version of the **Diabetes Reference Book** first published in 1985. The original was an excellent book but this is even better."

Professor Robert Tattersall, Diabetes in the news

"**Diabetes at your fingertips** is a guide, in lively question and answer form, to coping with diabetes. It is quite possible to lead a full life providing the sufferer understands and can control the disease."

Woman's Journal

"Has positive information to help both young and old lead active lives with the minimum of restrictions."

Good Housekeeping

"I would recommend it to people living with diabetes, but also to professionals in the diabetes field."

Professional Nurse

"The book is well presented, with good, clear illustrations and is reasonably priced. I highly recommend it for people newly diagnosed with diabetes and their families and as a source of reference for nurses dealing with diabetes."

Nursing Standard

"Woe betide any clinicians or nurses whose patients have read this invaluable source of down-to-earth information when they have not."

The Lancet

"Its strength is that it complements existing texts and is rooted in the practical day-to-day problems and care of people with diabetes. I am sure that it will be immensely useful to general practitioners and practice nurses as well as people with diabetes and their families."

Dr Colin Waine, former President of the Royal College of General Practitioners

Reviews of **Diabetes at your fingertips**

"Its question-and-answer format is easy to read and highly informative. Neither do the authors pull any punches – everything is factual and up to date. Nor is the book only of use to those with diabetes – it would make a very useful addition to General Practice bookshelves and hospital libraries. Look out doctors and nurses who have not perused this edition when confronted by someone who has."

Diabetes Wellness

"It seems that anything and everything about diabetes is mentioned in this book and the breadth of topics covered is highlighted in the 26-page index ... Overall this is a comprehensive, reasonably priced book that would be useful for anyone who lives or works with diabetes."

Practical Diabetes International

"This text would be of use to health care workers, teachers and people wanting to gain more knowledge about diabetes. It would also be a useful introductory reader for student nurses and I recommend a copy for all nursing and public libraries."

Journal of Community Nursing

Diabetes at your fingertips

THE COMPREHENSIVE AND MEDICALLY ACCURATE MANUAL WHICH TELLS YOU ALL ABOUT YOUR DIABETES AND HOW TO BEAT IT!

FOURTH EDITION

Peter Sönksen MD, FRCP
Professor of Endocrinology, Guy's, King's and St Thomas' Hospitals' School of Medicine, St Thomas' Hospital, London

Charles Fox BM, FRCP
Consultant Physician with Special Interest in Diabetes, Northampton General Hospital

Sue Judd RGN
Formerly Specialist Nurse in Diabetes, St Thomas' Hospital, London

CLASS PUBLISHING • LONDON

Printing history
First published 1985
Reprinted 1987
Second Edition, revised and expanded 1991
Reprinted with revisions 1991
Reprinted with revisions 1992
Third edition, revised and expanded 1994
Reprinted 1995, 1996
Reprinted with revisions 1997
Fourth edition, revised and expanded, 1998
Reprinted with revisions 1999
Reprinted with revisions 2001
Reprinted 2002

The authors and publishers welcome feedback from the users of this book.
Please contact the publishers.
Class Publishing, Barb House, Barb Mews, London W6 7PA, UK
Telephone: 020 7371 2119
Fax: 020 7371 2878 [International +4420]
Email: post@class.co.uk
www.class.co.uk

A CIP catalogue record for this book is available from the British Library

ISBN 1 872362 79 6

Designed by Wendy Bann

Edited by Michèle Clarke

Indexed by Valerie Elliston

Cartoons by Michelle Smith (ducks) and Christine Syme (foot care)

Line illustrations by David Woodroffe

Production by Landmark Production Consultants Ltd, Princes Risborough

Typesetting by DP Photosetting, Aylesbury, Bucks

Colour separation by Fotographics Ltd, Hong Kong

Printed and bound in Finland by WS Bookwell, Juva

Contents

Preface xi
Foreword by Sir Harry Secombe CBE xiii
Foreword by Professor Harry Keen CBE, MD, FRCP xv
Acknowledgements xvii

INTRODUCTION 1
How to use this book 2

CHAPTER 1 ***Diabetes***
Introduction 4
Symptoms 5
Types of diabetes 8
Causes of diabetes 9
Inheritance 14
Physiology 16

CHAPTER 2 ***Treatment without insulin***
Introduction 21
Diet 22
Overweight 33
Tablets 37
Non-medical treatments 44

CHAPTER 3 ***Treatment with insulin***
Introduction 48
Insulin 49

Diet and insulin 60
Injection technique 68
Injection sites 72
Insulin pens 75
Pumps and injectors 77
Practical aspects 80
Hypos 84

CHAPTER 4 ***Monitoring and control***
Introduction 92
Control and monitoring 94
Blood glucose 98
Urine 108
Haemoglobin A_{1c} and fructosamine 113
Diabetes clinics 116
Brittle diabetes 121

CHAPTER 5 ***Life with diabetes***
Introduction 123
Sports 124
Eating out 127
Holidays and travel 128
Work 134
Other illnesses 137
Hospital operations 142
Driving 143
Alcohol 147
Drugs 150
Smoking 153
Prescription charges and Social Security benefits 155
Miscellaneous 157

CHAPTER 6 ***Sex, contraception and HRT***
Introduction 162
Impotence 163
The pill, IUD and vasectomy 167
Thrush 170
Hormone replacement therapy (HRT) 171

Termination of pregnancy 173
Infertility 173

CHAPTER 7 ***Pregnancy***
Introduction 174
Prepregnancy 176
Management 178
Complications 182

CHAPTER 8 ***Diabetes in the young***
Introduction 187
The baby with diabetes 188
The child with diabetes 191
Diabetes and the adolescent 200

CHAPTER 9 ***Long-term complications***
Introduction 205
General questions 207
Eyes 211
Feet, chiropody and footwear 218
Kidneys 226
Nerves 228
Heart and blood vessel disease 232
Blood pressure 234
The mind 234

CHAPTER 10 ***Research and the future***
Introduction 236
Searching for causes and cures 237
Transplantation 240
Insulin pumps and artificial pancreas 242
New insulin and oral insulin 244
New technology 246

CHAPTER 11 ***Self-help groups***
Introduction 248
The British Diabetic Association 249
Tadpole Club 251

Youth Diabetes (YD) Project 251

CHAPTER 12 ***Emergencies***
Introduction 253
What every person on insulin must know 254
What other people must know about diabetes 254
Foods to eat in an emergency or when feeling unwell 255
Signs and symptoms of hypoglycaemia and hyperglycaemia 255

GLOSSARY 257

APPENDIX 1
Blood glucose meters 265

APPENDIX 2
Useful publications 268

APPENDIX 3 Useful addresses 270

INDEX 273

Preface to the Fourth Edition

The Diabetes Reference Book first appeared in 1985 and was republished after major revision as *Diabetes at your fingertips* in 1991. The book provides quick straightforward answers to the questions asked by people with diabetes and those who live with them and care for them. The time has come for a third revision, for although much remains stable in the field of diabetes care, there have been significant improvements in many of the technologies available to people with diabetes.

The results of a major American research trial on the relationship between diabetes control and outcome have also been published. In the Diabetes Control and Complications Trial (DCCT), it has been conclusively shown that good control does matter. Since our previous edition of *Diabetes at your fingertips*, diabetes care has partly moved away from specialist hospital centres towards family doctors and practice nurses. We support this trend provided of course the doctors and nurses keep themselves abreast of improvements in diabetes care. People with diabetes will also want to keep themselves up to date and well-informed and we hope this new edition will be of help to them.

We are not sure what ducks are doing in a book about diabetes but we like them and hope you do too.

Foreword

by Sir HARRY SECOMBE CBE

President, Diabetes UK

Everyone knows the importance of education in our lives, but if you have diabetes, then learning certainly becomes a way of life.

As someone with diabetes, I realise the more I know about the condition and the way it affects me, the healthier I stay.

So I have no hesitation in commending this book, compiled by people whose active involvement with diabetes is an example to everyone.

Harry Secombe

Foreword

by Professor HARRY KEEN CBE MD FRCP

Hon President International Diabetes Federation; Vice President Diabetes UK; Chairman WHO Expert Committee on Diabetes; Emeritus Professor and Consultant Physician, GKT School of Medicine, King's College, Guy's Hospital Campus, London

The message of the new edition of this diabetes 'enquire within' is that although many of the problems are still with us, medical science moves forward. Most of the questions stay the same but many of the answers have changed. The outlook for people with diabetes improves year by year. We can see real progress in the management of the diabetic state itself and in the treatment, control and prevention of its fearful complications: blindness, kidney failure, artery obstruction and nerve damage. These advances are clearly brought to the reader of *Diabetes at your fingertips*.

One thing remains unchanged, the absolute necessity for people with diabetes to learn and understand as much as they can about their disease. With diabetes, ignorance is often damaging and can sometimes be lethal. Understanding diabetes is, in itself, not enough; something must be done with that understanding – by doctors, nurses, dietitians and the whole team gathered to fight the diabetes, but most of all by the patient. He or she, young or not so young, makes a vital contribution to diabetes care. Without that contribution the work and efforts of the others are incomplete. *Diabetes at your fingertips* will help people with diabetes to take their proper place in the front rank of the fight for better health.

Harry Keen

Acknowledgements

We are grateful to all the people who helped in the production of past editions of *Diabetes at your fingertips* or the original *Diabetes Reference Book*: Maureen Brewin, Jenny Dyer, Anna Fox, Professor Harry Keen, Julia Kidd, Lis Lawrence, Pat McDowell, Sara Moore, Sheila Nicholass, Sir Harry Secombe, Michelle Smith and Peter Swift.

We should also like to thank the following people for their contributions to the third edition:

Gill Jowett for revising the section on feet;
Clara Lowy for contributing to the chapter on pregnancy;
Jill Metcalfe for the section on diet;
Suzanne Lucas at Diabetes UK for valuable comments;
Judith North and Janet Waterston for very helpful and practical suggestions;
Christine Syme for the cartoons on foot care.

Prue Richardson made a major contribution to this new fourth edition, and Dawn Kenwright gave us advice about running, for which we are very grateful.

We thank the companies who kindly provided illustrations:

Bayer Diagnostics
Becton Dickinson UK Ltd
LifeScan
Eli Lilly Diabetes Care Division
MediSense Britain Ltd
Novo Nordisk UK
Roche Diagnostics UK Ltd

We thank also the long-suffering patients at St Thomas' Hospital and Northampton General Hospital. They have asked many of the questions and have worked out solutions to most of the problems. We are simply passing on their experience to others. Finally, many thanks to all those who have written in for advice. Some of their questions have been incorporated.

Peter Sönksen
Charles Fox
Sue Judd

Introduction

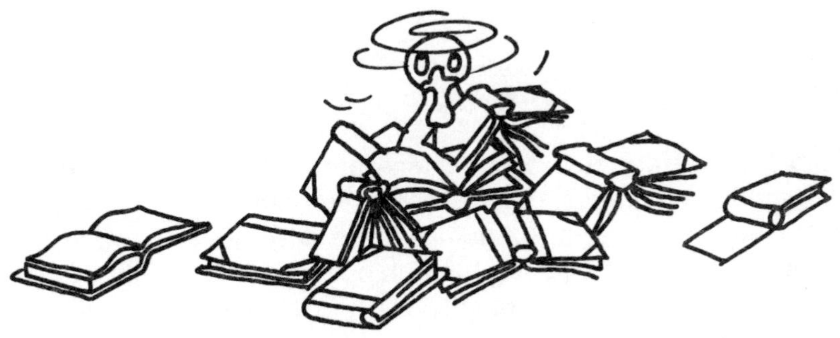

When diabetes suddenly hits you or a close relative, many unpleasant things come to mind ... injections, strict diets, urine tests, blindness. In fact most people with diabetes do not need injections, their diet is normal and wholesome, urine tests have gone out of fashion and eye disease can now be successfully treated. However, people do have to learn to control their diabetes and they can do this only by understanding the condition. Much advice and help comes from nurses, doctors, dietitians and others, but how well the condition is controlled is each individual's own decision. A lot of effort is being put into diabetes education and this book is part of that effort. There is a great deal of information for all of us to learn.

Diabetes is a complex disorder, and parts of this book reflect its complexity. Although some aspects of diabetes are hard to understand, most people manage to lead full lives by incorporating their condition into their normal work and activities. If you have just discovered that you (or a close relative) have diabetes, you will probably feel shocked and worried. This is not the time to try to learn about the most difficult aspects of the subject. But even at this early stage you, your partner, and your parents if you are a child, need to know certain basic facts. Once the initial shock reaction is over and your own experience with diabetes increases, you will be ready to learn about the frills. Remember that no one involved in this subject (including doctors and nurses) ever stops learning more about it.

How to use this book

This book is a series of questions and answers, and it is not designed to be read from cover to cover. Some of the sections do stand on their own, in particular those describing the nature of diabetes in Chapter 1, Chapter 4 on control of diabetes and Chapter 9 on long-term complications. A colour plate section on techniques for injection and blood glucose monitoring is included in the centre of the book.

If you are newly diagnosed, you may not be ready to come to grips with Chapter 10 on research but you may want to find out what is known about the causes of diabetes (in Chapter 1). If you have just started insulin injections you should read the following sections at an early stage:

Hypos (in Chapter 3)
Other illnesses (in Chapter 5)
Insulin (in Chapter 3)
Control and monitoring (in Chapter 4)
Blood glucose (in Chapter 4)
Driving (in Chapter 5)
Emergencies (in Chapter 12)

More experienced people will want to test us out in our answers in Chapter 5 on life with diabetes to see if our answers coincide with their own experience. Parents of children with diabetes will want to read Chapter 8 on diabetes in the young.

There is bound to be some repetition in a book of this sort, but we think it is better to deal with similar topics under separate headings rather than ask the reader to shuffle from one end of the book to the other. We hope that at least we are consistent in our answers.

Feedback is the most important feature of good diabetes care. This relies on people being honest with the doctor or nurse and vice versa. Not everyone will agree with the answers we give, but the book can only be improved if you let us know when you disagree and have found our advice to be unhelpful. We would also like to know if there are important questions we have not covered. Please write to us c/o Class Publishing, Barb House, Barb Mews, London W6 7PA, UK.

1
Diabetes

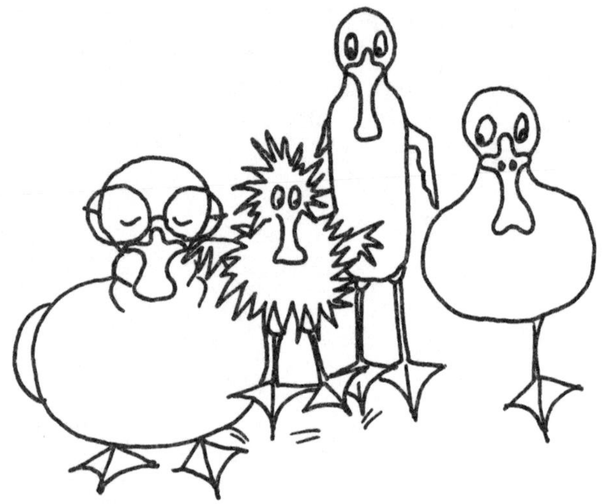

Introduction

This chapter opens with a description of how someone with diabetes might feel before the condition was diagnosed and treated. Once treatment has been started, people with diabetes should feel perfectly well. We also make the point that older people may have diabetes and yet feel quite well in themselves. In this case the condition will be discovered only if they have a routine blood or urine test for glucose, and diabetes may therefore exist for many years without being discovered. Unfortunately, undetected diabetes may, over a long period, lead to complications affecting eyes, nerves and blood vessels.

There are two main types of people with diabetes: younger people who feel unwell for a few weeks or months and who may become very ill if they do not receive insulin; and older people who may have had diabetes for many years before it was discovered and who do not feel particularly unwell. Diabetes in older people is often discovered by chance and commonly responds well to diet or tablets, although sometimes insulin is needed. There are other rare types of diabetes, and we also mention them in this chapter.

We also answer some very important questions about the central problem in diabetes, which is an increase in the amount of glucose (sugar) in the blood. We describe why this happens and why it may be dangerous.

Symptoms

Why does someone of my son's age (he is 11) feel thirsty when their diabetes is first discovered?

The first signs of diabetes in a young person are thirst and loss of weight. These two symptoms are related and one leads to the other (we deal in more detail with weight loss in the answer to the next question). The first thing to go wrong is the increased amount of urine. Normally we pass about 1½ litres (just over 2 pints) of urine per day but someone who has uncontrolled diabetes may produce five times that amount. This continual loss of fluid dries out the body. Feeling thirsty is a warning that, unless they drink enough to replace the extra urine, they will soon be in trouble.

Of course people who do not have diabetes may also pass large amounts of urine. Every beer drinker knows the effects of 5 pints of best bitter! In this case the beer causes the extra urine, whereas in diabetes the extra urine causes the thirst. The resulting thirst is usually mild in the early stages, and most people fail to realise its significance unless they happen to have a friend or relative with diabetes. Someone with undiagnosed diabetes may take jugs of water up to bed, wake in the night to quench their thirst and pass water, and still not realise that something is wrong. It would be a good thing if more people knew that unexplained thirst can be due to diabetes.

Why do people often lose weight before their diabetes is brought under control?

The main fuel for the body is glucose which is obtained from the digestion of sugary or starchy food. People with untreated diabetes have too much glucose in their bodies and this glucose overflows into the urine. Body tissues get broken down to form glucose and ketones, and this causes weight loss.

Someone who has uncontrolled diabetes may lose as much as 1000 g (just over 2 lb) of glucose (sugar) in their urine in 24 hours. Anyone trying to lose weight knows that sugar = calories. These calories contained in the urine are lost to the body and are a drain on its resources. The 1000 g of glucose lost are equivalent to 20 currant buns (4000 calories per day).

Why do I experience itching and soreness around my genitals?

A woman whose diabetes is out of control may be troubled by itching around her vagina. The technical name for this distressing symptom is *pruritus vulvae*. The equivalent complaint may be seen in men when the end of the penis becomes sore (*balanitis*). If the foreskin is also affected, it may become thickened (*phimosis*), which prevents the foreskin from being pulled back. This makes it impossible to keep the penis clean.

These problems are the result of infection with yeasts which thrive on the high concentration of glucose in this region. If you keep your urine free from glucose by good control of your diabetes, the itching and soreness will normally clear up. Anti-yeast cream from your doctor may speed up the improvement but this is only a holding measure while the glucose is cleared from your urine.

Can the eyesight be affected early on in diabetes?

Most of the serious eye problems caused by diabetes are due to damage to the retina (*retinopathy*). The retina is the 'photographic plate' at the back of the eye. Even minor changes in the retina take years to develop and are never seen early on in the disease in younger people. Older people may have diabetes for years without being aware of it, and in these cases the retina may already be damaged by the time the condition is discovered.

The lens of the eye which is responsible for focusing the image on the retina can also be affected in diabetes. However, this is usually a temporary change that causes blurred vision which can be corrected by wearing glasses. The lens of the eye becomes swollen when diabetes is out of control and this makes the person short-sighted. As the diabetes comes under control, so the lens of the eye returns to its normal shape. A pair of glasses fitted for a swollen lens at a time of uncontrolled diabetes will no longer be suitable when the diabetes is brought under control. A newly diagnosed person with blurred vision should wait until a few months after things have settled down before visiting an optician for new spectacles. The blurred vision will probably improve on its own, and glasses may not be necessary.

In very rare cases the lens of the eye may be permanently damaged (cataract) when diabetes is badly out of control.

You will find more information about the effect of diabetes on the eyes in the section on **Eyes** in Chapter 9.

Can diabetes be discovered by chance?

Yes, but this usually happens only in older people. In young people the diagnosis is usually made because someone feels unwell and goes to the doctor.

In older people with no obvious medical problems, diabetes is often discovered as a result of a routine urine test – sometimes during an insurance examination. Once the diagnosis is made, the person may admit to feeling slightly thirsty or tired or to having itching (pruritus), but these symptoms are often not very dramatic, and they may have been put down to 'old age'. So in older people diabetes can take a less obvious form. Even though this type of diabetes seems to be a minor problem, it must be taken very seriously, as so-called 'mild' diabetes can still lead to problems with vision and circulation. In any case, most people feel much better and more energetic once their diabetes is controlled. This can often be done by diet or by diet and tablets, although insulin injections are occasionally needed.

Types of diabetes

Are there different types of diabetes?

Yes, diabetes exists in many different forms. Two main groups are recognized.

- Younger people (under 40 years old) in whom the condition develops in a fairly dramatic way and for whom insulin injections are nearly always needed. About 30% of all people with diabetes fall into this category, known as type 1 diabetes (or insulin dependent diabetes, IDD for short; or juvenile-onset diabetes).
- At the other end of the scale is the older person who develops diabetes with less obvious symptoms and who is often overweight. In this group insulin by injection is not normally needed and these people are described as having type 2 diabetes (or non-insulin dependent diabetes, NIDD for short; or maturity-onset diabetes).

There are plenty of exceptions to this rule. Occasionally young people can be well controlled with diet or tablets and quite a large number of people who develop diabetes late in life are much better off on insulin injections.

What is diabetes insipidus?

The only connection between *diabetes insipidus* and the more common form of diabetes (where the full name is *diabetes mellitus*) is that people with both conditions pass large amounts of urine. Diabetes insipidus is a rare condition that is due to an abnormality in the pituitary gland and not the pancreas. One disorder does not lead to the other, and diabetes insipidus does not have the same potential for long-term complications as diabetes mellitus.

My wife has just given birth to a baby boy who weighed 4.3 kg (9 lb) at birth. Apparently she may have had diabetes while she was pregnant. Is this likely to happen again with her next baby?

Women who give birth to heavy babies (over 4 kg or 9 lb) may have had a raised blood glucose level during pregnancy. This extra glucose crosses into the unborn baby, who responds by producing extra insulin on its own. The combination of excess glucose and excess insulin makes the unborn baby grow fat and bloated. Once it has been born and cut off from its supply of glucose from the mother, the baby may then become *hypoglycaemic* (develop a low glucose concentration in the blood). These fat babies of mothers with diabetes are definitely at risk of hypoglycaemia.

Women like your wife who develop diabetes during pregnancy and who then return to normal after their babies are born have what is known as *gestational diabetes*. Now the problem has been identified she will have to keep a close check on her blood glucose during her next pregnancy. Providing it is kept strictly normal (insulin may be needed for this), the baby will be a normal weight and will not be at risk.

Women who have diabetes during pregnancy are slightly more likely to develop diabetes later in life.

Causes of diabetes

Why have I got diabetes?

The short answer is that your pancreas is no longer making enough insulin for your body's needs. The long answer as to why this has happened to you is not so well understood. However, there are a few clues. Diabetes may run in families (see the next section on ***Inheritance***). Other possible causes are discussed here in this section. It is not a rare condition. In England, about 1 in 50 of the population is known to have diabetes and perhaps an equal number of people actually have the disease but are unaware of it. We say this because, whenever a whole population is carefully screened for diabetes, many new patients are discovered, usually in the proportion of one new patient for every patient that is known already. About 3 children per 1000 have diabetes and there is good evidence that the risk is increasing, particularly in very young children below the age of 5 years.

Is diabetes caused by a virus?

Despite a vast amount of research throughout the world the cause of diabetes is not known. It is known that in some families there is a tendency towards diabetes (see the next section on ***Inheritance***) and that the disease in young people often develops when triggered off by some infection such as a cold. Some people suspect that a certain virus could actually cause diabetes but there is no proof. If a virus is the cause, it is probably a common one (like Coxsackie B) which leads to diabetes only in susceptible people (i.e. those who have inherited some tendency towards diabetes). Research workers have suggested that full-blown diabetes may not be discovered for several years after the 'trigger' infection has occurred.

There is certainly no 'diabetes virus' and you cannot catch diabetes like chicken-pox. Diabetes in older people is probably nothing to do with a virus infection.

Can fatness cause diabetes?

If the tendency towards diabetes is present, then fatness (obesity) may bring on the disease. This does not happen often in young people, but it is a common cause of diabetes in middle-aged or older people. In most cases this type of diabetes can be controlled by dieting and weight loss. Many fat people with diabetes find it hard to lose weight; others find that strict dieting alone is insufficient to lower the blood glucose and have to take tablets or insulin injections. This is second-best as the sensible and safe treatment for an overweight older person is weight loss.

You will find more information about diet and diabetes and being overweight in Chapter 2.

Can a bad shock bring on diabetes?

Sometimes diabetes develops soon after a major disturbance in life, such as a bereavement, a heart attack, or a bad accident and the diabetes is blamed on the upset. This is not really the case, as insulin failure in the pancreas takes a long time to develop. However, a bad shock may stress someone's system and bring on diabetes a bit earlier if the insulin supply is already running low.

Do large babies cause their mother to develop diabetes?

No, it's the other way round. In pregnancy even very 'mild' diabetes, which may not be detected without special tests, may result in an overweight baby. In any woman who has given birth to a baby weighing more than 4 kg (9 lb), the possibility of diabetes should be considered by her doctors. If a mother has diabetes during pregnancy but recovers soon after her baby is born, she does carry an increased risk of diabetes for the rest of her life. The baby itself does not carry this risk.

Diabetes and pregnancy are dealt with in detail in Chapter 7.

Can diabetes be prevented?

No. At the present time, if you are going to get diabetes, you get diabetes. It is possible, under certain circumstances, to identify some people who do not have diabetes but who have a very high risk of developing it within a year or so. Various drugs have been tried to prevent diabetes in these high-risk people, but so far with no lasting success.

Can tablets or medicines cause diabetes or make diabetes worse?

Yes, there are several drugs in common use that can either precipitate diabetes as an unwanted side effect or make existing diabetes worse. The most important group of such medicines are hormones.

Hormones are substances produced by special glands in the body and insulin from the pancreas is itself a hormone. Some hormones have an anti-insulin effect and one of these, a steroid hormone, is sometimes used in treating medical conditions, such as severe asthma or rheumatoid arthritis. The most commonly used steroid is prednisolone which opposes insulin and therefore tends to cause the level of glucose in the blood to rise. Steroids in large doses will often precipitate diabetes which usually gets better when the steroids are stopped.

The contraceptive pill is another type of steroid hormone with a very mild anti-insulin effect. Sometimes people on insulin find they have to give themselves more insulin if they are on the pill.

Glucagon is a hormone from the pancreas with a very strong anti-insulin effect. It is used to correct a severe insulin reaction (see the section on ***Hypos*** in Chapter 3 for how and when to use glucagon).

Apart from other hormones, certain medicines may have an anti-insulin effect. In particular, water tablets (diuretics) which make people pass extra amounts of urine sometimes precipitate diabetes.

I have recently been given steroid treatment (prednisone) for severe arthritis. My joints are better but my doctor has now found sugar in my urine and tells me I have diabetes. Is this likely to be permanent?

Steroids are very effective treatment for a number of conditions but they may lead to side effects, as you have just discovered. One of these side effects is to cause diabetes which can usually be controlled with tablets (e.g. glibenclamide). Insulin is not normally required. When you stop steroid therapy there is a good chance that the diabetes will go away completely.

However, you may have had diabetes without knowing it before you started on steroids, in which case you will always have diabetes and will need to continue some form of treatment for it indefinitely.

I am told that other hormones apart from insulin may cause diabetes. Is this true?

It is a deficiency of the hormone insulin that leads to diabetes. If certain other hormones (chemical messengers) are produced in excessive amounts in the body then diabetes may result. Thus someone who produces too much thyroid hormone (*thyrotoxicosis*) may develop diabetes which clears up when their thyroid is restored to normal. Thyrotoxicosis and diabetes tend to run together in families, and people with one of these conditions are more likely to develop the other.

Sometimes a person will produce excessive quantities of steroid hormones (*Cushing's disease* or Cushing's syndrome), and this may lead to diabetes (see the previous two questions for the connection between steroids and diabetes). *Acromegaly* is a condition where excess quantities of growth hormone are produced and this too may lead to diabetes.

Can a severe illness cause diabetes?

Any serious condition (e.g. coronary thrombosis or severe injuries from a traffic accident) may lead to diabetes. This is because most of the hormones produced in response to stress tend to have the opposite effect to insulin and cause the glucose level in the blood to rise. Most people simply produce more insulin to keep the blood glucose stable. However, in some cases, if the reserves of insulin are inadequate, the blood glucose level will climb. Such a person has temporary diabetes, and the glucose level will usually return to normal once the stress is over. However, he or she will have an increased risk of developing permanent diabetes later on in life.

I have had to go to hospital for repeated attacks of pancreatitis and now have diabetes. I am told these two conditions are related – is this true?

Pancreatitis means that your pancreas has become inflamed and this can be a very painful and unpleasant illness. The pancreas is the gland which, among other things, produces insulin and if it becomes badly inflamed and scarred it may not be able to produce enough of this hormone. Sometimes someone – like you – develops diabetes during or after an attack of pancreatitis and they then need tablets or insulin to keep their blood glucose controlled. This form of diabetes is usually, but not always, permanent.

Do other diseases increase the chances of getting diabetes?

Yes, and they fall into four groups.

- The first group is glandular disorders, in particular thyrotoxicosis (overactive thyroid), acromegaly (excess growth hormone) and Cushing's disease or syndrome (excess steroid hormone).
- The second group is diseases of the pancreas, including pancreatitis, cancer of the pancreas, haemochromatosis (iron overload) and cystic fibrosis (a serious inherited childhood

disorder). Surgical removal of the pancreas (for either pancreatitis or cancer) also causes diabetes.

- The third group is virus diseases such as rubella (German measles) and mumps, but these rarely lead to diabetes. Another type of virus, Coxsackie virus, just may be involved as a possible cause of diabetes.
- The fourth and final group includes problems which put stress on the body, such as heart attacks, pneumonia, and major surgical operations. The diabetes usually clears up when the stress is removed.

You will find more information about the relationships between these disorders and diabetes in other questions earlier in this chapter.

Inheritance

Does diabetes run in families?

Diabetes is a common disorder which in this country has been diagnosed in about 1 in 100 people (which means that it affects about 1 in 50 people, but in half of them it has not yet been diagnosed). So in any large family more than one person may be affected, simply by chance alone. However, certain families do seem to carry a very strong tendency for diabetes. The best known example of this is a whole tribe of American Indians (the Pima): over half its members develop diabetes by the time they reach middle age.

Genes are the parts of a human cell that decide which characteristics you inherit from your parents. The particular genes that you get from each parent are a matter of chance – in other words, whether you grow up with your father's big feet or your mother's blue eyes. Similarly it is a matter of chance whether you pass on the genes carrying the tendency for diabetes to one of your children. It is *only* the tendency to diabetes which you may pass on – the full-blown condition will *not* develop unless something else causes the insulin cells in the pancreas to fail. If you are a father with diabetes there is probably a 1 in 20 chance that your child will develop diabetes at some stage. If you are a mother with diabetes the risk lessens to about 1 in 50.

If diabetes is known to be in the family, can other members of the family take any preventive action?

The inheritance of diabetes is a complicated subject – indeed different sorts of diabetes appear to be inherited in different ways. For instance, a tendency for one sort of diabetes (type 1) can be inherited, but only a small proportion of the people who inherit this tendency will go on to develop diabetes. It is now possible to tell if these people at risk have inherited the family of relevant genes, and to a certain extent their chances of developing diabetes can be predicted.

The more common type 2 diabetes, often treated by diet or by diet and tablets, is only rarely associated with known single gene abnormality but is thought to be strongly inherited in many cases. Indeed when we have learnt more about it, it may well prove that there are several different sub-types which cannot be distinguished from one another – all inherited in different ways. We do know that many of these people are overweight and that obesity not only makes diabetes worse but it may even lead to its appearance in susceptible people.

There is no really effective action other family members can take except to follow the usual health advice to keep physically active, eat a balanced diet and avoid becoming overweight. It is worth bearing in mind the slight possibility that someone else in your family may develop diabetes – especially if they ignore this advice. Their urine or blood should be tested as soon as they develop any symptoms which you may think relevant, so that the diabetes can be detected and treated early on.

I am 16 and have had diabetes for five years. Why has my identical twin brother not got diabetes?

A large study has been carried out in which examples of identical twins with diabetes have been collected for over 20 years. These results show an interesting difference between young people who need insulin and older people who usually manage on diet alone or on diet and tablets. If you have an identical twin who is a young person on insulin, then you only have a 50% chance of developing diabetes yourself. On the other hand, the identical twin of a middle-aged person with diabetes who does not need insulin is almost 100% certain to get the same sort of diabetes. So in your case your twin brother has an evens chance of developing diabetes.

Physiology

What is the pancreas?

The pancreas is a gland situated in the upper part of the abdomen and connected by a fine tube to the intestine (see Figure 1.1). One of its functions is to release digestive juices which are mixed with the food soon after it leaves the stomach. They are needed for food to be digested and absorbed into the body. This part of the pancreas has nothing to do with diabetes.

The pancreas also produces a number of hormones which are released directly into the blood stream, unlike the digestive juices

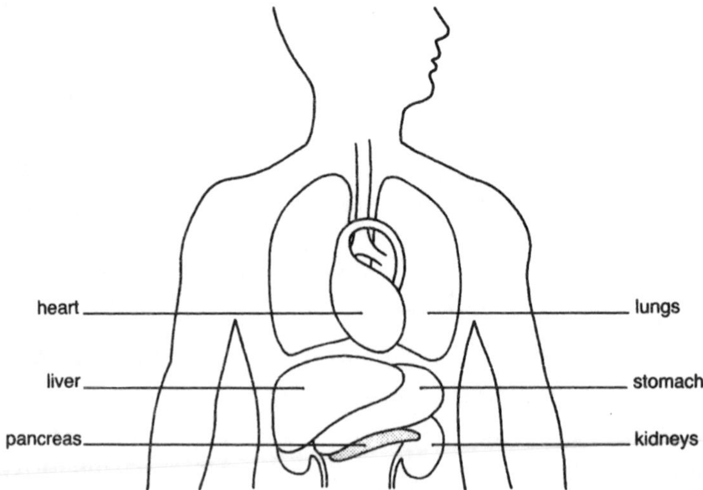

Figure 1.1 Location of the pancreas

which pass into the intestine. The most important of these hormones is insulin, lack of which causes diabetes. The other important hormone produced by the pancreas is glucagon which has the opposite action to insulin and may be used in correcting serious hypos (see the section on ***Hypos*** in Chapter 3 for more information about this). Both of these hormones come from a part of the pancreas known as the islets of Langerhans.

Is diabetes a disease of modern times?

No. The earliest detailed description of diabetes was made 2000 years ago. Diabetes appears to be more common now than in the past, partly because cases which would not have been picked up then are nowadays detected by routine check-ups. There is a suggestion that diabetes in younger people may be occurring more frequently.

Why does the body need insulin?

Without insulin the body cannot make full use of food that is eaten. Normally, food is eaten, taken into the body and broken down into simple chemicals (one of which is glucose) which then provide fuel for all the activities of the body. These simple chemicals also provide building blocks for growth or replacing worn-out parts, and any extra is stored for later use. In diabetes food is broken down as normal, but because of the shortage of insulin the excess glucose produced is not stored but accumulates in the blood stream and spills over into the urine. Insulin ensures the correct balance between glucose production in the body and its utilization.

How does insulin control the supply of fuel?

Food is a mixture of complex materials which are absorbed into the body and broken down to various simple chemicals. This takes place in the liver which can be regarded as a food processing factory. Glucose is one of the simple chemicals made in the liver from all carbohydrate foods. In the absence of insulin, glucose pours out of the liver into the blood stream. Insulin switches off this outpouring of glucose from the liver and causes glucose to be stored in the liver as starch or glycogen. Insulin also helps glucose to get inside some cells where it is used as a fuel.

So, if there is not enough insulin, glucose will pour out of the liver into the blood stream and have difficulty getting into some cells. This causes a build-up of glucose in the blood. Insulin has a similar effect on amino acids and fatty acids which are the breakdown products of protein and fat respectively.

How do people who do not have diabetes get their insulin?

Insulin is stored in the pancreas and is released into the blood stream immediately the blood glucose level starts to rise after eating. It is taken straight to the liver where it has the important effect of stopping glucose production and promoting the storage of glucose as glycogen. The level of glucose in the blood then falls and, as it does so, insulin production is switched off. So people who do not have diabetes have a very sensitive system for keeping the amount of glucose in the blood at a steady level.

The slightest rise in blood glucose causes insulin to be produced. This in turn brings down the glucose level, and the insulin is switched off (see Figure 1.2).

In diabetes this system is faulty. People with less severe diabetes have some insulin but the pancreas cannot produce it fast enough or in sufficient amounts, so the blood glucose level goes up. Other people have little or no insulin of their own and need injections of insulin to try to keep the blood glucose level normal.

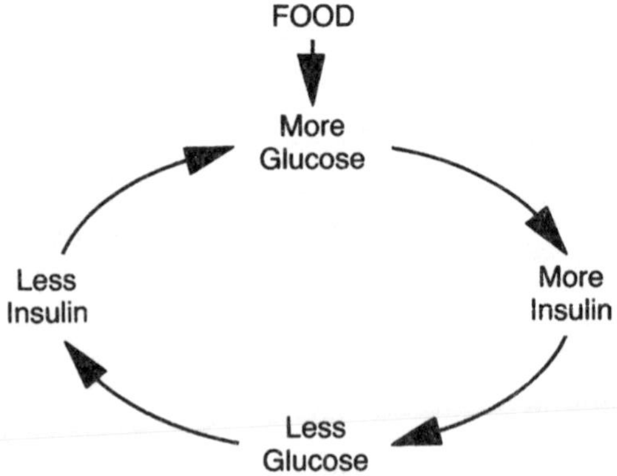

Figure 1.2 Insulin production system

Obviously, an injection of insulin once or twice a day is not as efficient at regulating blood glucose as the pancreas which can switch insulin supply on or off at a moment's notice in response to mild fluctuations.

I take insulin. Can I keep my blood glucose at a normal level?

Yes, although it may not be easy and can only be done by means of a balancing act.

There are three main things which affect your blood glucose: (i) food (which puts it up); (ii) insulin; and (iii) exercise (which both bring it down). Any form of stress, in particular an illness like flu, puts up your blood glucose. The only way of learning how to balance your blood glucose level is by trial and error. This means you making a lot of measurements and discovering how various foods and forms of exercise alter your blood glucose.

In the past, people were brought into hospital to be 'stabilized' on a certain dose of insulin. Experience has shown that the insulin needed in the artificial surroundings of a hospital ward may bear little relation to the amount needed in someone leading an active life in the outside world. Nowadays, you can 'stabilize' your own diabetes at home yourself. You will find information to help you do this in Chapter 3 on ***Treatment with insulin*** and Chapter 4 on ***Monitoring and control***.

How can diabetes cause 'fatty liver'? What treatment should be given and is there anything one can do to help reverse the situation?

The liver may sometimes be enlarged in cases of poorly controlled diabetes, owing to a build up of fatty tissue within the substance of the liver. The reason for fat accumulation is not understood but the liver responds in this way to a number of insults (such as alcohol). Insulin plays an important part in the metabolism of fat and, when the insulin supply is deficient, the levels in the blood of both glucose and fat may rise very high. This in turn may cause fat to be laid down in the liver.

'Fatty liver' is more common in children and young people with poorly controlled diabetes and sometimes the liver may become greatly enlarged. The only treatment is to improve control of the diabetes, following which the liver will steadily shrink back to its normal size.

2
Treatment without insulin

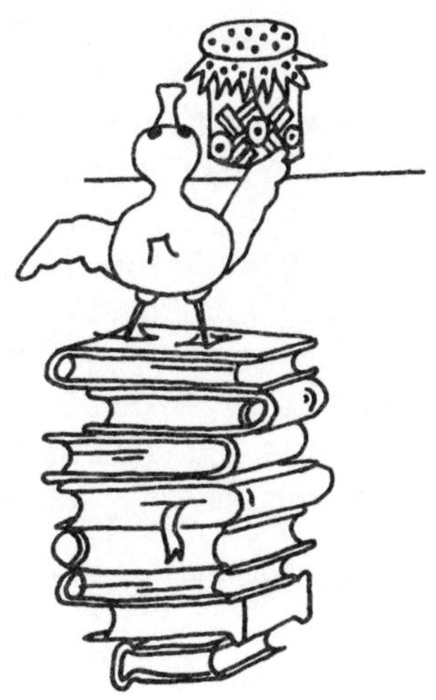

Introduction

In this chapter and the next we describe different ways of treating diabetes. In younger people there is usually no choice and they need to start insulin injections fairly soon, but in older people found to have diabetes, the eventual form of treatment that they will need may not be obvious at the outset. Provided they are not feeling terribly ill they are usually given advice to change the type and quantity of food that they eat. This alone may have a dramatic effect on their condition, especially in overweight people who manage to get their weight down. If changing the diet fails to control diabetes, tablets are usually tried next by adding them to the diet. These may be very effective but tablets do not always work and in such cases insulin is the only alternative. Treatment with insulin is discussed in Chapter 3.

Knowing about the right type of food and the amount that you can eat is important. Most of the questions we have included help explain the general principles but people's diets are very individual, so do ask for help and further explanations from your own diabetes advisers and dietitians. It is particularly important to have an opportunity to review what you are doing about food regularly every few years. If you are looking for new ideas for meals, then there are now many helpful recipe books produced written especially for people with diabetes, most of which are available from Diabetes UK. A list of current titles can be found in Appendix 2.

Most people with diabetes and, especially, parents who have a child with diabetes, long for a miracle cure. This explains why we have been sent so many questions about unorthodox methods of treatment. We have tried to answer these questions in a sensitive manner but there is no escaping the fact that, for a child, insulin is the only miracle cure and that is how it was regarded when it was discovered in 1921.

Diet

There must be many people like me who have diabetes but who are not on insulin. Why have I been told to control my weight?

Probably because you are overweight! People who develop diabetes later in life are often overweight. They do not usually need treatment with insulin injections – instead their treatment is by diet alone or by diet and tablets.

If you are overweight, the insulin produced by your pancreas is less effective because of the excess fat in your body. This is known as 'insulin resistance', and you overcome it by losing that excess fat. Achieving and maintaining a sensible weight therefore helps you improve your control of your diabetes. An additional benefit is that it also reduces all the other health risks associated with being overweight, such as high blood pressure and heart disease.

Why do people put on weight?

Your body needs energy from food and drink to fuel your body processes, such as breathing, which go on even when you are sleeping. All forms of physical activity (such as walking, shopping, typing and so on) require additional energy. This energy is measured in calories (see the next question for more information about calories).

Ideally your calorie intake from the food you eat should balance the amount of energy used by your body. When this happens you will neither gain nor lose weight. If the amount of food and drink you consume provides more energy (calories) than you use in your daily activities, then the extra food will be converted into body fat and you will put on weight. If you are overweight you need to reduce your daily intake of calories so that you are taking in less energy than your body needs. Your body will make up the difference by using up the fat stored in your body and you will then lose weight.

What are calories or joules?

These are both measures of the energy that your body can obtain from the food and drink you consume. In this country we usually refer to calories, but in some countries they use joules as the unit. One calorie is equal to 4.2 joules.

Strictly speaking, we should really be talking about kilocalories (often abbreviated to kcal) and kilojoules (abbreviated to kjoules or kJ), and these are the units that you will probably see on the nutritional information labels on food packaging. But most people simply use the shorthand term 'calorie' when they mean kilocalories, and that is what we have used in this book.

I have diabetes which is controlled by diet alone. Do I have to keep to strict mealtimes?

People on medication for diabetes (tablets or insulin) are usually advised to keep fairly closely to regular mealtimes to avoid getting a low blood sugar (hypo). As you are on diet alone, your risk of a hypo is very low, so you do not need to keep to strict mealtimes. However, it is worth remembering that everyone finds their diabetes easier to control if they have three or so small meals a day rather than one or two large ones.

My husband's diabetes is controlled by diet alone. Since being diagnosed two years ago, he has kept strictly to his food plan. In the past year he has not had a positive urine test and his clinic blood glucose measurements have been normal. Does this mean he no longer has diabetes?

Once you have developed diabetes, you always have diabetes. This applies to almost everyone and exceptions to this are extremely rare. Your husband has obviously done very well by keeping to his food plan, and this is the reason his diabetes is so well controlled. If he went back to his old eating habits and started putting on weight, it is very likely that all his old symptoms would return and his blood glucose would be high again.

Do people on diet alone need to eat snacks in between meals?

No, not usually. The reason that people taking insulin injections are sometimes advised to eat a snack between their main meals is to balance the effect of the insulin they take. People on diet alone or diet and tablets do not usually have this problem and so do not usually need to have snacks. Too many snacks can cause a problem with weight gain!

Remember that not eating snacks is *not* the same thing as missing meals. Some people on diet alone can go hypo if they go without food – there is a question about this in the section on ***Hypos*** in Chapter 3.

Can I eat as many diabetic foods as I like?

No, you most certainly cannot, and we would recommend that you do not even include them in your food plan! They are no lower in fats or calories than ordinary food and they are also expensive.

The main selling point for most of these so-called 'diabetic foods' is that they replace ordinary sugar with a substitute. This substitute may be another type of sugar called fructose, but is often a chemical called sorbitol, excessive intake of which causes loose bowels (diarrhoea). Fructose and sorbitol both contain as many calories as ordinary sugar.

Today the recommended food plan for most people with diabetes allows you to include some sweetened foods, especially if you choose products with a higher fibre and lower fat content. If you are of normal weight (or even underweight) you will be able to eat modest amounts of ordinary extras or treats, such as biscuits, cakes or confectionery. These should form part of your food plan and should preferably be eaten at the end of a meal. There is therefore no need for you to buy diabetic foods just to give yourself a treat.

The only 'special' foods we recommend for people with diabetes are the ones labelled as 'diet' or 'low calorie', especially soft drinks, reduced sugar preserves, diet yogurts and sugar-free jellies. These are not marketed specifically for people with diabetes, but for everyone who wants to keep their weight under control or avoid eating too much sugar. They are usually sweetened with artificial sweeteners such as saccharin or aspartame (trade name NutraSweet) which are virtually calorie-free. These artificial sweeteners can also be used to replace sugar in your tea or coffee, or you can get them in granular form to sprinkle on your breakfast cereal.

Be careful to check the labels on foods marked 'sugar-free' to see which type of sweetener has been used. Sugar-free chewing gum and pastilles are often sweetened with sorbitol, which means that they are not low-calorie. You can include them in your food plan (but be careful – remember the side effects of sorbitol!) but you will need to count their calories.

Where or how do I find out about the carbohydrate or calorie content of foods?

The publishers of the many slimming magazines on the market also produce booklets for slimmers listing the calorie contents of foods, and you may find that your local newsagent stocks one of these.

You could also look at the labels on the food you buy, as most foods are now labelled with their carbohydrate and calorie content (as well as with other nutritional information). Your dietitian can teach you how to use the information on these labels if you are not quite sure what something means. Some manufacturers label their foods more clearly than others!

I have just started tablets for my diabetes. Does this mean I can relax my diet?

No. You will have been prescribed tablets because treatment with diet alone was not enough to bring your blood glucose level down. If you start on your tablets and then relax your diet, your blood glucose levels may climb even higher. Remember, it's treatment with diet *and* tablets, not just with tablets.

If it has been a while since you have seen a dietitian, it might be worthwhile to make an appointment to review your diet now that you are on tablets to see if there are any changes that can be made.

How does a person with diabetes get an appointment with a dietitian?

Everyone agrees that food plays a crucial part in the way people look after their diabetes. Soon after diagnosis and at other stages of diabetes, people with diabetes need expert advice from a dietitian and this is recommended in Diabetes UK booklet *What diabetes care to expect* (see Appendix 2). The availability of dietitians varies considerably and most diabetes centres have a dietitian as part of the team. Some general practitioners provide dietitian sessions in their own health centres, but in other places, the patient will have to wait for an appointment at the local hospital.

I have many family celebrations in the summer and would like advice on the choice of drinks. I have managed to lose weight and my control has improved so much that I have been taken off my tablets.

We assume that you are asking about alcoholic drinks. Drunk in moderation, alcohol has been shown to be good for people with or without diabetes. You will need to remember that it is a major source of calories (one small glass of wine is equivalent to a slice of bread) but even on a weight-reducing diet most people are allowed some alcohol for special occasions. As your control of your diabetes is so good, there will be no problem about you enjoying a drink at your family celebrations.

You can choose from all types of wine, red or white, but you should probably avoid the very sweet wines and sherries because of their high sugar content. Spirits are sugar-free (but not calorie-free) and are best enjoyed with sugar-free ('diet' or 'slimline') mixers or soda water.

If you prefer a pint, you can choose beer, lager or cider. You are best to avoid the 'strong' brews which are often labelled as being low in carbohydrate, as these are higher in alcohol and calories than the ordinary types. Low-alcohol and alcohol-free beers and lagers often contain a lot of sugar, so if you enjoy these you should look for the ones which are also labelled as being low in sugar.

Drinking alcohol affects your blood glucose level and you should be aware of this. You will find more information about this in the section on ***Alcohol*** in Chapter 5.

Which scales do you recommend for weighing food?

You don't need to weigh your food on a daily basis. In most cases you can measure food portions with enough accuracy using handy household measures, and you should have been shown how to do this when you were first diagnosed as having diabetes. If no one showed you how, we suggest that you make an appointment to see a dietitian to ask for advice.

A few foods (such as rice, pasta and jacket potatoes) can be a little difficult to judge at first, and for these it might be worth weighing out your portions on your ordinary kitchen scales until you get an idea of what the portion size looks like. After that, you shouldn't need to bother about scales any more than the average cook!

I have a number of queries about my diet. Can you advise me how I can get advice about it?

Good advice on diet is essential in the proper care of diabetes and it needs to be tailored to fit every individual person. Diabetes UK offers helpful literature and advice but this is not really a substitute for personal advice from a properly trained person.

You can arrange to see a professionaly qualified dietitian through either your hospital or your GP. Most hospitals have a professional dietitian attached to the diabetes clinic, and you could make an appointment to be seen on your next clinic visit. Some general practitioners organize their own diabetes clinics, and they may arrange for a dietitian to visit this clinic. Many of the nurses and health visitors who are specially trained in diabetes will also be able to give you good basic dietary advice.

I have had diabetes for 22 years and have only recently come back under the care of my local hospital. When I talked about my diet to the dietitian she was keen to make some changes saying that there were quite a lot of new ideas and diet recommendations. What are these and is it worth me changing?

Advice on diet for people with diabetes has certainly changed since you were first diagnosed. Much more is now known about nutrition, and a diagnosis of diabetes no longer means eating differently from everyone else. In fact, the advice on a healthy diet for people with diabetes is exactly what has been recommended for the population as a whole – eating less fat and sugar, and more fibre and fresh fruits and vegetables. It's an eating plan which your whole family could, and should, follow if they want to eat healthily and well. Changing to a diet with more fibre and a lot less fat is certainly very worth while and may reduce your risks of developing heart disease in later life.

One of the things which we now know much more about is carbohydrate, found in both sugary and starchy foods. The carbohydrates found in sugary foods are very rapidly absorbed by the body, and make your blood glucose levels rise very quickly – not a good thing if you have diabetes! Starchy, high-fibre carbohydrate foods are absorbed more slowly, make blood glucose levels rise more slowly, and so are more suitable.

The dietary fibre found in these starchy carbohydrate foods is of two main types: 'fibrous' fibres, which are typically found in wholegrain cereals, wholemeal flour or bran; and 'viscous' fibres found in pulses (peas, beans and lentils) and some fruit and vegetables. Viscous fibres (especially those found in beans) appear to be of particular benefit because they slow down food absorption and hence the rate at which carbohydrate present in a meal will be absorbed into the blood stream. All plant foods, especially those which are eaten raw or only lightly cooked, are digested very slowly because the plant cell walls have to be broken down before their carbohydrate content is released. As well as this slow absorption (which means a slower rise in blood glucose levels), another major benefit of including more fibre-rich foods in your diet is the prolonged effect that these foods can have in maintaining blood glucose levels. This helps to reduce unexpected hypos if your meals or snacks are delayed or missed.

So yes, it is worth updating your diet. Your dietitian will give you full details, but the main recommendations can be summed up as follows:

1. Too many calories in your diet worsens your control of your diabetes. Everyone with diabetes therefore requires a food and eating plan, based on their own individual needs, which does not contain a surplus amount of food energy. (We have discussed balancing calories taken in and used up in more detail in the questions at the very beginning of this section.)
2. To reduce your risk of developing coronary heart disease and arterial disease (and also to help you keep your weight under control) you should reduce the amount of fat in your diet. You can do this easily by substituting semi-skimmed or skimmed milk for whole milk; using less butter or margarine or replacing them with low fat spreads; greatly reducing your intake of cream and cheese; grilling rather than frying foods; choosing fish or poultry (skin removed) rather than meat; and having smaller portions of meat and buying the leanest cuts you can afford. You should not eat too much protein and people with diabetes should not follow high protein/low carbohydrate food plans.
3. Whilst you should still avoid adding sugar to food or drinks or eating very sugary foods as much as possible, you can now include them in your diet plan on an occasional basis. They are

best eaten at the end of a meal which has included plenty of fibre-rich starchy carbohydrates, as then they will be absorbed more slowly. You should eat plenty of starchy carbohydrates – in fact they should provide about half your daily total of calories. Choose foods such as fruit, vegetables and beans. Eat wholemeal bread rather than white whenever possible, and pick high-fibre breakfast cereals such as Weetabix, Shredded Wheat, Bran Flakes, All-Bran or porridge. Use some wholemeal flour in baking, and substitute brown rice for white rice and wholemeal pasta for ordinary pasta.

4. If you need to lose weight, you should not follow a diet which is low in carbohydrate: you should include some bread or potatoes or pasta or rice or breakfast cereal at each meal. A high carbohydrate/low fat diet is particularly suitable if you want to lose weight as it contains plenty of bulk and so you are less likely to feel hungry.
5. Special 'diabetic foods' are not worth including in your food plan because they are expensive and are usually high in calories. Low calorie 'diet' foods and drinks can be usefully included in your diet, especially if you need to lose weight. (We have talked about diabetic and diet foods in more detail in an earlier question.)
6. You can drink a moderate amount of alcohol provided you take its energy contribution (the number of calories it contains) into account. Beers and lagers specially brewed to be low in carbohydrate have a high alcohol and calorie content and are not recommended. (Again we have discussed this subject in more detail in an earlier question in this section.)

I am gradually losing my desire for sweet foods. When I do have them I follow my dietitian's advice and make sure that it is at a time when they are least likely to result in a high blood glucose. However, I really do not enjoy my selection of high-fibre breakfast cereals without some sweetener – I was a Sugar Puff fan before! Can I put a little sugar on?

Nowadays the experts do accept that your food plan can include a little sugar, preferably eaten at the end of a high-fibre meal. However, a much better choice for your cereal would be one of the granulated sprinkle-type sweeteners which are virtually calorie-free. Primarily aimed at slimmers, they are readily available in chemists and supermarkets. Brand names to look for include Canderel, Sweetex granulated, Sweet 'n' Low, Hermesetas Sprinkle and Sweet 'n' Lite. Not only will these not have any effect on your blood glucose, they won't rot your teeth either!

I come from the Caribbean and rice is part of my way of life. Since I have developed diabetes my doctor has told me not to have it any more. If I wash it well, won't I get all the 'fatness' out of it?

I am afraid you are both wrong! Your doctor should let you have some rice – it is no worse than bread and potatoes at putting up the blood glucose and putting on the weight.

The key to the problem is how much you eat in any one go and how you cook it. About a cupful of cooked plain-boiled rice contains only 150–200 calories, the same as a large potato or two slices of bread. There are very few food plans that could not fit this in at a main meal, especially as people with diabetes are now being encouraged to eat more carbohydrates. Of course you should not add any extra oil or fat during the cooking, and it would be better for you if you could change from white to brown rice.

Washing rice before or after cooking may remove a little of the loose starch it contains but it does not really reduce the overall content by more than a fraction.

As a single parent I really find it hard to make ends meet. I know that very often I do not buy the foods I should to help control my diabetes. Is there any way I can eat healthily but cheaply?

You are far from alone in wanting to eat well but cheaply nowadays. The sort of food plan advised for most people with diabetes should not cost more than the foods most people are eating before diagnosis, but there is no doubt that when people are on very limited incomes the amount they have to spend on food is often less than is required to buy a healthy diet. The following tips may help, and you could also ask your dietitian for some more ideas – it is a problem which will have often been encountered before.

For breakfast, have porridge, which is very cheap and an excellent breakfast cereal from the point of view of your diabetes control. When it's too hot for porridge, try home-made muesli, which you make by mixing some rolled oats (the type you use to make porridge) with some fruit (perhaps a chopped apple) and some cold skimmed milk. You need enough milk to make the mixture about the same consistency as porridge, and you can also add some plain unsweetened low-fat yogurt if you like. Leave it to stand overnight and it will be ready to eat in the morning.

A sandwich lunch can be very healthy, especially if you can use wholemeal bread. Tinned fish such as sardines, mackerel, or pilchards are excellent choices for sandwich fillings and can work out very inexpensive. You do not really need large helpings of meat at your main meals, and you can often extend it with extra tinned, frozen or fresh vegetables. Diet yogurts make excellent desserts and are good value for money. You can cut costs further by buying a large pot of plain natural yogurt (which is usually cheaper than the fruit varieties) and adding chopped or purèed fresh or tinned fruit in natural juice with a little extra artificial sweetener if needed. Another quick and healthy home-made dessert is a low sugar jelly (available from most supermarkets) made up with milk or yogurt.

Children love crisps as snacks but these can work out expensive, which cuts down the money you have to spend on main meals. A cheaper, healthier snack for you all would be home-made popcorn. A half-pound bag that you pop yourself would make well over the equivalent of a dozen packets of crisps and cost considerably less!

The dietitian says that my high blood glucose levels during the morning may be caused by the pure fruit juice that I drink at breakfast. It is unsweetened juice, so how can this happen?

Pure unsweetened fruit juice will put up your blood glucose levels, whether it comes from a bottle or a carton or from fresh fruit that you have squeezed yourself at home. All fruit contains natural sugar. If you eat it as the whole fruit then it takes time to be digested and the effect on blood glucose is quite slow. If you take away all the flesh (which contains the dietary fibre) and just drink the juice, then the sugar will pass into your blood stream very quickly indeed.

Nearly all dietitians suggest that people with diabetes limit the amount of fruit juice they drink to just a very small glass, and preferably drink it diluted with mineral water or diet lemonade. The juice is also best taken at the end of a meal. If, after following this advice, you still find it difficult to improve your blood glucose control in the morning then it is probably best for you to avoid even this small amount of juice, or perhaps to drink it later in the day.

I have read in a recently published book about diabetes that I can use urine testing strips to test drinks to judge their sugar content. Everything I test, including the diet drinks, test positive. Do they all contain sugar?

The answer is no! You should not test drinks or foods with these strips – it simply does not work. This is not a new idea, but one which first appeared in the late 1970s. It was not correct then and it is not correct now!

Overweight

I have just been told that I have diabetes. Is it true that if I lose weight I will probably not need insulin injections?

Possibly not, if you were overweight at the time of diagnosis, but as with so many questions we have to qualify this by saying that it all depends!

Most of the people in the UK who have diabetes do not need insulin, especially those who are over 40 years old at the time of diagnosis and who are overweight. People who are of normal weight at the time of diagnosis are more likely to need treatment with insulin or with diet and tablets rather than just with diet alone. If you are overweight, it is impossible to predict how much weight you will need to lose in order to control your diabetes. In some people the loss of half a stone (3 kg) is enough to restore the blood glucose to normal, while in other people the blood glucose remains high even after they lose several stones in weight. These people may then need tablets or insulin but, provided they do not become too thin, they will still be better off for shedding the excess weight.

I am trying to lose weight. How much should I lose a week?

It rather depends on how much you weigh, how active you are, and what you were eating before you decided to tackle your weight problem. As a general rule people should be quite happy with a weight loss of anything between 1–2 lbs (½–1 kg) a week. This doesn't sound very much, especially when you can read about diets which claim to offer you a rapid weight loss of several pounds a week. But losing weight slowly and steadily really is the healthiest way – if you lose weight too fast you will not only lose your fat but also the types of body tissue that you need to keep, such as muscle tissue. And not only is it the healthiest way, it's also the most efficient, as people who lose weight too quickly tend to put it all back on (and more!) within just a few years.

Most people can manage to lose weight simply by modifying the quantities and types of food they eat, particularly by cutting down the amounts of fat, sugar and alcohol they consume. By doing this they 'save' about 500 calories a day, which leads to a weight loss of about 1 lb (½ kg) a week.

I eat very small amounts of food and am constantly on a diet but cannot seem to lose any weight. My friend who is the same age eats four times the amount of food I do but remains as slim as a reed. Why is this?

This happens because your metabolic rate is different from your friend's metabolic rate. Your metabolic rate is the rate at which you 'burn up' your food (convert it to energy that your body can use). The rate depends on your make up (which is largely inherited) and, although it seems very unfair, some people burn up their food very fast and remain slim, while others eat the same amount of food and put on weight.

The metabolic rate can be altered under certain circumstances.

For example, people subjected to long periods of starvation slow their metabolic rate right down to conserve energy, whilst those who take regular, vigorous exercise speed up their rate of metabolism so that they are able to eat more food and not put on extra weight.

The only way *you* will lose weight is by eating less food than *your* body needs, so that you burn up the stores of fat in your body. A dietitian will be able to give you specific advice about this, and you will find information about consulting a dietitian in the previous section on ***Diet***.

I have been dieting on and off since I had my last child 15 years ago. The diabetes that I developed in that pregnancy has now returned despite not taking sugar in my drinks. What more can I do?

The answer probably lies in your dieting 'on and off'. If you are still overweight you are going to have to reduce – and maintain the reduction in – your energy (calorie) intake until you lose the excess weight. Once you have lost the weight, you will then need to follow a sensible eating plan that balances the amount of energy you take in with the amount you use up in your daily activities, and you will then be able to keep your weight steady.

To lose weight, try to concentrate on reducing the amount of fat you eat, and cut down on foods that contain both fat and sugar, especially biscuits and confectionery. If this does not work, seek help from a dietitian who will take a dietary history and work out where else you can save calories. Finally, increasing the amount of regular exercise you take can help speed up the rate at which you burn up food (your metabolic rate), which often slows down as the result of long-term dieting.

Why are both my dietitian and diabetes specialist nurse so against my family buying me diabetic foods? I find my diet very hard to keep to and never lose weight anyway. So why can't I have diabetic foods as a treat?

In all probability the reason why you are not losing weight is that you are eating these 'diabetic foods' on top of your diet! Unfortunately foods labelled as 'diabetic' are, with very few exceptions, foods which are very high in calories. Bars of 'diabetic' chocolate and 'diabetic' biscuits contain just as many calories as the ordinary varieties. This is because the only change in the recipe is a swap – the ordinary sugar is replaced with either sorbitol or fructose. But both these substitutes contain just as many calories as sugar! To make things worse, the manufacturers of 'diabetic' foods often find they have to add a little more of some of the other ingredients (such as fat, flour or milk powder) to improve the taste, and these again add extra calories.

Why not ask your dietitian to increase your diet plan a little to make it easier for you to actually keep to it? She would probably be prepared to allow you the occasional treat in your food plan if you promised to stick to it in the future, and also promised to avoid the diabetic foods. If you did this, you would be much more likely to lose weight.

I am very overweight and trying hard to lose about 3 stone (20 kg). I love ice-cream and most of the cheaper varieties in the supermarket contain non-milk fat. Will this be suitable for me?

It would probably be acceptable to have a small bowl (1–2 scoops) of ice-cream as a treat now and again, as part of your reduced fat and sugar food plan. Non-milk fat does not mean that it is fat-free or low calorie, just that the manufacturers have used vegetable fats (which have just as many calories as milk fat) because they are cheaper. Most standard ice-cream is about 7–10% fat and around 80–100 calories per scoop, and Cornish ice-cream is more. You can buy reduced calorie ice-cream but it is more expensive and the saving in calories does not really justify it for occasional use.

Are there any appetite suppressants on the market that are suitable for people with diabetes?

Most appetite suppressants contain substances which, if used for more than a few weeks, become addictive but cease to be effective in curtailing your appetite. For this reason, they are not recommended for anyone (not just people with diabetes), except under special circumstances.

I have heard that tablets for diabetes can make you fat. Is this true?

Tablets can only make you fat if used wrongly. If you are overweight but not in urgent need of insulin, then you should first get down to your normal weight and only then go on to tablets if your blood glucose level is still raised. If you start on tablets straight away without first trying the effect of diet alone, then you will find it difficult to lose weight and you might become even fatter. In other words, tablets should not be used as a substitute for diet treatment and weight reduction.

Tablets

I understand that there are different sorts of 'diabetic' tablets. Can you tell me what they are and what the difference is between them?

There are three main types of tablets which may be prescribed for people with diabetes. They work in different ways.

- *Sulphonylureas* (including glibenclamide, chlorpropamide, gliclazide, glipizide and tolbutamide): they act by increasing the amount of natural insulin produced by the pancreas.
- *Biguanide* (metformin or Glucophage): this works by reducing the release of glucose from the liver and increasing the uptake of glucose into muscle.
- *Alpha glucosidase inhibitor* (acarbose or Glucobay): this slows the digestion of carbohydrates in the intestine and suppresses the rise in blood glucose after meals.

What are the lengths of action of the various 'diabetic' tablets?

The two most commonly used tablets belong to the same group (sulphonylureas): they are glibenclamide and chlorpropamide. Glibenclamide tablets act for about 18 hours and are taken once or at the most twice daily. Chlorpropamide has a very long action of 36 hours or more. For this reason it never needs to be taken more than once a day. This long action of chlorpropamide can be dangerous in the elderly: if for some reason they are unable to eat, they may have a very low blood glucose level for several days.

Can taking too much glibenclamide cause slight dizziness?

Glibenclamide could be causing your blood glucose level to be too low so your dizziness could be a mild hypo, particularly if you get this feeling when taking exercise or before meals. You can easily find out by checking your blood glucose at a time when you feel dizzy. If your blood glucose level is above 4 mmol/l then something apart from the glibenclamide must be causing the dizziness. There are of course other causes of dizziness which have nothing to do with diabetes!

I find I am dropping off to sleep all the time and never feel refreshed. I take 500 mg Diabinese (chlorpropamide) and 500 mg metformin a day. Could I be taking too much?

Diabinese 500 mg is quite a large dose and your sleepiness could be due to a hypo. You should check that your blood glucose is not too low (below 4 mmol/l). On the other hand, people with a high blood glucose often feel drowsy and lacking in energy. So your complaint could be due to either a low or a high blood glucose, and the best way of finding out is to do a blood glucose test.

Can one get withdrawal symptoms when taken off Diabinese (chlorpropamide)?

Some medicines, especially certain sleeping tablets and painkillers, become necessary to the body if taken regularly for long periods of time. When these drugs are stopped the body reacts violently, causing withdrawal symptoms. Tablets for diabetes do not have these effects and can be stopped quite safely – provided, of course, that you no longer need them to keep your blood glucose under control. If your blood glucose begins to rise, the symptoms of thirst, itching, and so on will return but these cannot be described as withdrawal symptoms.

My chemist tells me that some tablets for diabetes react badly with alcohol. Can you please enlarge on this?

A number of people who take chlorpropamide (Diabinese) experience a hot flush in the face when they drink alcohol. It seems that flushing caused by the combination of chlorpropamide and alcohol may run in families. Fortunately none of the other 'diabetic' tablets have this effect of causing flushing when combined with alcohol. If you are taking chlorpropamide and are troubled by this problem you could take an equivalent dose of glibenclamide instead.

Alcohol may have other effects on the blood glucose in people with diabetes, and we discuss these in the section on ***Alcohol*** in Chapter 5.

Since taking Glucophage (metformin) I have had feelings of nausea and constant diarrhoea and have lost quite a lot of weight. Is this due to the Glucophage?

Nausea and diarrhoea are possible side effects of Glucophage. The loss of weight could either be due to poor food intake because Glucophage has reduced your appetite or else because your diabetes is out of control. Either way you should stop Glucophage or at least reduce the dose and see if the nausea and diarrhoea disappear. If your diabetes is then poorly controlled with high blood glucose levels (more than 10 mmol/l) you may need a different sort of tablet or perhaps insulin injections in addition to diet, and you should consult your doctor.

My elderly mother has been taking gliclazide to control her diabetes for five years. Recently her sugars have been high and her doctor has asked her to take metformin as well with good results. Are there concerns about the long-term safety of metformin?

Metformin is a very good drug and I am not surprised that your mother's diabetic control has been better since she started taking it in addition to gliclazide. The down side is that metformin frequently causes side effects, mainly affecting the stomach or guts (diarrhoea, constipation, nausea, loss of appetite). These may develop after metformin has been taken for several years. Metformin causes one serious but very rare side effect, namely lactic acidosis. As a general rule, this only occurs when the person taking metformin has suffered some other medical condition such as a heart attack, severe infection or kidney failure. Lactic acidosis can be difficult to treat and is a feared complication of treatment with metformin.

What is the cause of a continuous metallic burning taste in the mouth? I am 62 years of age with diabetes, controlled on tablets for the last four years.

You are probably taking metformin (Glucophage) tablets as these sometimes do cause a curious taste in the mouth. If the taste is troublesome (and it sounds unpleasant) you should stop taking these tablets. Other tablets for diabetes (e.g. glibenclamide or chlorpropamide) do not cause this side effect. You should consult your doctor for advice.

I have diabetes controlled on tablets. My dose was halved, and my urine was still negative to glucose. Would it be all right to stop taking my tablets altogether to see what happens? Obviously I would restart the tablets if my urine showed glucose.

Your idea is probably a good one but you should also check your blood glucose level as urine tests can sometimes be misleading. Provided your blood glucose remains controlled (less than 8 mmol/l) you would be better off without any tablets. If you no longer need tablets, diet becomes even more important for controlling your diabetes and you must avoid putting on weight. Some people think that if they come off tablets they no longer have diabetes but this is not so. There is always the chance that they will need tablets or even insulin at some stage in the future.

I have been taking Euglucon tablets to control my diabetes for the past three years. This week my doctor gave me Daonil instead and the chemist tells me it is the same substance. Could you please let me have a list of the tablets for diabetes?

Your chemist is correct in saying that Daonil and Euglucon are identical. It is confusing because different manufacturers market the same substance under different trade names. The different sulphonylurea tablets used in the treatment of diabetes are listed in Table 2.1. The main difference between them is their length of

Table 2.1 Sulphonylurea tablets

NAME	TRADE NAME	DOSE RANGE (mg)
gliquidone	Glurenorm	15–180
glipizide	Glibenese, Minodiab	2.5–40
tolbutamide	Rastinon	500–2000
gliclazide	Diamicron	80–320
glibenclamide	Daonil, Euglucon, Libanil, Diabetamide, Calabren, Malix	2.5–15
tolazamide	Tolanase	100–1000
chlorpropamide	Diabinese	100–500

action which varies from a few hours (e.g. gliquidone) to up to 36 hours or longer (e.g. chlorpropamide). Metformin (Glucophage) and acarbose (Glucobay) are from different groups of drugs and are not included in this list.

I have just started taking Glucobay tablets for my diabetes. Could you explain how Glucobay works?

Glucobay, the trade name for acarbose, acts by slowing the digestion of starch and related foodstuffs. Acarbose (Glucobay) slows the breakdown and absorption of many dietary carbohydrates, reducing the high peak of blood glucose which can occur after eating a meal containing carbohydrate. It is an addition to diet treatment and has been shown to be effective in many people with diabetes who do not require insulin treatment.

My doctor has suggested that I try a new form of treatment for my diabetes called Glucobay. I already take glibenclamide and I feel perfectly well although my blood glucose is often high. I am not keen on being a guineapig for the new drug.

Glucobay was launched in the UK in May 1993 and has been used extensively over many years in other European countries, particularly in Germany. It has been subjected to extensive trials and you have no reason to be worried about it – you are not being used as a guineapig. Many people with diabetes have found Glucobay very helpful.

However, Glucobay may lead to side effects when you first start taking it. These side effects are related to its action in the body (see the previous question). Because Glucobay slows down the breakdown of carbohydrates, complex sugars may then reach the lower part of the gut where they may cause a bloating sensation giving rise to wind (flatulence) and occasional transient diarrhoea. There are two ways of reducing this problem.

- Start with a very small dose of one 50 mg tablet of Glucobay a day, taken with your largest meal. Increase the dose slowly, in consultation with your doctor, until the optimum dose is reached. This may be up to 100 mg three times a day.
- Try and exclude sucrose from your diet. Sucrose is the ordinary sugar which we add knowingly to sweeten food. It is also added to many foodstuffs by the manufacturers.

I gather there is a completely new type of tablet for treatment of diabetes and it is called 'rosiglitazone' – could you please tell me something about it?

Rosiglitazone (trade name Avandia from SmithKline Beecham Pharmaceuticals) is an entirely new type of medication designed for people with type 2 diabetes. It has just been launched in the UK but has been available for some time in the USA and elsewhere. It acts by reducing the body's resistance to insulin. It has been tested extensively in the UK and elsewhere in clinical trials in patients with type 2 diabetes and is recommended as an additional therapy in combination with either metformin or a sulphonylyurea (e.g. glibenclamide or glucazide) when metabolic control is not adequate. The newly formed NHS 'National Institute of Clinical Excellence (NICE)' has reviewed all the information available on the drug and has recently given it their 'seal of approval'. Because it is a new drug, certain precautions with its use are advised.

I am a 65-year-old and remain a bit overweight despite my best efforts to reduce my weight through strict dieting and increasing the amount of exercise I take. I know my

metabolic control is not good and I am on what my doctor says is a maximum dose of metformin. Today she suggested I add a new tablet called 'rosiglitazone' to my treatment regime. She says that it is a new type of tablet and because of this I will need to have regular blood tests to check on my liver. This all sounds a bit formidable – should I go ahead and try these new tablets?

It sounds as though your doctor is right up to date and is giving you sound advice. Rosiglitazone is a new drug and it has been shown to be effective and safe in improving metabolic control in people such as yourself. Extensive trials have shown the drug to be quite safe but, as a precaution, because it shares certain similarities with a previous drug that occasionally exhibited toxic effects on the liver (troglitazone – introduced in the previous reprint of this book), regular liver function tests are recommended in the initial stages of treatment. Should these blood tests become abnormal then discontinuation of the drug will result in complete recovery.

Please tell me what is the maximum dose of tablets before insulin is required?

We have listed the minimum and maximum doses of tablets that you can take each day in Table 2.1.

Many people continue to use the maximum dose of tablets for years with rather poor control of their diabetes (blood glucose consistently greater than 10 mmol/l). Although these people often feel fairly well in themselves they are usually much better off when they change to insulin. After the change to insulin people notice that they have more energy and can usually manage on a less strict diet.

What should I do if I have an intercurrent illness while on tablets?

This can be a really difficult problem. Of course if you are ill enough to need hospital admission, you will often be given insulin while your sugars are running high. At home, this is not as simple because there is no way of knowing what dose of insulin you will need and an inadequate dose of insulin is of no benefit to you. So although in a perfect world you would have insulin for the duration of your illness, in reality it is acceptable to run high sugars for a day or so, in the expectation that they will soon settle down spontaneously. In a longer-lasting illness there is, of course, time to adjust the insulin dose in response to the results of blood glucose measurements.

My doctor has advised me to change from tablets to insulin. Would I be right in thinking that I could avoid doing this if I cut down my intake of carbohydrate?

No, you would probably not be right. If you are overweight you *might* be able to avoid insulin by dieting strictly and losing weight but only if you are eating more than you need at the moment. If your present food intake is the amount you need, then reducing this will only make you lose weight and in due course become weak – and you may already be suffering from thirst, weight loss and fatigue. So if you are eating too much, eat less and try to improve your control that way. If you are already dieting properly do not try to starve yourself. Accept insulin and you will probably be very grateful.

My diabetes has been treated with tablets for two years and now my doctor has said I need insulin injections. Is my diabetes getting worse?

If your blood glucose can no longer be controlled with tablets, then your pancreas is becoming even less efficient in producing insulin, and in that sense your diabetes is worse. However, it does not mean that you are going to suffer any new problems from the disease. Once you have got over the initial fear of injecting yourself (and most people manage this very quickly) then going on to insulin should not alter your life – in fact it will probably make you feel much better.

My mother is quite elderly. Should she go on insulin? I believe that there are new ways of giving insulin which make it simpler.

I agree that insulin pens have made it easier for old people to administer insulin. However, it is often difficult to predict whether an older person will be better off on insulin rather than tablets. The factors in the decision are as follows:

- How unwell or thirsty does she feel while on tablets?
- What side effects are the tablets causing?
- How high are her blood sugars?
- How active and dexterous is she?
- How keen is she to start insulin?

Of all these questions, the last one is the most important and we must not pressurize older people to start a form of treatment which they may dread. One way round this is to try insulin for a specified period of say two months and allow her to decide after that time whether or not she wishes to continue with insulin or revert to her previous treatment with tablets.

Non-medical treatments

Recently I saw a physical training expert demonstrating a technique of achieving complete relaxation. She concluded by saying 'Of course, this is not suitable for everyone, for example people with diabetes'. Is this true and, if so, why?

This sounds like an example of ignorant discrimination. There is no reason why people with diabetes should not practise complete relaxation if they want to. If the session went on for a long time you might have to miss a snack or even a meal but as you are burning up so little energy in a relaxed state, perhaps it would not matter.

My back has troubled me for many years and a friend has suggested that as a last resort I should try acupuncture. Would there be any objection to this, given that I have diabetes? Might it even help my diabetes?

Acupuncture has been a standard form of medical treatment in China for 5000 years. In the last 20 years it has become more widely used in this country. In China acupuncture has always been thought of as a way of preventing disease and is considered less effective in treating illness. In the UK acupuncture tends to be used by people who have been ill (and usually in pain) for a long time. It is most often tried in such conditions as a painful back, where orthodox medicine often fails to help. Even practitioners of the art do not claim that acupuncture can cure diabetes. But it will not do it any harm either, providing that you do not alter your usual diabetes treatment while you are having your course of acupuncture.

Do you think that complementary or alternative medicine can help people with diabetes?

Alternative medicine suggests a form of treatment that is taken in the place of conventional medical treatment. As such this could potentially be very dangerous, particularly if your diabetes is treated with insulin.

However, there may be a place for complementary therapies that can be tried alongside conventional medicine. Although there is no scientific evidence to show that complementary therapies such as yoga, reflexology, hypnosis or aromatherapy can benefit someone with diabetes, some people who have tried them report that they feel more relaxed. As stress can have a detrimental effect on blood glucose control it may mean that their diabetes improves as a result.

We must emphasize that these therapies should always be used in addition to, not instead of, your usual diabetes treament. You should not alter your recommended diet or stop taking your tablets or your insulin, nor would a reputable complementary practitioner suggest that you do any of these things.

I have heard that there are herbal remedies for diabetes. Could you enlarge on these?

There are many plants which have been said to reduce the high level of blood glucose in people with diabetes. One of these is a berry from West Africa and another a tropical plant called karela or bitter gourd. These only have a minimal effect on lowering blood glucose and, as the bitter gourd lives up to its name and tastes disgusting, you will find conventional tablets more convenient, more reliable and safer. Herbal remedies have no effect on diabetes that requires insulin treatment.

My little girl has just contracted diabetes at the age of three. I would do anything to cure her. Would hypnosis be worth a try?

Most parents have a desperate desire for a cure when their child develops diabetes. In one sense, insulin injections are a cure in that they replace the missing hormone, but this is not much consolation to a distressed parent. Although a sense of desperation is natural, it is best for your child's sake for you to try to accept that she will always have diabetes. In this way she is more likely to come to terms with the condition herself. It is normal to grieve but at some stage you must face facts as a family and make use of all the help that is available for you and your daughter. In that way she will be less upset about her diabetes than you are. Hypnosis will not help her insulin cells to regenerate.

An evangelistic healing crusade claims to heal among other diseases 'sugar diabetes', malignant growth and multiple sclerosis, etc. Are these claims correct?

There are, of course, a handful of (unproven) reports of miracle cures of various serious diseases like cancer but these are few and far between. A mildly overweight person might be persuaded to lose weight by a faith healer and so it might appear that his diabetes was 'cured', but no person on insulin has ever benefited from a healing crusade except in the strictly spiritual sense.

I recently read an article on ginseng which said it was beneficial to people with diabetes. Have you any information on this?

Ginseng comes from Korea and the powdered root is said to have amazing properties. There is no scientific evidence to suggest that it is of any help to anyone whether they have diabetes or not.

3
Treatment with insulin

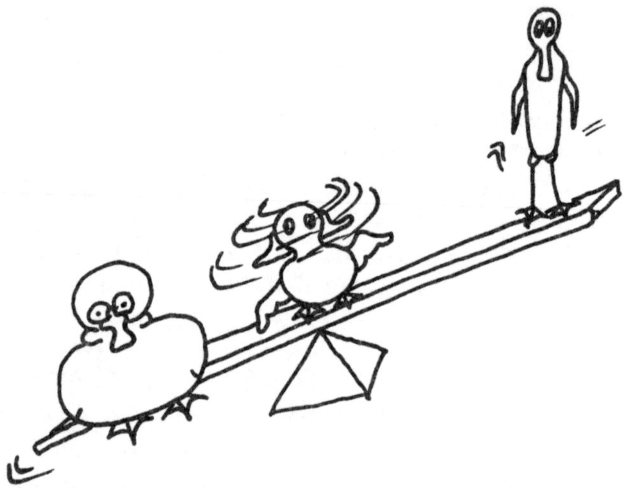

Introduction

The discovery of insulin by Banting and Best in Toronto in 1921 heralded the most important step in the history of diabetes. Within a very short time the good news that an effective treatment for diabetes had been discovered spread throughout the world. Dr Robin Lawrence was in Florence when he heard the news, waiting to die from diabetes. Instead he lived on and, with H. G. Wells, went on to found the British Diabetic Association (now called Diabetes UK).

Insulin treatment replaces the insulin normally produced by the pancreas gland, which becomes severely deficient in most people whose diabetes develops before they are 30 years old. In people in whom diabetes develops later in life, the deficiency of insulin is much less marked and forms of treatment other than insulin injections usually work for some time, if not indefinitely. Treatment without insulin is covered in Chapter 2.

Insulin still has to be given by injection because it is inactivated if it is taken by mouth. About a quarter of all people with diabetes are treated with insulin. Virtually everyone who develops diabetes when they are young needs insulin from the time of diagnosis. People diagnosed in later life may manage quite satisfactorily for many years on other forms of treatment but eventually many of them will need insulin to supplement their diminishing supply from their pancreas.

Everyone dreads the thought of having to inject themselves but the modern needles and syringes or insulin pens are so good that in nearly all cases this fear disappears after the first few injections, and daily injections become no more of a hassle than brushing your teeth!

People on insulin still have to watch what they eat. There is a section on ***Diet and insulin*** in this chapter, but we suggest that you also read the section on ***Diet*** in Chapter 2, as the information there is relevant whatever your form of treatment.

The section on ***Hypos*** (low blood glucose) is one of the most important parts of this book. They usually affect people on insulin but can happen to those taking certain tablets. It is the fear of hypos that prevents some people from controlling their blood glucose tightly. Diabetes care teams are often criticized for not giving people who are newly diagnosed enough information on hypos. So if you have just started insulin treatment, read this section carefully.

Insulin

When was insulin discovered?

Insulin was discovered by Frederick Banting and Charles Best in the summer of 1921. The work was carried out in the Physiology Department of Toronto University while most of the staff were on their holidays. The first human to be given insulin was a

14-year-old boy named Leonard Thompson who was dying of diabetes in Toronto General Hospital. This was an historic event, representing the beginning of modern treatment for diabetes. It was then up to the chemists to transform the production of insulin into an industrial process on a vast scale.

Where does insulin come from?

Since the discovery of insulin in 1921, countless people with diabetes have injected themselves with insulin extracted from the pancreas of cows and pigs. In the last 10 years or so human insulin has become widely available. This human insulin cannot be taken from human beings in the same way as beef and pork insulin is extracted. A great deal of research went into producing 'human' insulin by means of genetic engineering. This means that the genetic material of a bacterium or a yeast is reprogrammed to make insulin instead of the proteins it would normally produce. The insulin manufactured in this way is rigorously purified and contains no trace of the original bacterium. Human insulin has also been made on a commercial scale with a pig insulin chemically altered so that it becomes identical to the human variety. However, the method of genetic engineering will probably become standard as it is cheaper in the long run and does not depend on a supply of pancreas from pigs.

How is long-acting insulin made?

The first insulin to be made was clear soluble insulin. Injected under the skin, this lasts for about six hours and is called short-acting insulin. Various modifications were made to this original insulin so that it would last longer after injection. When protamine or zinc was incorporated into the insulin, a single injection could last from 12 up to 36 hours. For many years a single daily injection was advised by many doctors but people realized that this was not a good way of controlling the variations in blood glucose that occur during the day. Nowadays many people who need insulin have a mixture of short- and long-acting insulin twice a day and an increasing number have insulin four times a day which they inject with an insulin pen (there is a section on ***Insulin pens*** later in this chapter).

I have been on ordinary pork insulin for seven years and my doctor has just changed me over to human insulin. I feel upset because I was given no real explanation. Can you please help?

There has been a gradual switch to human insulin since it was introduced in 1982. Many doctors felt that human insulin was generally better because it led to less antibody formation than pork insulin. However, these antibodies probably do no harm and they may even be of some benefit by making the insulin injection last longer. There are also commercial pressures as insulin manufacturers would prefer to make only the human variety which would in turn reduce production costs.

Most people are able to swap from pork to human insulin without any difficulty but it is usual to reduce the dose by about 10% to be on the safe side and to compensate for the reduction in antibodies. This may be a gradual process lasting up to six weeks. Obviously during this transition period you will need to be especially careful to do frequent blood checks and if necessary to adjust the dose of insulin.

If the new type of insulin causes any problems, you can always ask to go back on pork insulin.

Since changing to human insulin my hypos have changed. There is less warning and on several occasions I needed help from my wife to get me back to normal. Have other people had the same experience?

This is a fairly common complaint and is very worrying because people rely on their warning signs to help them cope with the problem of hypos. Before human insulin was introduced, exhaustive tests were performed to try and find ways in which it differed from animal insulin. By and large these tests failed to show any significant differences apart from the lower levels of antibodies to insulin. It came as a surprise when a few people reported that their hypos were different on the new insulin and no real explanation has been found for this observation, but you may find it worthwhile to try the pork insulin again. (Please see the section on ***Hypos*** later in this chapter for more information.)

A self-help group exists for people who are treated with insulin, and their carers. The Insulin Dependent Diabetes Trust has highlighted a number of problems connected with insulin and the delivery of care. It has been an effective pressure group over the question of human insulin. See Appendix 3 for details.

I have had problems with human insulin and would like to go back to pork insulin. However, my chemist tells me that Actrapid is only available in the human form. Any suggestions?

It is true that pork Actrapid and Monotard are no longer manufactured. However, the same company still makes Velosulin in both pork and human form. This is a highly purified soluble insulin comparable to Actrapid. You should be able to substitute porcine Velosulin for your original dose of porcine Actrapid.

There is no pork zinc insulin the same as Monotard, but Insulatard is often a good substitute, and this is available in both human or pork forms. For the record, Mixtard is also available in both forms, as is Mixtard 30. Cartridges for the insulin pen are available as human, bovine, or porcine insulin (see the list of insulins in Table 3.1).

My diabetes has been well controlled on beef insulin (soluble and isophane) for the past 22 years. Should I use human insulin instead?

Provided you are doing well on your present insulin, there is no need to change back. Although the major insulin companies have not made beef insulin for many years, a firm called CP Pharmaceuticals supplies beef and pork insulin under the brand names Hypurin Bovine and Hypurin Porcine. They produce Bovine Neutral, Isophane, Lente and PZI, and Porcine Neutral, Isophane and 30/70 Mix. All of these except Lente and PZI are available in cartridges as well as vials, and the company provides free pens for those using their cartridges.

I have been taking beef insulin for many years and am worried about the possibility of this insulin being contaminated with BSE. Is this possible?

The manufacturers of beef insulin consider that the risk of any BSE (bovine spongiform encephalopathy) agent remaining after the intensive purification processes used to extract insulin is either negligible or non-existent. In addition, beef insulin used in the UK is derived from cattle originating in countries considered to have a negligible incidence of BSE, so that the risk of coming into contact with BSE through beef insulin is very small indeed.

I have seen a programme on television which says that human insulin may be dangerous. My 14-year-old son has just developed diabetes and I see that the doctor has put him on human insulin. You can imagine how worried I am about it.

Yes, it is unfortunate that this programme appeared at such a bad time for you. The people who make these programmes do not realise the fear and anxiety that they can cause.

First you must believe that your son needs insulin – without it he would soon become very ill. It does not really matter at this stage what sort of insulin he has although most doctors in this country start people who need insulin on the human variety. The only problems with human insulin seem to be caused by the change over from animal to human insulin. As your son has been on human insulin from the start he should not run into any difficulties. Perhaps you should talk to a family in which one of the children has had diabetes for a few years. They would probably be able to give the reassurance you need. You could try the local Diabetes UK voluntary group as a contact. Even if the Parents Group is not attached to Diabetes UK, they should be able to give you a contact number.

I was changed from pork to human insulin four years ago and I have not really noticed any difference. I have recently heard that human insulin can be dangerous. Should I be worried?

There has been adverse publicity about human insulin, which has been mentioned in the preceding questions. A number of people changing from animal to human insulin have noticed that they get less warning of hypos. This change of awareness may result from other factors (see the section on ***Hypos*** later in this chapter) but some people are convinced that the problem was caused by human insulin.

There have also been reports of unexpected deaths in people who have changed to human insulin. These deaths *may* have been due to hypoglycaemia but this has not been proved. Nor has it been shown that the numbers involved have increased since human insulin was introduced. Diabetes UK has been carrying out research into these vital questions but so far no cause for alarm has been found.

Can I get AIDS from human insulin?

Definitely not. Human insulin is either made from bacteria or yeast 'instructed' to produce insulin that has the same structure as human insulin, or from pork insulin modified to resemble human insulin. It is rigorously purified and cannot be a source of infection.

My doctor is considering changing me from one to two insulin injections per day. Will the second interfere with my social life – eating out, and so on?

No, instead the second injection should make your life more flexible. Most people on one injection a day find they need a meal in the late afternoon, around 6.00 to 7.00 p.m. With a second injection, this meal can be delayed for several hours with the insulin given shortly beforehand. With an insulin pen, it is easy to give yourself insulin even when eating out.

I have heard that there is a new fast-acting insulin which is even faster acting than Actrapid. Does it have any advantages?

You are quite right, Humalog is a new synthetic 'designer' insulin from Lilly. It is the first of what will be a series of new insulins (known as insulin analogues) which will be produced in the years to come, as we forecast in the last edition of this book. Humalog is designed not to aggregate when injected under the skin (a process which occurs to a varying extent with other insulins), thus facilitating its absorption and action. Its big potential advantage is that it doesn't need to be injected until immediately before the meal, and its action more closely matches the digestion of the meal than that of conventional clear insulins. This results in better control of the rise in blood glucose following meal digestion and absorption with lowering of the peak glucose concentration. It has another advantage stemming from its short action: when injected before breakfast, it has less tendency to cause hypos before lunch as its effects wear off more quickly.

It is ideally suited for the popular 'basal + bolus' regimes and is available in both vials and cartridges.

Is it possible to be allergic to insulin?

Very occasionally people may develop an allergy to one of the additives to insulin such as protamine or zinc, but the insulin itself is unlikely to cause an allergy.

When I was first diagnosed I was put on insulin, but now the dosage has been decreased. The doctor tells me I am in the 'honeymoon period' of diabetes. What does this mean?

Like you, most people need a reduction in their insulin dose soon after diagnosis is made. This is due to partial recovery of the insulin-producing cells of the pancreas. During this period hypos are often a problem but on the whole it is easy to control the blood glucose during this 'honeymoon'. The honeymoon period usually comes to a sudden end within a few months, often when the person has a bad cold or suffers some other stress to the insulin-producing cells. However, the honeymoon period is a good thing and will improve your chances of successful long-term control of your diabetes.

When I developed diabetes I was started on insulin but kept having hypos, and three months ago I came off insulin. Why was I given it in the first place?

Presumably you were given insulin because your doctors thought you needed it. Most people under 40 years old who have ketones in their urine are likely to need insulin and tend to be started on this without any delay. When insulin has been given for a week or so, it is quite common for people to be troubled by hypos, in which case the insulin has to be reduced. Sometimes even tiny doses of insulin cause hypos during this 'honeymoon period' (see the previous question) and the injections have to be stopped completely. The honeymoon period may occasionally last as long as a year.

What should I do if I suddenly realise I have missed an injection?

It is quite easy to forget to give yourself your injection or – even worse – to be unable to remember whether or not you have had your injection. If this happens you should measure your blood glucose to help you decide what to do next.

If your blood glucose is high (more than 10 mmol/l) you probably did forget your injection and you should have some insulin as soon as possible. The dose depends on how close you are to the next injection time.

If your blood glucose is normal or low (7 mmol/l or less) you probably did have your injection even if you have forgotten doing it. It would be safest to check your blood glucose again before your next meal and if it is high to have an extra dose of short-acting insulin.

Does the timing of the injections matter? Can a person who is on two injections a day take them at 10.00 a.m. and 4.00 p.m.?

Unless you are taking Humalog, which is a very quick-acting insulin and should be taken immediately before a meal, it is best to have your insulin about 30 minutes before a meal, and we discuss this further in the next section on ***Diet and insulin***. If you have your main meals in the middle of the morning and in the afternoon, then you could try giving insulin at the times you suggest. You may find that an afternoon injection may not last the 18 hours until the next morning – that is why most people try to keep their two injections approximately 12 hours apart.

I have had diabetes for nine months and attend the diabetes clinic every month to have my insulin dose adjusted. How long does it usually take before doctors get you balanced?

This is an interesting question as it assumes that it is up to the *doctors* to balance *your* diabetes. Of course the doctors and nurses in the clinic must provide you with all the help and information that you need but, in the end, it is *your* diabetes for *you* to control. Good control depends not just on the dose of insulin but the site you choose for your injections, the timing and type of food that you eat and the amount of exercise you take. These are things over which your doctor has no direct control. Most people begin to get their blood glucose under control in a few weeks.

Is my insulin requirement likely to vary at different times of the year because of the weather?

Several people have remarked that their dose of insulin needs to be altered in very hot weather – some need to give themselves more insulin and others less. This is probably because people react in different ways to a heat wave. There is a tendency to eat less and take less exercise in tropical conditions. However, because blood flow to the skin is increased in warm temperatures, this could speed up the absorption of the injected insulin and mean that a given dose will not last as long. Everyone is different and you will have to find out for yourself how hot weather affects your own blood glucose.

If my insulin requirements decrease over the years, does this mean that the pancreas has gradually started to produce more natural insulin than when I was younger?

No. It is most unlikely that after many years of diabetes your pancreas will start to produce natural insulin. However, this reduction in dose in older people is well recognized. It could be that you were having more insulin than you really needed in the past. Since the introduction of blood glucose measurement many people are found to be having too much insulin – or sometimes too much at one time of the day and not enough at another. Other possible explanations for older people needing less insulin are that they eat less food, they become thinner, or because of hormonal changes.

There seem to be a lot of different types of insulin on the market. Can you give me some details?

The range of insulins available can be confusing, although they do fall into three separate groups as we have shown in Table 3.1.

Table 3.1 Insulins available

1 SOLUBLE INSULIN which is clear and lasts from 4–6 hours with a peak action at 2–3 hours

NAME	MANUFACTURER	SOURCE	VIAL OR CARTRIDGE
*Humalog	Lilly	human	vial & cartridge
Actrapid	Novo Nordisk	human	vial
Actrapid Pen	Novo Nordisk	human	preloaded pen
Actrapid Penfill	Novo Nordisk	human	cartridge
Human Velosulin	Novo Nordisk	human	vial
Pork Velosulin	Novo Nordisk	human	vial
Humulin S	Lilly	human	vial & cartridge
Humaject S	Lilly	human	preloaded pen
Hypurin Porcine Neutral	CP Pharmaceuticals	pork	vial & cartridge
Hypurin Bovine Neutral	CP Pharmaceuticals	beef	vial & cartridge

* very rapid action – onset within 15 minutes, peak of action is 30–70 minutes and duration of action is 2–5 hours.

2 MEDIUM- AND LONG-ACTING INSULIN which is cloudy and lasts 6–24 hours with a peak at 8–12 hours

NAME	MANUFACTURER	SOURCE	VIAL OR CARTRIDGE
Human Insulatard	Novo Nordisk	human	vial
Human Insulatard Penfill	Novo Nordisk	human	cartridge
Human Insulatard pen	Novo Nordisk	human	preloaded pen
Pork Insulatard	Novo Nordisk	pork	vial
Monotard	Novo Nordisk	human	vial
Ultratard	Novo Nordisk	human	vial
Lentard MC	Novo Nordisk	pork & beef	vial
Humulin I	Lilly	human	vial & cartridge
Humaject I	Lilly	human	preloaded pen
Humulin Lente	Lilly	human	vial
Humulin ZN	Lilly	human	vial
Hypurin Porcine Isophane	CP Pharmaceuticals	pork	vial & cartridge

Hypurin Bovine Isophane	CP Pharmaceuticals	beef	vial & cartridge
Hypurin Bovine Lente	CP Pharmaceuticals	beef	vial
Hypurin Bovine PZI	CP Pharmaceuticals	beef	vial

3 MIXED INSULIN containing both short- and longer-acting insulin. This is designed to have an early peak of action at 2 hours with a total action of more than 8 hours

NAME	MANUFACTURER	SOURCE	VIAL OR CARTRIDGE
Human Mixtard 30*	Novo Nordisk	human	vial
Pork Mixtard 30*	Novo Nordisk	pork	vial
Human Mixtard 10* Pen	Novo Nordisk	human	preloaded pen
Human Mixtard 20* Pen	Novo Nordisk	human	preloaded pen
Human Mixtard 30* Pen	Novo Nordisk	human	preloaded pen
Human Mixtard 40* Pen	Novo Nordisk	human	preloaded pen
Human Mixtard 50* Pen	Novo Nordisk	human	preloaded pen
Mixtard 10* Penfill	Novo Nordisk†	human	cartridge
Mixtard 20* Penfill	Novo Nordisk	human	cartridge
Mixtard 30* Penfill	Novo Nordisk	human	cartridge
Mixtard 40* Penfill	Novo Nordisk	human	cartridge
Mixtard 50* Penfill	Novo Nordisk	human	cartridge
Human Mixtard 50*	Novo Nordisk	human	vial
Humulin M1 10/90*	Lilly	human	vial & cartridge
Humulin M2 20/80*	Lilly	human	vial & cartridge
Humulin M3 30/70*	Lilly	human	vial & cartridge
Humulin M4 40/60*	Lilly	human	vial & cartridge
Humaject M1	Lilly	human	preloaded pen
Humaject M2	Lilly	human	preloaded pen
Humaject M3	Lilly	human	preloaded pen
Humaject M4	Lilly	human	preloaded pen
Hypurin Porcine‡ 30/70* mix	CP Pharmaceuticals	pork	vial & cartridge

* The numbers refer to the percentage of soluble (short-acting) to isophane (medium-acting) insulin, e.g. Mixtard 20 is 20% soluble to 80% isophane, Humulin M4 40/60 is 40% soluble to 60% isophane.

† All NovoNordisk Penfills are available in 1.5 and 3.0 ml sizes.

‡ All Hypurin packaging is marked with Braille.

Please note that the times of insulin action vary greatly from one person to another and those given here must only be regarded as a rough guide.

The vials mentioned in the table are bottles of insulin for use with a syringe, and cartridges are for use with an insulin pen.

I am taking a mixture of short- and intermediate-acting insulin twice a day and do not understand which insulin is working at which time of day.

Many people are confused by the length of action of their insulin particularly when taken more than twice a day. The diagram in Figure 3.1 gives a representation of some commonly used regimens. If you are still unclear about it have another word with your doctor or diabetes specialist nurse.

Diet and insulin

I have been told that I am going to have to start insulin after many years of diet and tablets. Will my diet need to change?

Possibly, and in any case it would be helpful for you to have the opportunity to discuss your present eating habits with your dietitian before you start on insulin. If you have been trying to avoid going on to insulin by restricting the amount of carbohydrate you eat, you may well be advised to increase your intake.

Why do thin people taking insulin injections need a 'diet'?

The word 'diet' can often be misleading, as many people think of a diet only in terms of a weight-reducing diet. In fact, the word diet just means a way of eating or a prescribed course of food, and for a person with diabetes it simply means planned eating. It might be better if we all used the terms 'food plan' or 'eating plan' instead, but most of us just continue to use the word 'diet' in our everyday conversation!

The reason everyone with diabetes needs a food plan is to help them balance the amount of food that they eat against the amount

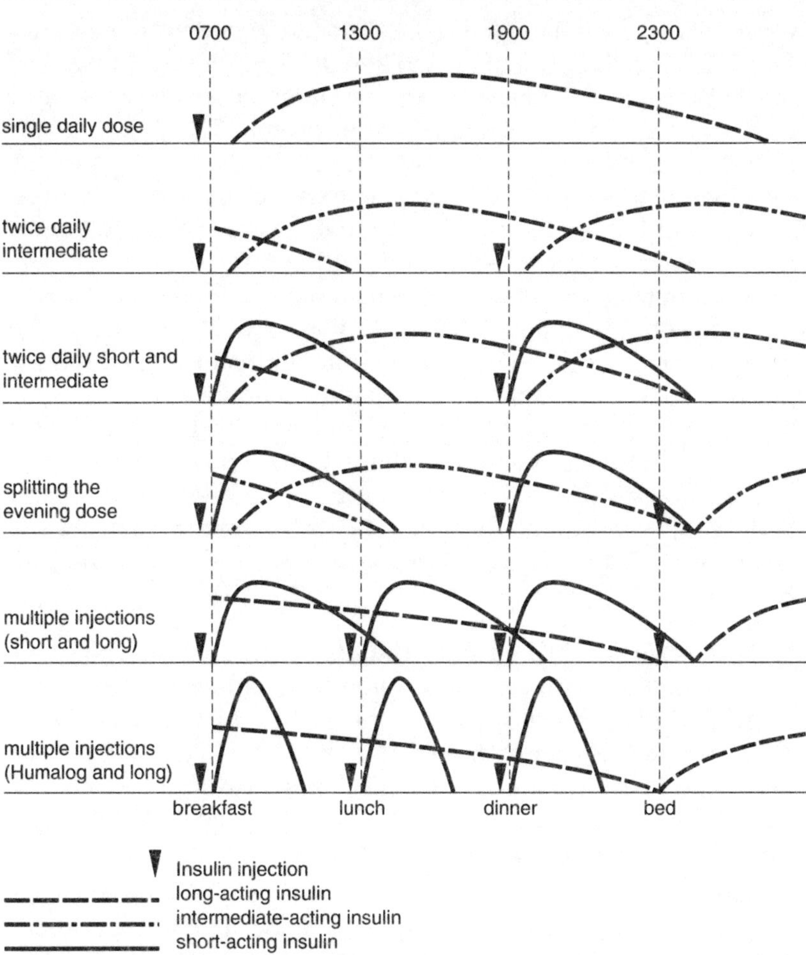

Figure 3.1 Representation of five common insulin regimens

of insulin and exercise they take. The simplest plan just encourages you to eat some carbohydrate foods at each meal. Carbohydrate foods are starchy or sugary foods such as bread, biscuits, crackers, crispbreads, pasta, potatoes, rice, fruit, ice-cream, and so on.

A more detailed plan would tell you about the amounts of proteins and fats you should eat. Proteins are an essential part of everyone's food intake but are only needed in moderate amounts. Foods high in proteins include meat, fish, eggs, cheese, pulses and nuts. Fats are used for energy and are a more concentrated source of calories than either carbohydrate or protein. They should only be eaten in small amounts as excess fat in the diet can lead to you being overweight and may contribute to heart disease in later life. Examples of fats are butter, cream, margarine, cheese and cooking oil. Cakes and pastries are also high in fats.

Most people eat roughly the same amount of food each day and so, when you are trying to balance food, insulin and exercise, it makes sense to keep your carbohydrate and calorie intake fairly constant, so that only your insulin and the amount of exercise you take need to be adjusted. The aim of your food plan is to eat roughly the same amounts of carbohydrate and calories at much the same time every day. The dietitian will firstly assess your previous diet and then advise you on the essential changes you need to make whilst trying to retain as much as possible of your previous eating pattern.

My 16-year-old son has had diabetes since he was six. We have managed quite well but since he has been transferred to the diabetes clinic we have seen more of the dietitian. I am confused – why doesn't she seem to stress the exchanges? She spends time urging us to eat more fibre-rich foods and cut down the fats. He's not overweight and has never had a problem with his bowels.

Nowadays we know that it is not just the number of exchanges that matter (an exchange = 10 g of carbohydrate). Different foods or meals affect blood glucose levels in varying ways even when their carbohydrate content is the same. We also know that it's the total number of calories you eat (not just the amount of carbohydrate) that affects whether or not you are overweight, and that a fibre-rich diet is good for all of you, not just your bowels.

There is now a lot more emphasis on the type and quality of the carbohydrate foods we eat. Carbohydrates that are rich in fibre usually take longer to digest, do not raise the blood glucose quite so much or so quickly, and keep blood glucose at a steady level for longer, which helps to prevent hypos. They also contain more vitamins and minerals and are believed to prevent the build up of excess fat in the arteries. The amount of heart disease amongst people with diabetes (and the general population) worries the experts and this is why there is much more emphasis on the whole diet, particularly in eating more of the fibre-rich foods and cutting back on fatty foods.

How long before eating should I have my insulin injection?

People who do not have diabetes start to produce insulin at the very beginning of a meal. Since it takes some time for injected insulin to be absorbed, you should ideally aim to have your insulin injection about 30 minutes before your meal, unless you are taking Humalog which should be given immediately before a meal. If your blood glucose level is low at the time of the injection there should be less delay between your insulin and your food.

I am on two injections a day. Sometimes I find it inconvenient to take my evening injection. Can I skip it and have a meal containing no carbohydrate?

No, you cannot skip your evening injection. When the effect of your morning injection wears out, your blood glucose levels will rise even if you have no carbohydrate to eat. Nowadays you can use an insulin pen which makes injections much less inconvenient.

Do people taking insulin need to eat snacks in between meals?

Sometimes, yes. When your pancreas functions normally, it produces insulin 'on demand' when you eat and 'switches off' when the food has been used up. Injected insulin does not 'switch off' in this way. As injected insulin has a peak effect at certain times of the day, it is important for you to cover its action by eating a certain amount of carbohydrate, or you will have a hypo. It is worth remembering that the carbohydrate you eat will last longer if it is rich in fibre as it is then more slowly absorbed.

If you find it difficult to eat between meals it may be possible to cut down the number of snacks you need by changing from a short-acting insulin to an intermediate-acting insulin, although some people still need to eat snacks even when taking a longer-acting insulin, particularly if they are very active. Alternatively, you could try a new very short-acting insulin analogue. There are many ways in which you can adjust your insulin regimen to suit the life you want to lead, and your doctor or diabetes specialist nurse will be able to advise you about these.

As I have to take insulin should I eat a bedtime snack?

Generally speaking, no, unless you have a blood glucose of less than 7 mmol/l at bedtime. If it is lower than this, or if you have hypos during the night (blood glucose tends to fall during the night) then you might need a bedtime snack. Something like a bowl of cereal, a piece of bread or toast, sandwiches, or some wholemeal crispbreads will last you better through the night than a rapidly absorbed milk or fruit juice drink with biscuits. If you are on insulin, you may do better by adjusting your dose – there is a question about this in the section on ***Hypos*** later in this chapter.

Should I increase my insulin over Christmas to cope with the extra food I shall be eating?

Yes, you can take extra insulin to cover the extra carbohydrate that you eat on any special occasion, not just Christmas. At Christmas everyone (including people with diabetes) eats more and it is best to accept this – but remember that if you do this too often you will be very likely to put on too much weight!

Extra food does need extra insulin and it is up to you to try to discover how much to increase your dose. You will probably need to work this out by trial and error, but firstly we would suggest that you do not increase the insulin by more than 4 units at a time, best taken in a quick-acting form shortly before your meal.

Don't forget the effect of exercise on your blood glucose – the traditional afternoon stroll after Christmas lunch is probably a good idea.

Is it all right for me, as someone who takes insulin, to have a lie-in on Sunday or must I get up and have my injection and breakfast at the normal time?

As with many of the answers in this book, the best advice we can give is try it and see on a couple of occasions. Try the effect of delaying your morning injection and breakfast and measure your blood glucose when you get up three or four hours late. If it is well below 10 mmol/l, all well and good, but if your blood glucose is higher than 10 mmol/l it means that you should not have missed your insulin. Alternatively try to persuade someone else to give you your morning injection and bring you breakfast in bed!

I have two injections a day: morning and evening. I keep regular times for breakfast and evening tea but I would like to vary the time I take lunch. What effect would this have on my control of my diabetes?

This is a difficult problem for someone on insulin. Because of your morning injection, you may tend to feel hypo if you are late for lunch. If your morning injection is mainly intermediate-acting insulin (e.g. Monotard or Insulatard), you may be able to delay your lunch a little provided you have a mid-morning snack. Have you thought of having multiple injections using an insulin pen? There is a section on ***Insulin pens*** later in this chapter.

Sometimes I suffer from a poor appetite. Is it all right for me to reduce my insulin dose on such occasions?

Yes, that is perfectly acceptable provided that you do not miss out completely on a main meal. You will have to find out for yourself (by measuring your blood glucose) by how much you should reduce your insulin for a particular amount of food. If you are underweight do not reduce your food intake too drastically. On the other hand, overweight people need to reduce both food intake and insulin.

My daughter has had diabetes for four years and has had no problems with her diet. She takes part in most school sports but, since she has taken up running longer distances, she finds that she has a hypo about two hours after she has finished running. She has no problems during the run so what should she do to counteract this?

The effect of exercise on the body can last well after the exercise has stopped, as the muscles are restocking their energy stores with glycogen. Your daughter is obviously taking in enough food to last her during her run, but not enough to keep her going through this 'restocking' process. She would probably find it helpful to eat an extra carbohydrate snack, such as a sandwich or two, after her run has finished. It might also be a good idea for her to reduce her morning dose of insulin on the days she is running. We talk more about balancing insulin, food and exercise in the section on ***Sports*** in Chapter 5.

My son has been putting on weight since being diagnosed as having diabetes three months ago. What are the reasons for this?

Most people lose weight before their diabetes is diagnosed and treated. In uncontrolled diabetes body fat is broken down and many calories are lost as glucose in the urine (this is discussed in more detail in the section on ***Symptoms*** in Chapter 1). As soon as the diabetes is brought under control, the body fat stops being broken down, the calories are no longer lost and the weight loss stops. Many people, like your son, begin to put weight back on again.

If your son starts to put on too much weight he should discuss this with his diabetes specialist nurse and his dietitian. They will advise him about his diet and, if he is on insulin, about reducing his food intake and his insulin simultaneously.

I have been taking insulin for eight years and over this time I have put on a lot of weight. My doctor says that insulin does not make you fat, but if that is so, then why have I put on so much weight?

People tend to lose weight if their diabetes is badly controlled, mainly because they are losing a lot of calories as glucose in their urine (this is discussed in more detail in the section on ***Symptoms*** in Chapter 1). Once the diabetes is controlled, the calories are no longer lost in this way, the weight loss stops, and there will be a tendency for a person starting treatment to put on weight. Insulin in the right dose does not make you fat, but if you are having too much insulin you will have to eat more to prevent hypos, and these extra calories will increase your weight.

When you are on insulin and become too fat, then losing the extra weight can be a slow business. You cannot afford the luxury of sudden, drastic dieting (not that this is recommended for anyone – it is not the best way to lose weight) but can only lose weight by careful reduction of both food and insulin. This can be a delicate balance but many people manage it successfully. It is obviously better if you can avoid putting the weight on in the first place!

There is a particular risk of weight gain when children stop growing. Children need enormous amounts of food when they are actually growing taller, but once fully grown they need to make a conscious effort to reduce their total food intake. Girls usually stop growing a year or two after their first period and unless they eat a lot less at that stage they will almost certainly become fat – and will find that it is much easier to put on weight than to take it off.

Since I went onto multiple injections to improve my control and fit in with my hectic work schedule I have put on quite a lot of weight. I am really pleased with my control but I know in part it is because I take my insulin now whereas I often didn't before because of the fear of hypos. Why do I keep on getting fatter?

The new system is helping you control your diabetes in your hectic lifestyle but it is important to realize that now you are taking your insulin at the right time all the food you eat is going to be used, and the excess is going to be stored as fat!

To control your weight you need to balance the food you eat with the amount of energy you use up. You should aim for a weight loss of between 1–2 lbs (½–1 kg) a week. Start by looking at the amounts of fat and alcohol in your diet, as these are both very concentrated sources of calories. Try to cut back on fatty foods, perhaps by having fruit or a diet yogurt instead of crisps or biscuits, and by choosing lean rather than fatty meat or replacing it with fish or poultry with the skin removed. If your weight loss slows up or stops, then be prepared to trim back a little on your starchy foods.

Before you start to notice a drop in weight your control might well improve further, so do be prepared to monitor your blood glucose and reduce your insulin as necessary. Regular exercise will help burn off some of the fat and stop the problem developing in the future. If your weight continues to be a problem be prepared to record all your meals and snacks for three or four days and then ask the dietitian to go over them with you to see where further changes can be made.

My 18-year-old daughter has diabetes and is trying to lose weight. She eats a low-carbohydrate diet and sticks to this rigidly. I cannot understand why she does not lose any weight.

Just reducing the amount of carbohydrate in her diet will not necessarily result in her losing weight. When you are trying to lose weight it is important to reduce the total number of calories in your diet, and this involves reducing the amounts of fat, protein, and alcohol you consume – particularly fat as it is such a concentrated form of calories. Your daughter should avoid fried foods, sugary foods and alcohol, cut down her cheese intake, substitute skimmed milk for ordinary milk and allow only a scraping of butter or margarine on her bread. She will find a diet that contains plenty of high-fibre carbohydrate will be more satisfying and cause less fluctuation in her blood glucose, and as a result it will be easier for her to follow. Ask your daughter to seek help from her doctor, dietitian and diabetes specialist nurse so that they can work together to prevent hypoglycaemia.

Injection technique

Is it necessary to use spirit before or after injecting myself?

We do not advise you to use spirit or alcohol for cleaning your skin as it is not necessary and it tends to harden the skin. If you feel you must clean the injection site (say after playing football) use soap and water only.

Is it dangerous to inject air bubbles that may be in the syringe after drawing up insulin?

The only reason you are taught to get rid of large air bubbles from the syringe after drawing up insulin is because the air takes the place of the insulin and therefore the dose will not be accurate. Very large quantities of air injected directly into the circulation could be dangerous and produce an airlock in the blood stream, but these amounts are far larger than could possibly be introduced when injecting insulin. Tiny air bubbles, even when introduced into a vein, would not do any harm and would quickly be absorbed.

Can two types of insulin be mixed in the same syringe?

Yes, many people these days are taking mixtures of insulin. Unless instructed otherwise by your doctor, you should inject mixtures of insulin immediately after they are drawn up, particularly if you are using a zinc-based insulin such as Monotard, Ultratard or ZN.

The rule for drawing up two types of insulin is to draw up the clear (short-acting) insulin first followed by the cloudy (long-acting) insulin. The reason for this is to prevent the clear bottle of insulin becoming 'contaminated' by the cloudy insulin. If this happens the clear (short-acting) insulin loses its quick-acting properties. The correct way of mixing insulins in the same syringe is illustrated in Plate 9 in the colour section in the middle of the book.

When drawing up my insulin I sometimes find that the insulin gets 'sucked back' into the bottle. Why is this?

This is due to a vacuum developing and it can be overcome by injecting a little air into the bottle before drawing the insulin out. Many people routinely put the same amount of air into the bottle as the amount of insulin they draw out to overcome the problem. Plates 8 and 9 in the colour section in the middle of the book show you how to do this. Research has shown that it may not be necessary to inject air into the bottle, but it is a simple procedure and cannot do any harm.

I have been giving my insulin injections at an angle of about 45 degrees for many years but have been told that this is incorrect. What do you advise?

Insulin is designed to be given into the deep layer of fat under the skin but not into the muscle. In the past, when longer needles were in use, people taking insulin injections were taught to pinch up their skin and then inject at an angle of 45 degrees. With the introduction of shorter 8 mm needles, teaching gradually changed, and many people gave their injections at right angles to the skin without first pinching up the skin. However, recent reports have suggested that thin people who use this perpendicular injection technique may sometimes inject into the muscle leading to an erratic absorption of insulin, and as a result teaching methods have changed yet again.

The current advice is to give the injection by first pinching up a generous amount of skin (do not squeeze too tightly as this may cause bruising), and then pushing the needle in quickly at right angles to the skin. If the needle is pushed through the skin quickly the injection should be virtually painless. Injection technique is shown in Plate 10 in the colour section in the middle of the book.

My young daughter spends a very long time giving her injection and complains that it is painful. Is there any advice you can give?

One of the reasons that she finds it painful is because she is probably pushing the needle slowly through the skin. The sensitive nerve endings lie virtually on the surface of the skin and are more likely to be stimulated if the needle enters the skin very slowly. Try to encourage her to push the needle through the skin as quickly as possible. The use of Micro-Fine needles will also make things easier, particularly if she is using the 8 mm 30G needle. If she still experiences difficulty then the ice cube technique may be helpful. She can hold a cube of ice against her skin for about 10 seconds – this 'freezes' the skin just long enough for the injection to be given. This method can be used until she has gained more confidence in giving herself her injections.

Sometimes after giving my injection I find that a small lump appears just under the skin. What is the cause of this?

It sounds as though you are giving your injection at too shallow a depth. If the insulin is injected into the skin (intradermally) a small lump will appear. Apart from being more painful, the insulin will not be absorbed properly. Try giving your injection more deeply by injecting at right angles to the skin (see Plate 10 in the colour section) and this will not happen.

Should I draw back on the plunger after inserting the needle to check for blood?

It used to be common practice to teach people to draw back on the plunger before injecting insulin to check that the needle had not entered a blood vessel. These days this is not usually taught as the chances of insulin entering a blood vessel are extremely slight, and pulling back on the plunger could make the injection more difficult for some people. The majority of people are now using pens and are unable to 'draw back'. If you are in the habit of drawing back before giving insulin by all means continue but it is not strictly necessary.

Sometimes after giving my injection I notice that the injection site bleeds a lot. Does this do any harm?

This may happen if you puncture a blood capillary (a very small blood vessel) which means that the needle goes straight through the capillary. You may then bleed from the injection site and probably see a bruise the following day, but it does no harm. It helps to press quickly with your finger or a tissue over the site. Occasionally this might lead to a slightly faster absorption of insulin.

When I have given my injection I sometimes see some insulin leaking out from the injection hole after taking out the needle. Should I give myself extra insulin later and how much should I give?

Insulin does sometimes leak out immediately after an injection. This can often be avoided by moving the skin to one side immediately after withdrawing the needle or, alternatively, moving the skin to one side before inserting the needle. This effectively means that the needle channel closes after the needle has been withdrawn. If either of these methods fails then have a tissue handy at injection time ready to press straight on the spot after giving the injection. Extra insulin should not be given if you lose a little because you will not know how much has been lost and will probably overcompensate, give too much and risk hypoglycaemia. Having taken too little insulin may mean that your blood glucose levels will be just higher than normal that day.

Injection sites

Where is the best place to give an injection of insulin?

Insulin is designed to be given into the deep layers of fat below the skin and basically can be given in any place where there is a reasonable layer of fat (Plate 10). The recommended places are the fronts and sides of the middle or upper thighs, the abdomen and the buttocks. The upper arms may also be used, but some women prefer not to use the arms in the summer months in case they have marks at the injection sites which may be noticeable when they wear summer dresses. It is very important not to develop 'favourite' injection areas, and to change to new sites regularly. Suitable sites for injection are shown in Figure 3.2.

I have unsightly lumps on my thighs where I inject my insulin. Could I have plastic surgery to make my thighs smooth again?

If you inject your insulin into the same area every time there is a strong chance that these lumps will appear. Some people have similar lumps on their abdomen from repeated injections into the same spot. If you carefully avoid the lumps and inject insulin somewhere else, then the lumps will eventually disappear although this may take a long time. Apart from looking odd these lumps may cause problems with your blood glucose control by altering the rate at which you absorb your insulin.

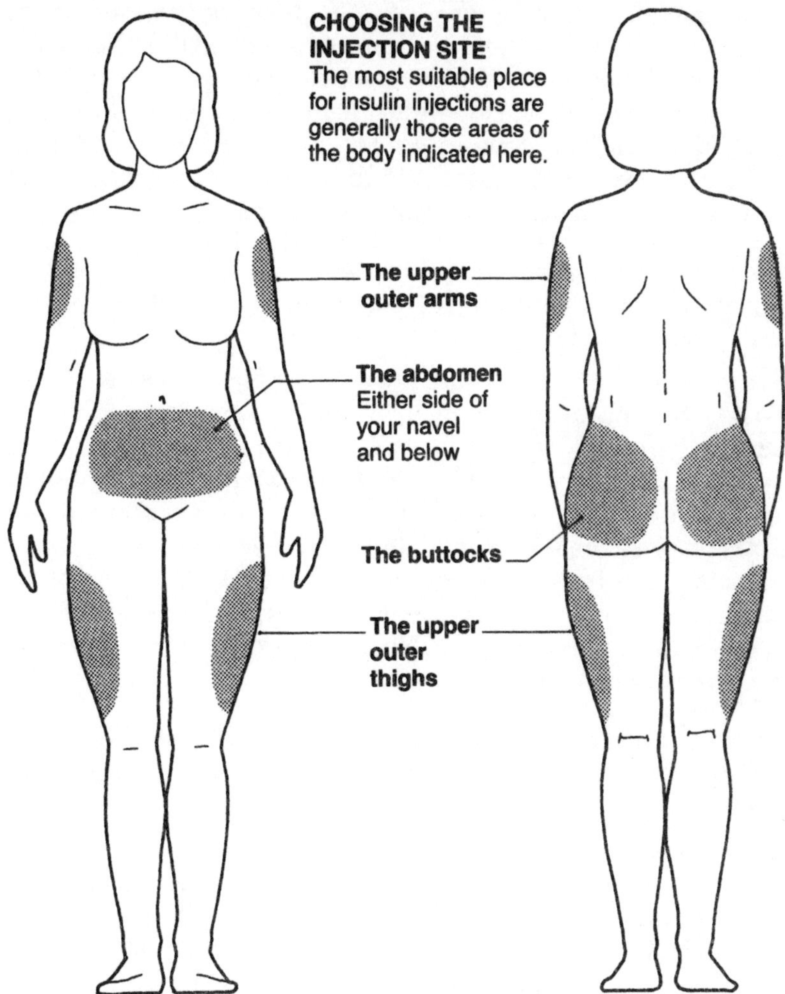

Important
Do not give injections in the same small area. This may lead to lumpiness of the skin.

Figure 3.2 Injection sites

So you can see that it is worth you changing to new sites for your injections – the sites you can use are shown in Figure 3.2. Sometimes it can be difficult to persuade people to change sites to avoid the lumps as injecting into them is less painful. Unfortunately they will only tend to get larger if you keep using them. Plastic surgery would leave a scar and is not recommended, although liposuction has had varying degrees of success.

The layer of fat beneath the surface of the skin of my thighs is very hard and I find it difficult to inject myself. Have you any suggestions?

This could be because you are not rotating injection sites and are reusing the same place too many times. This causes your flesh to become hard and as a result leads to erratic absorption of the insulin. These over-used areas should not be injected for about a year and new areas should be found instead (you will find suggestions for suitable sites in Figure 3.2).

Another possible cause for hard skin is the use of spirit for swabbing the skin. This is unnecessary and makes the skin tough and difficult to inject. Stop swabbing your skin and try softening it by rubbing in hand cream at night.

I have been taking insulin for 18 years and have unsightly bulges at the top of my thighs where I give my injections. How can I get rid of them?

These bulges are known as lipohypertrophy and are due to the build-up of fat below the skin. This is almost certainly caused by your constantly injecting insulin into the same site over several years. Insulin will not be absorbed properly from these areas and you should not use these sites again for at least a year. Instead inject into your abdomen, buttocks and upper arms until your thighs have been 'rested'. When you return to using your thighs, use a much larger area than before, and try to avoid the top of the thigh.

I have to increase my dose of insulin by 4 units when injecting into my arms and by 6 units when injecting into the abdomen to maintain control. Can you tell me why this is, and should I inject only into my thighs?

It is known that insulin is absorbed at different rates from different areas of the body. The fastest rate of absorption is from the abdomen and arms, and the slowest from the thighs and buttocks. For many people this will not make much difference to their control, but for others the difference may be significant, and you may be one of these people. You may wish to see if injecting into different areas affects your control by taking several blood glucose measurements at different times of the day each time you choose a new area.

Insulin is also more quickly absorbed from the thighs and buttocks if exercise is taken immediately after the injection. Heat also influences the rate of absorption of insulin, and it will be more quickly absorbed following a hot bath, after sunbathing in a hot country or after using a sun bed.

After using the tops of my thighs for my injection for many years I have recently started using my abdomen but now seem to have hypos every day. Why is this?

This is probably due to insulin being poorly absorbed in the past from your much-used injection areas. We normally suggest that people reduce their dose of insulin when changing to a new or rarely used area because the insulin is usually more effectively absorbed from these new areas, particularly if the dose has slowly increased over the years owing to the injection being given in the same place continually.

Insulin pens

What is an insulin pen, and what are the advantages of using one?

An insulin pen consists of a cartridge of insulin inside a fountain pen type case which is used with a special disposable needle. After you have dialled the required number of units of insulin, you press a button and the pen will release the correct dose of insulin.

Several makes of pen are now available and your specialist nurse or doctor will show you current models. They may be used with any of the cartridges listed in Table 3.1. Novopens are available on request from Novo Nordisk. B-D pens are obtainable from Becton Dickinson and can be fitted with replacement night and day caps (featuring a sun and a moon), if two different pens are being used. B-D can supply free magnifiers called B-D Pen Magniguides which can be clipped over the numbers of the B-D pens if your eyesight is a problem. The Autopen is obtainable from Owen Mumford (medical shop). All these pens should be available free of charge from your diabetes clinic. Addresses of manufacturers are listed in Appendix 3.

Insulin cartridges for all these pens can be prescribed by your doctor but unfortunately pen needles are not yet available on prescription.

Preloaded disposable pens which contain 300 units of insulin are obtainable on prescription. They are available with Human Actrapid, Insulatard, the full range of Mixtards, as well as the Humaject range made by Lilly. The preloaded pens are listed in Table 3.1.

The great advantage of the pen is that you do not need to carry around syringes and bottles of insulin. It is easy to give an injection away from home, e.g. in a restaurant or when travelling. If you are visually impaired, or if you suffer from arthritis in your hands, then you may find the dial-a-dose clicking action is easier to use than drawing up insulin in a conventional syringe.

All these pens rely on ordinary finger pressure for the injection, i.e. they are not automatic injectors.

If you have problems giving your injections but would like to use a pen, Lilly have introduced a pen that delivers the insulin via an automatic injector. After the dose has been dialled and the clip on the pen pressed, the needle (which is hidden from view) quickly penetrates the skin and automatically injects the insulin. It takes the standard 1.5 ml Humulin cartridge, uses B–D Micro-Fine+ pen needles, and has a two year guarantee. There are two models – the Diapen 1 which delivers up to 18 units of insulin at a time with 1 unit adjustments, and the Diapen 2 which delivers up to 36 units at a time with 2 unit adjustments. They can be purchased from Lilly Diabetes Care – if you contact them, they will tell you the current price.

Addresses for all the companies mentioned in this answer can be found in Appendix 3. Some of the pens are illustrated in the plate section.

What is the advantage of taking four injections a day with an insulin pen?

The idea of using a multiple injection regimen is to try to mimic the normal pancreas, and to give small doses of short-acting insulin to cover meals with a longer-acting insulin taken at bedtime to act as a background insulin. Now that most people are using insulin pens to give insulin, this system should really be called basal/bolus, i.e. long acting 'basal' insulin at night with a 'bolus' of short-acting insulin before each meal.

Some people who lead rather erratic lives find the insulin pen regimen more convenient. They have a little more flexibility over the timing of their meals, as the insulin is not taken until just before the meal is eaten. In practice they may also need some longer-acting insulin taken in the morning to act as a background insulin. Another advantage of using an insulin pen is that bottles of insulin do not need to be carried around during the day, and it is easy to give the injection very discreetly.

Pumps and injectors

I have heard about insulin pumps for treating diabetes. Doctors in my own clinic never seem very keen on the idea. How do pumps work and are they a good form of treatment?

First, an explanation of why insulin pumps have been developed. People who do not have diabetes release a very small amount of insulin into the blood stream throughout the day and by night. This insulin prevents the liver from releasing glucose into the blood-stream. Whenever the glucose level rises after a meal the pancreas immediately produces extra insulin to damp the level down. This is a simple feedback system designed to keep the level of blood glucose steady. Without the 'background' insulin in between meals, the level of blood glucose would slowly rise.

Insulin pumps are an attempt to copy this normal pattern. They consist of a slow motor driving a syringe containing insulin which is pumped down a fine-bore tube and needle. The needle is inserted under the skin and strapped in place. There is also a device for giving mealtime boosts of insulin.

Many people have successfully controlled their blood glucose with an insulin pump. However, they are cumbersome devices which have to be carried about all day long, and they also need a great deal of professional back-up.

You will see that pumps are not all plain sailing and they also require extra blood tests and adjustments in the dose of insulin. They are a good way of achieving tight control of diabetes in people with a high degree of commitment. Since the introduction of insulin pens, pumps have become less popular, although this may change again since the publication of the results of the DCCT (Diabetes Control and Complications Trial). There is more about the DCCT in the section on ***Control and monitoring*** in Chapter 4.

My diabetes is well controlled. Should I be thinking of buying a pump?

Probably not, if your diabetes really is well controlled. Pumps are only used in a small number of diabetes clinics throughout the UK. Insulin pumps require an expert team who can provide 24-hour cover in case of emergencies. Without such technical back-up, it is not really feasible to embark on pump therapy. However, since the publication of the DCCT (see the section on ***Control and monitoring*** in Chapter 4) pumps may be introduced into more centres in the future.

Research has shown that, if you are the sort of person who achieves good control by giving insulin with a standard insulin syringe, then you would probably be able to do slightly better using a pump, but if your control is normally erratic then equipping you with a pump is not likely to improve matters.

What are the main difficulties of using a pump for giving insulin?

The main problem with pumps is that, like all machines, they are capable of going wrong. One reason for the high cost of insulin pumps is the need to build a warning system into the design to alert the user to a mechanical fault. If the pump suddenly stops, the user will rapidly go into a state of complete insulin lack and may quickly develop ketoacidosis.

Because the needle remains under the skin it acts as a foreign body and may set up a focus of infection leading to an abscess. The needle must only be inserted after careful cleaning of the skin.

From the user's point of view, the main disadvantage of the pump is the fact that it has to be worn day and night. This is obviously more inconvenient than the ordinary injections which are over and done with. Many people dislike the pump which they find a constant reminder of their diabetes.

My son has trouble giving himself injections and has asked me if he can use an injector. What type of injector should he use?

With insulin pens and fine gauge disposable needles injections are rarely a problem if the correct technique is used. Most people find injectors more trouble than they are worth, and they are something extra to carry around, but they may help people like your son who are going through a difficult patch.

There are several injectors around which work on a similar principle of pushing the needle very quickly through the skin, whilst hiding the needle from view. The Injectomatic is for use only with Monoject syringes, comes in two sizes (one specifically for 1 ml and one for 0.5 ml syringes) and is obtainable from D.E.P.T.H. As well as offering fast needle penetration the Auto-Injector also automatically delivers the insulin at speed with a conventional syringe. Its disadvantages are that it is rather noisy and oversized. It is obtainable from Owen Mumford (Medical Shop), or D.E.P.T.H. (addresses in Appendix 3). The latest addition to the range is the B-D Automatic Injector (Inject-Ease) which fits all the B-D insulin syringes and is extremely easy to use. It pushes the needle through the skin but does not inject the insulin. It is available either through healthcare professionals or retail pharmacies. None of these injectors is available on prescription.

If your son would like to use an insulin pen, Lilly have introduced a pen that delivers the insulin via an automatic injector. You will find information about it in the first question in the section on ***Insulin pens*** earlier in this chapter.

What is the 'jet' injector?

This is an injector which works by firing liquid, such as insulin, through the skin from very high pressure jets. It is not entirely painless, is very bulky, very expensive, unsuitable for those who mix insulins and has not yet been proved to be harmless when multiple injections are given. These injectors are no longer marketed in the UK. Until more is known about the long-term effects, we would not advise its use.

Practical aspects

When I was discharged from hospital with newly diagnosed diabetes I was given a few disposable syringes and needles for my injections. How do I obtain more?

Disposable insulin syringes and needles are available free on prescription. Your GP can supply you with a prescription for any make of insulin syringe you choose and they can then be obtained free from the chemist. Alternatively you can buy them directly from the chemist without a prescription (although you will have to pay for them), or you can send for them by post from suppliers such as D.E.P.T.H. or Owen Mumford (Medical Shop). Their addresses are in Appendix 3. Alternatively you may consider changing to an insulin pen.

What is the best way of disposing of insulin syringes and needles?

There is a device available called the B-D Safe-Clip which cuts the needle off the top of the syringe and retains it in the device. The clipped syringes can then be disposed of in a used bleach bottle (or similar) which should have the cap replaced and sealed with tape before being thrown into the dustbin. Some local authorities provide special containers and a collection service for people who are treated with insulin.

The B-D Safe-Clip is obtainable on prescription from your GP.

I have heard that disposable syringes and needles can be reused. How many times can they be reused and how can they be kept clean in between injections?

Although the manufacturers state that disposable syringes and needles are for single use only, they may be reused. (The Department of Health has stated that insulin syringes should be marked for Single Patient Use to avoid confusion about the reusability of syringes.)

The most commonly used insulin syringes come complete with a fixed needle on the end of the syringe and therefore will only last as long as the needle. We do not recommend that these are used for more than about four or five injections as the needles become blunt. Some cloudy insulins tend to clog the fine gauge needles when they are reused frequently.

Disposable syringes should be kept dry between injections with the protective cover placed over the needle, and preferably kept in a clean place. They must never be boiled and should not be kept in any type of spirit as the marks rub off.

There is a bewildering array of syringes and needles on the market. Which are the best types to use?

In this country there are three sizes of syringe for use with U100 insulin: the more commonly used 0.5 ml syringe marked with 50 single divisions for those taking not more than 50 units of insulin in one injection; the 1 ml syringe marked up to 100 units in 2 unit divisions for those taking more than 50 units of insulin in one injection; and the most recently introduced (from B-D) 0.3 ml syringe which has been designed for children, or those taking less than 30 units of insulin in one injection. All these syringes are marked with the word INSULIN on the side of the syringe, and no other type should be used when giving an insulin injection. They are all shown in Figure 3.3.

Note that one division on the 0.3 ml and 0.5 ml syringes is equal

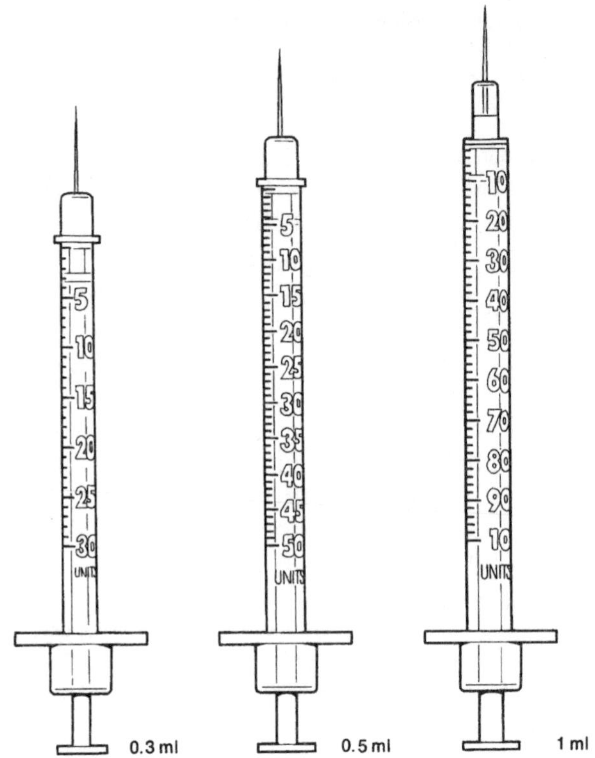

Figure 3.3 Insulin syringes – 0.3 ml, 0.5 ml and 1 ml

to 1 unit of insulin, while on the 1 ml syringe one division is equal to 2 units of insulin.

The most popular syringe is the B-D syringe which comes complete with a fixed Micro-Fine+ ½″ (12.7 mm) needle, but there are several other makes available. B-D have recently introduced an 8 mm 30G needle which is the finest gauge available.

I am partially sighted. What syringes are available for people like me, or for people who are blind? Are there any gadgets which would help me with my injections?

Most visually impaired people would be advised to use an insulin pen but, if you wish to use a syringe, B-D and Sherwood can supply

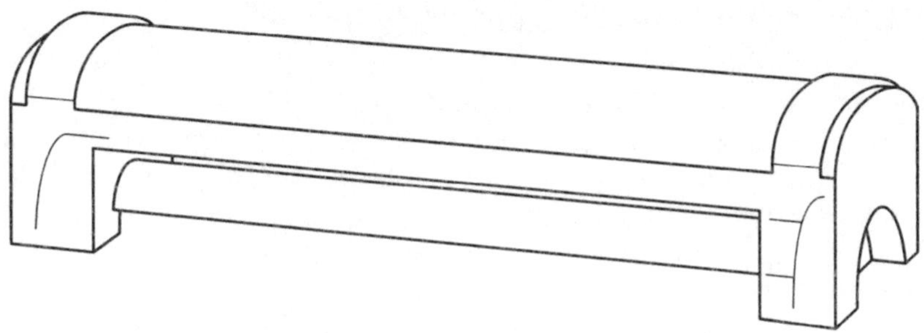

Figure 3.4 B-D magnifier to clip over plastic syringes

magnifiers which clip over their plastic syringes which may make the marks easier to read. Scale magnifiers for syringes may also be obtained from D.E.P.T.H. B-D also supply plastic gauges for use with their syringes but, as they have to be cut off at the correct dose by a sighted person, they would be of little use for people requiring frequent changes in their dose of insulin.

An insulin pen is probably the best choice for people like you who are visually impaired. It is quite easy to use once the technique has been mastered, and offers a good choice of insulin regimens. This should be discussed with your physician or diabetes specialist nurse. There is a section about ***Insulin pens*** earlier in this chapter.

I am using a glass insulin syringe but do not know the best way of sterilizing it. I have been told that boiling is not good.

We do not recommend that you boil glass syringes as they may crack after being boiled several times. It also takes time and the syringes wear out more quickly. It is better to store the glass syringe (and needle) in a syringe carrying case that is half filled with industrial methylated spirit (*not* surgical spirit) and change the spirit in the case about once a week. Before the insulin is drawn up the plunger should be worked up and down several times to remove the spirit. Industrial methylated spirit and syringe carrying cases are obtainable on prescription from your GP. Alternatively you may wish to consider changing to an insulin pen (see previous question).

Where should I keep my supplies of insulin?

Stores of insulin should ideally be kept in a refrigerator, but *not* in the freezer or freezing compartment. The best place is the vegetable compartment or the door of the fridge, which will ensure that there is no possibility of the insulin freezing. If you do not have a fridge, then insulin may be stored for about a month at room temperature but keep it away from direct heat such as radiators and strong sunlight. Many people prefer to keep their insulin bottle and/or their insulin pen in current use at room temperature as it may make the injection more comfortable.

Should I wipe the top of the insulin bottle with spirit before drawing up the required dose?

Although some clinics teach people to clean the tops of the insulin bottles, we do not think that it is necessary.

Hypos

Since my wife has been started on insulin she has had funny turns. What is the cause of this?

Your wife's funny turns are likely to be due to a low blood glucose. The medical name for this is hypoglycaemia and most people call it *hypo* for short.

The feelings people have when they are hypo are due to two things. First, the brain itself cannot work properly when the blood glucose falls below a certain level (usually 3 mmol/l), and secondly the body reacts to a low blood glucose by producing hormones (mainly adrenaline) which increase the blood glucose. When the brain is affected by a low blood glucose level, it may cause weakness of the legs, double or blurred vision, confusion, headache and, in severe cases, loss of consciousness and convulsions. The adrenaline causes sweating, rapid heartbeat and feelings of panic and anxiety. Children often describe a 'dizzy feeling' or just 'tiredness' when they are hypo. Most people find it hard to describe how they feel when hypo but the proof is that the blood glucose is low. If there is any doubt about the accuracy of readings, it is always safer to take glucose or sugar. A list of hypo symptoms is given in Table 3.2.

Table 3.2 Symptoms of hypo in groups

CAUSE	SYMPTOM
Due to adrenaline response	Sweating Pounding heart Shaking/trembling Hunger Anxiousness Tingling
Due to brain lack of glucose	Confusion/difficulty in thinking Drowsiness/weakness Odd (stroppy) behaviour Speech difficulty
Non-specific	Nausea Headache Tiredness

What is the best thing to take when I have a hypo?

This very much depends at which stage you recognize the hypo is developing. In the early stages the best treatment would be to have a meal or snack if one is due. If it is some time before your next meal, then it would be best for you to have an extra snack, such as fruit, sandwiches, or biscuits.

If your hypo is fairly well advanced then you need to take some very rapidly absorbed carbohydrate. This is best taken as sugar, sweets or fruit juice or, for even greater speed, a sugary drink such as ordinary (*not* 'diet') Coke, lemonade or Lucozade. The best things to carry in your pocket are glucose tablets such as Dextro-Energy as they are absorbed very quickly (three tablets of Dextro-Energy contain 10 g of glucose). They are also less likely to be eaten when you are not hypo than ordinary sweets!

I am taking soluble and isophane insulin twice a day and am getting hypos two to three hours after my evening meal. As I live alone this has been worrying me. What can I do?

Anyone who is having frequent hypos at a particular time of day can easily put this right by adjusting their insulin. In this case you are having hypos at the time when your evening dose of soluble insulin is working. You should reduce the amount of soluble insulin you take in the evening until you have stopped having hypos at that time. Hypos *before* your evening meal could be corrected by reducing your morning dose of intermediate-acting (isophane) insulin.

My teenage daughter has diabetes and sometimes turns very nasty and short-tempered. Is this due to the insulin?

Yes, probably – although it is not the only cause of bad moods in teenagers! The only way to find out is try to persuade her to have a blood glucose measurement during her bad moods. If it is low (3 mmol/l or less) then some glucose should restore her good nature. Because the brain is affected by a low blood glucose level, irrational behaviour is common during a hypo. Your daughter may forcibly deny that she is hypo and resist taking the glucose her body needs. If you are firm and do not panic you will be able to talk her into taking the glucose (Lucozade can be useful here) and she will soon be back to normal.

Children can also become irritable if their blood glucose is very high.

My 8-year-old son often complains of feeling tired after recovering from a hypo. Is this usual and what is the best way to overcome it?

It is unusual to feel tired for a long time after a hypo but if your son does so, you should first check his blood glucose. If this is more than 4 mmol/l you will just have to let him rest until he is back to normal. It is not uncommon for hypos to trigger headaches and migraine attacks, which may be the problem here.

My teenage son refuses to take extra carbohydrate when he is hypo and insists that we let him sleep it off. Is this all right?

Hypos should always be corrected as quickly as possible. Your son is right in thinking that the insulin will eventually wear off and that his blood glucose will return to normal. However, if his blood glucose falls to very low levels, it could cause problems and he may even become unconscious. His refusal to take sugar is part of the confusion that occurs during a hypo and, if he can be persuaded to take glucose, he will get better more quickly.

I have been taking insulin for 38 years and my hypos have always been mild. Recently I suffered two blackouts lasting a minute which I presume were hypos. Why has this started?

Blackouts tend to occur in children who have not yet learned to recognize the warning signs of a hypo but, on rare occasions, anyone on insulin can be caught unawares and have a sudden hypo, which makes them black out.

Sometimes as people get older the 'adrenaline' warnings of a hypo fail to operate. This failure may be due to the natural ageing process or to damage (caused by diabetes) of the involuntary nerve supply which transmits the warning signs. Recent studies have suggested that keeping blood glucose levels above 4 mmol/l can help to restore lost hypo warnings. 'Make 4 the floor' is the latest advice.

A number of people have reported that after changing to human insulin they have less warning of hypos. So far there is no explanation for this. We have discussed human insulin in the section on ***Insulin*** at the beginning of this chapter.

I have recently lost my warning signs for hypos. Is it likely that they will return?

Very tight diabetic control is known to reduce hypoglycaemic awareness. In a recent study, carried out with the help of patients who had lost their warning symptoms, the results showed that when they ran their diabetic control so as to prevent low blood glucose levels altogether for three months, partial or complete restoration of warning symptoms was experienced by all patients who had managed to avoid dropping to blood glucose levels of 3 mmol/l or less. Do you think that you may fall into this category?

If so, it may be worth discussing this with your diabetes team and reducing your dose of insulin.

My father has had diabetes for 20 years. Recently he had what his doctor calls epileptic fits. Would you tell me how to help him and if there is a cure?

A bad hypo may bring on a fit and it is important to check your father's blood glucose during an attack. If it is low then reducing his insulin should stop the fits. If the fits are not related to his diabetes then it should be possible to control them by taking tablets regularly – ask your doctor for more details about these.

Can insulin reactions eventually cause permanent brain damage?

This question is often asked and is a great source of anxiety to many people. The brain quickly recovers from a hypo and there is unlikely to be permanent damage, even after a severe attack with convulsions. Very prolonged hypoglycaemia can occur in a patient with a tumour that produces insulin, and if someone is unconscious for days on end then the brain will not recover completely. This is not likely to occur in people with diabetes, in whom the insulin wears off after a few hours.

I have heard that there is an opposite to insulin called glucagon. Is this something like glucose and can it be used to bring someone round from a hypo?

Glucagon is a hormone which, like insulin, is produced by the pancreas. It causes glucose to be released into the blood stream from stores of starch in the liver. It can be used to bring someone round from a hypo if they are too restless or unconscious to swallow glucose. Glucagon cannot be stored in solution like insulin but comes in a vial in a plastic pack. This contains the glucagon powder plus a syringe and sterile fluid for dissolving the powder. The process of dissolving the glucagon and drawing it into the syringe may be a bit difficult especially if you are feeling panicky. It is worth asking the diabetes specialist nurse to show you and your likely helper how to draw up glucagon.

It is usually stated that glucagon only has a short-lasting effect and it is therefore important to follow it up with some glucose to prevent a relapse of coma. However, in children the blood glucose may rise very high after glucagon and, as they often feel sick, it seems silly to force more sugar down them. It is best to do a blood test to help decide whether more glucose is needed immediately. Longer-acting carbohydrate (such as bread or biscuits) should be given as soon as they feel well enough to eat it as the blood glucose can fall again later.

Is it normal to vomit shortly after a glucagon injection?

Some people do vomit after regaining consciousness after a glucagon injection, particularly children. If only half the contents of the vial are given, it will usually be enough to correct the hypo but be less likely to cause sickness.

My diabetes was controlled by tablets for 20 years but two years ago my doctor recommended that I begin insulin treatment. I am well controlled but my sleep is often disturbed by dreams, or I wake up feeling hungry. Can you advise me what to do if this happens?

You may be going hypo in the middle of the night. It has been shown that many people have a low blood glucose in the early hours of the night and provided they feel all right and sleep well this probably does not matter. However, if you are regularly waking with hypo symptoms (such as hunger) or having nightmares you should first check whether you are hypo by measuring your blood glucose at around 3.00 a.m. when your blood glucose is usually lowest. If the reading is below 4 mmol/l you need to reduce your evening dose of medium-acting insulin. If your blood glucose is then high before breakfast the next day, an injection of medium-acting insulin taken before going to bed instead of before your evening meal may solve your problem.

What can I do if my son has a bad hypo and is too drowsy to take any glucose by mouth?

You should try giving him Hypostop. This is a jelly loaded with glucose which comes in a container with a nozzle. It can be squirted onto the gums of someone who is severely hypo and in many cases it leads to recovery within a few minutes. Hypostop is available on prescription from your GP, or can be obtained from Bio Diagnostics Ltd (the address is in Appendix 3). If Hypostop fails, you should next try injecting your son with glucagon – there are some questions about glucagon earlier in this section.

Am I correct in thinking that only people on insulin can have hypos?

No. Some of the tablets used for diabetes cause hypos. The commonly used ones are glibenclamide (Euglucon, Daonil) and chlorpropamide (Diabinese). These hypos will improve with glucose in the normal way but, because the tablets have a longer action than insulin, the hypo may return again after several hours. Chlorpropamide is particularly dangerous in this respect, as the hypos may return at any time for up to 36 hours. Anyone having hypos on tablets probably needs to reduce the dose. Metformin does not cause hypos.

My diabetes is treated by diet alone and I have headaches and a light-headed feeling around midday if I have been busy in the morning. I am all right after eating something. Why is this?

It seems surprising but some people on diet alone can go hypo if they go without food. This is because they produce their own insulin but too late and sometimes too much. Ideally you should try to arrange a blood glucose measurement at a time that you feel odd in order to prove that you are actually hypo. If so, you could avoid the problem by eating little and often, especially on days when you are busy.

My daughter aged 21 takes insulin for her diabetes and is moving down to London where she hopes to rent a flat on her own. In view of the risk of hypoglycaemic attacks, would you advise against this?

By the age of 21 your daughter will be ready to be independent and live in a flat by herself. All parents worry when their children leave home, and diabetes adds to their anxiety, but sooner or later, young people have to lead separate lives. We know that night hypos are common and that people either wake up and sort themselves out or else their blood glucose returns to normal as the insulin wears off and they wake up next morning unaware of any problem. However, there has been a handful of cases when people on insulin are found unexpectedly dead in bed, and presumably this is due to hypoglycaemia. This must be a cause of concern but considering the hundreds of thousands of people on insulin, the risk of this tragedy is equivalent to being struck by lightning and young people on insulin have a right to independence.

Your daughter should be aware of the risk of hypo when driving or swimming and be encouraged to tell her close friends and companions about diabetes. They should be told that, if she ever behaves oddly, she must be given some form of sugar, even if she protests. People often fail to take this simple precaution; it can avoid a lot of worry to their friends who may find them hypo and yet have no idea how to help.

4

Monitoring and control

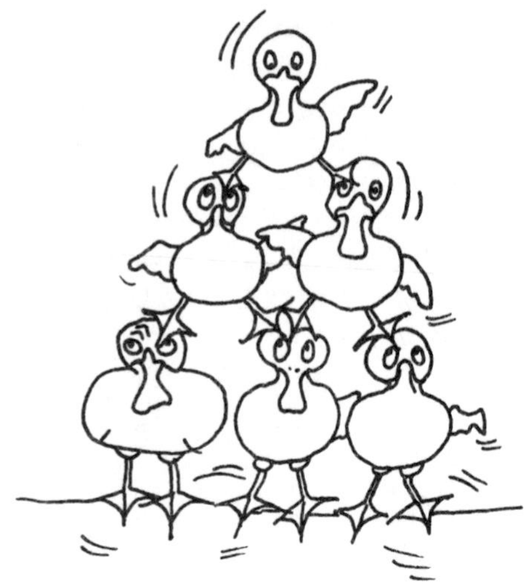

Introduction

The key to a successful life with diabetes is achieving good blood glucose control. Your degree of success can be judged only by measurements of your body's response to treatment as, unfortunately, if you have diabetes the fact that you feel well does not mean that you are well controlled. It is only when control goes badly wrong that you may be aware that something is amiss. If your blood glucose is too low you may be aware of hypo symptoms which, if left untreated, may progress to unconsciousness (hypoglycaemic coma). At the other end of the spectrum, when the blood glucose concentration rises very steeply, you may be aware of increased thirst and urination – which, if left untreated, may progress to nausea, vomiting, weakness, and eventual clouding of consciousness and coma. It has long been apparent that relying on how you feel is too imprecise, even though some people may be able to 'feel' subtle changes in their control. For this reason, many different tests have been developed to allow precise measurement of control and as the years go by these tests get better and better.

The involvement of the person with diabetes in monitoring and control of their own condition has always been essential for successful treatment. With the development of blood glucose monitoring this has become even more apparent: it allows you to measure precisely how effective you are at balancing the conflicting forces of diet, exercise and insulin, and to make adjustments in order to maintain this balance. In the early days after the discovery of insulin, urine tests were the only tests available and it required a small laboratory even to do these. Urine tests have always had the disadvantage that they are only an indirect indicator of what you really need to know, which is the level of glucose in the blood. Blood glucose monitoring first became available to people with diabetes in 1977 and since then has become widely accepted. As anyone who has monitored glucose levels in the blood will know, these vary considerably throughout the day as well as from day to day. For this reason, a single reading at a twice yearly visit to the local diabetes clinic is of limited value in assessing long-term success or failure with control.

The introduction of haemoglobin A_{1c} (glycosylated haemoglobin or HbA_{1c}) and fructosamine measurements has given a very reliable test for longer-term monitoring of average blood glucose levels (taking into account the peaks and troughs) over an interval of two to three weeks in the case of fructosamine, and of two to three months with HbA_{1c}. Attaining a normal HbA_{1c} or fructosamine level indicates that the blood glucose concentration has been contained within the normal range, and also that (providing there are no unacceptable attacks of hypoglycaemia) balance is excellent and no further changes are required. It can be seen that attaining a normal HbA_{1c} or fructosamine level and maintaining it as near normal as possible is an important goal. Not everyone can achieve this, but it is undoubtedly the most effective way of eliminating the risk of long-term complications, as has been proven in the Diabetes Control and Complications Trial in the USA (see the second question in the section on ***Control and monitoring*** for more information about this trial).

Monitoring other aspects of health is also an important part of long-term diabetes care. Regular checks on eyes, blood pressure and feet are a good way of picking up conditions that require treatment at a stage before they have done any serious damage (long-term complications are covered in Chapter 9). The control of your diabetes is important and so is the detection and treatment of any complications, so make sure you are getting the medical care and education you need to stay healthy. Diabetes UK have published a guide called *What diabetes care to expect*, which we have reprinted in the section on ***Diabetes clinics*** later in this chapter.

Control and monitoring

I am an 18-year-old on insulin. When my glucose is high I do not feel any ill effects. Is it really necessary for me to maintain strict control?

It is quite true that some people do not develop the typical thirst or dry mouth, frequency of passing water (urination), or tiredness which usually occur if the blood glucose is high and diabetes out of control. It sounds as if you are one of these people, which makes it much more difficult for you to sense when your control is poor and take steps to improve it. Yet even without these symptoms, control of your blood glucose is still important. The development of complications after many years is much less likely (and may possibly even be eliminated) if you can maintain blood glucose concentrations within the normal range. We know that it is difficult at 18 to be concerned about things which may only happen a long time ahead in your future, but good control really is worth it in the long run.

My 17-year-old daughter has had diabetes for six years. She is finding it very difficult to keep her diabetes under control at present and doesn't seem to care if her sugars run high most of the time. Do you think she is doing herself any real damage?

Until recently there was no hard proof that good control of blood glucose made any difference to the risk of developing the complications of diabetes (which are dealt with in Chapter 9). However, in September 1993 the findings of the Diabetes Control and Complications Trial (known as the DCCT) were published. In this painstaking study in the USA over 1400 people with type 1 diabetes were divided into two groups, depending on how closely they controlled their blood glucose, and followed up for an average of seven years.

The group with good control, with an average HbA_{1c} of 7.2% (see the section on ***Haemoglobin A_{1c} and fructosamine*** later in this chapter for an explanation of this measurement) benefited from a 60% reduction in disease of the eyes, kidneys and nerves compared with the group with less good control. To achieve this degree of control the people in this group had four daily injections or gave insulin with a constant infusion pump. They also had considerable support from a team of diabetes specialists, including nurse educators, dietitians, psychologists and doctors. This improvement in control was accompanied by a threefold increase in the risk of hypos, and occasionally these hypos required help from a third party to bring the person round.

Thus your daughter is faced with a difficult decision. If she carries on with poor control, she increases her chance of developing long-term problems from her diabetes. If, on the other hand, she decides to try and improve her blood glucose levels, she may have more hypos. In practice, it is worth spending time with your daughter discussing the problem with sensitivity rather than facing her with a stark choice. She needs to be given time to make up her own mind, but remember that occasional hypos do not do any lasting harm and, so long as they are not frequent or severe, are almost always experienced by those with good control.

Whenever I go to the clinic I always feel guilty for not doing enough blood tests. In fact I sometimes feel like writing in some make-believe tests into my testing book just to keep the doctors happy.

Writing make-believe tests in your book won't keep your doctors happy and, more importantly, won't help you stop feeling guilty about not doing your blood tests. What might help is looking at some possible reasons why you are not doing the tests.

When you first went on insulin you were probably the centre of attention with support from your family, school friends or workmates. You probably had close contact with a diabetes specialist nurse to help you through a difficult time. During this period, measuring your blood glucose became a routine occurrence so that you could adjust your dose of insulin. After a few months, this phase of intense attention passed and you may have decided on a fixed insulin dose, only to be varied in unusual circumstances.

It can be depressing when the initial interest fades and you have to come to terms with the realization that the routine of diabetes is for keeps. This is a time when people may give up testing their blood glucose except when they feel ill. We have interviewed a number of people who have given up testing and the most common reasons they gave for giving up are as follows:

- Testing is messy and bloody.
- I haven't got time/can't be bothered to test my blood.
- There is no need to test if you feel all right.
- Testing my blood brings it home to me that I have diabetes.
- It is inconvenient/embarrassing testing in public or at work.
- Insulin injections are essential, blood tests are not.
- A bad test makes me feel even more depressed about my diabetes.
- There is no point in testing my blood as I don't use the information.

These are the opinions of people living with diabetes and they must be respected. You might like to think where you stand on this subject, and perhaps discuss it with someone on your next clinic visit. We feel that if you need insulin you will only achieve good control by doing regular blood tests as the only way of finding out how you are getting on.

In the past 12 months I have had to increase my insulin dosage several times yet I was still unable to get a blood test result that was near normal. I have had diabetes for 25 years and until last year I have always been well controlled. What has gone wrong?

Here are a few reasons why your blood glucose levels may have crept up and why you need more insulin after many years of good control.

- Less exercise will mean that more insulin is needed for your food intake.
- An increase in your diet.
- Increased stress or emotional upsets.
- Any illness which tends to linger on may lead to a need for more insulin.
- Technical problems with injections such as the appearance of lumps from repeated doses of insulin into the same site.
- Increase in weight and middle-aged spread.

Having said all that, some people do find that the dose of insulin that they need may vary by quite large amounts for no obvious reason.

Can stress influence blood glucose readings?

Yes, but the response varies from one person to another. In some people stress tends to make the blood glucose rise whereas in other people it may increase the risk of hypoglycaemia.

Would I be able to achieve better control if I went onto three injections a day?

Possibly. Most people on multiple injections use an insulin pen which is very convenient. In some cases this has improved control, but studies carried out so far show that not all people have necessarily shown an improvement. However, people like the insulin pen because it makes mealtimes more flexible and frees them from having to eat at fixed times. There is a section on ***Insulin pens*** in Chapter 3.

Blood glucose

What is the normal range of blood glucose in a person who does not have diabetes?

Before meals the range is from 3.5 to 5.5 mmol/l. After meals it may rise as high as 10 mmol/l depending on the carbohydrate content of the meal. However long a person without diabetes goes without food, the blood glucose concentration never drops below 3 mmol/l, and however much they eat, it never goes above 10 mmol/l.

My blood glucose monitor is calculated in millimoles. Can you tell me what a millimole is?

In the 1960s, international agreement led to scientists in most parts of the world using a standard system of metric measurements. The units are called SI units, an abbreviation of their full name – the 'Système International d'Unites'. There are several units, many of which you probably use without thinking about them, such as the metre. The unit for an amount of a substance is called a mole; the prefix milli- means one thousandth, so a millimole is one thousandth of a mole. Blood glucose is measured in millimoles of glucose per litre of blood, and this is abbreviated to mmol/l.

Before SI units were introduced, blood glucose was measured in milligrams per 100 millilitres of blood (abbreviated to mg% or to mg per dl) and this measurement is still used in the USA. The table below shows how one set of units relates to the other.

1 mmol/l = 18 mg%	9 mmol/l = 162 mg%
2 mmol/l = 36 mg%	10 mmol/l = 180 mg%
3 mmol/l = 54 mg%	12 mmol/l = 216 mg%
4 mmol/l = 72 mg%	15 mmol/l = 270 mg%
5 mmol/l = 90 mg%	20 mmol/l = 360 mg%
6 mmol/l = 108 mg%	22 mmol/l = 396 mg%
7 mmol/l = 126 mg%	25 mmol/l = 450 mg%
8 mmol/l = 144 mg%	30 mmol/l = 540 mg%

Is blood glucose monitoring suitable for people whose diabetes is controlled by tablets?

Yes, it is. Everyone with diabetes, whether controlled by diet, diet and tablets, or insulin, should strive for perfect control. Traditionally this has been achieved by regular urine tests at home. Since 1977 there has been a move towards encouraging people to do their own blood glucose measurements. This form of monitoring was first thought to be most suitable for insulin-treated people. However, further experience has shown that it is equally suited to those treated with diet and tablets. The disadvantage of having to prick your finger to obtain a drop of blood is more than compensated for by the increased accuracy and reliability of the readings so obtained.

Should I keep my sticks for blood glucose monitoring in the fridge with my insulin?

No. It is important to keep them dry as any moisture will impair their activity. You must put the lid back on the container immediately after removing a strip (unless the strips are individually foil-wrapped). The strips contain enzymes which are biological substances that do not last forever, and the sticks should never be used beyond their expiry date. The bottle of sticks should be kept in a cool, dry place, and should not be exposed to extremely high temperatures. If you have any reason to suspect the result of a blood test the best thing is to repeat the test using a new bottle of strips.

I had a glucose tolerance test and my highest blood glucose was 17 mmol/l. However, my urine analysis was negative for glucose. Is there a way I could test my blood for glucose without going to the laboratory?

You appear to have a 'high renal threshold' to glucose (see the section on ***Urine*** later in this chapter for more information about this) which means that it is only at very high concentrations of glucose in the blood that any glucose escapes into your urine. In your case urine tests are unhelpful and blood tests essential. Nowadays most people monitor their blood glucose quite simply at home.

There are several different blood testing techniques, most of them based on reagent strips containing enzymes that react to the glucose in the blood and produce a colour which is deeper as the concentration of glucose in the blood rises. Although the colour that develops on the strip can be read by eye, it is possible to make this reading more effective by use of a specially designed meter. Some strips which do not change colour can only be used with a specific meter.

Most hospital diabetes clinics will be able to show you the various strips and meters that are available, and your choice should be made after discussion with your diabetes specialist nurse or doctor in the clinic. All the different methods give good results provided they are used sensibly and after proper instruction. The blood glucose meters are not available on prescription, but the strips are.

There is more information about both strips and meters later in this section, and a list of meters currently available in Appendix 1. Plates 1–7 in the colour section in the middle of the book show how to use them correctly.

When I am in a hypo I cannot read the colours on the blood test strips. What do you advise?

In your case it would be preferable for you to have a meter that will give you a direct reading of your blood glucose. People vary in their ability to read the colours on the strips, but when the blood glucose levels are low, colour vision often deteriorates. Concentration also fails which makes the timing of the procedure less accurate and increases the risk of error. If you are unable to test have something to eat and try again later.

I feel hypo when my blood glucose is normal and only well when it is high. I feel very ill when my doctor tries to keep my blood glucose normal. Am I hooked on a high blood glucose?

In someone who has had poor control for several years, the brain and other tissues in the body can adjust themselves to a high concentration of glucose in the blood. As a result they may feel hypo at a time when their blood glucose is normal or even high. The long-term outlook for such people is not good unless they can re-educate themselves to tolerate normal blood glucose levels without feeling unwell. This is possible but requires determination and an understanding of the long-term dangers of a high blood glucose.

Your problem can be overcome by regular measurement of blood glucose, but you must accept that however unwell you feel no harm will be done if your blood glucose remains above 4 mmol/l. It may take up to six months of good control for this feeling to wear off, but it will be worth it.

Apart from the initial day or two after diagnosis I have had no glucose in my urine at any time since I have been on treatment with a diet and metformin tablets. I feel lost without an occasional blood glucose for guidance, so can you suggest any guidelines for me?

If you check your urine two hours after a meal and your tests consistently remain negative for glucose, then you need to ascertain what sort of levels the blood glucose reaches before you show any glucose in the urine. You can do this either by making a note of the results of the blood tests that you had when you went to the diabetes clinic or to your GP and relating those to your urine tests, or alternatively by learning how to do your own blood glucose readings and making a study yourself at home.

Consistently negative urine tests used to be regarded as an indication of satisfactory diabetes control. We now know that this is not always the case and that some people can still have negative urine tests at a time when their blood glucose is quite high. Our criteria for good control is blood glucose readings within the range 4–10 mmol/l with an average of approximately 5 mmol/l and a haemoglobin A_{1c} of less than 6.0% (depending on the range of the local laboratory). If you can achieve this by monitoring your urine then that is all that is strictly necessary but it sounds as if you would feel happier if you gave up urine testing and adopted blood testing as your regular monitoring routine.

Is there a way of knowing how much extra Actrapid insulin to give depending on my blood glucose level so I can maintain a better blood glucose?

The answer is yes, but it will require some experimenting on your part. The particular type and dose of insulin most suited to *you* can best be judged by repeated measurements of *your* body's response to the insulin you are taking. If you find, for example, that your blood glucose always goes very high after breakfast then you may be able to prevent this by taking more Actrapid before breakfast but, before making any adjustment in insulin dosage, it is important to see that the blood glucose changes you see are part of a regular pattern. This is part of the process of balancing insulin, diet and exercise, and we would caution against taking an extra dose of insulin if you come across a rather high blood glucose reading as an isolated finding. It is usually far better to try to work out a routine whereby you can prevent your blood glucose from rising too high rather than to take an extra injection of insulin after it has happened. There are exceptions to this rule, of course. If you suddenly become unwell and your blood glucose goes very high, repeated extra injections of a short-acting insulin such as Actrapid are the most effective way of preventing the development of ketoacidosis (see the ***Glossary*** for an explanation of this serious condition).

Are there any general guidelines for insulin adjustment?

This will really depend on the type of insulin you are taking, and the number of injections you have each day. We give three examples in Table 4.1.

The general rule is to increase one insulin at a time, by 2 units at a time, and to leave the dose as it is for a few days to see if the results improve. The exception to this is at times of illness and infection, when the dose may need to be increased by 4–10 units, sometimes with additional doses of short-acting insulin given between the usual injection times until the blood glucose levels start to improve.

The dose of insulin will need to be reduced if hypos occur regularly.

Table 4.1 Insulin adjustment

Intermediate-acting insulin (e.g. Humulin I, Insulatard, Monotard) taken twice a day

IF YOUR BLOOD GLUCOSE IS TOO HIGH

BEFORE BREAKFAST	BEFORE LUNCH	BEFORE DINNER	BEFORE BED
Increase p.m. insulin	Increase a.m. insulin	Increase a.m. insulin	Increase p.m. insulin

Short-acting insulin (e.g. Actrapid, Velosulin, Humulin S) taken with intermediate-acting insulin twice a day

IF YOUR BLOOD GLUCOSE IS TOO HIGH

BEFORE BREAKFAST	BEFORE LUNCH	BEFORE DINNER	BEFORE BED
Increase p.m. intermediate insulin	Increase a.m. short insulin	Increase a.m. intermediate insulin	Increase p.m. short insulin

Short-acting insulin taken three times a day, before meals, with intermediate- or long-acting insulin at bedtime

IF YOUR BLOOD GLUCOSE IS TOO HIGH

BEFORE BREAKFAST	BEFORE LUNCH	BEFORE DINNER	BEFORE BED
Increase bedtime insulin	Increase breakfast short insulin	Increase lunchtime short insulin	Increase dinnertime short insulin

I find that my control is only good for one week a month and that is the week before my period. Why is this and what should I do about it?

In some women the dose of insulin required to control diabetes varies in relation to the menstrual cycle. Your question implies that you become more sensitive to insulin in the week before you menstruate and you probably require more insulin at the other times in your cycle. There is no reason why you should not try to work out a pattern where you reduce your insulin dose in the week before your period and increase it at other times.

The variation is due to different hormones coming from the ovaries during the menstrual cycle. Some of these hormones have an anti-insulin effect. The same sort of effects may occur when a woman is taking oral contraceptive tablets (the pill) or is pregnant. The correct thing to do is to make adjustments in the insulin dose in order to compensate for these hormonal changes and to keep the balance of the blood glucose where it should be.

I have noticed that there are much greater fluctuations in my blood glucose level when I am having a period. I have great difficulty in keeping my blood glucose balanced then. I have read many books on diabetes but I have never seen this mentioned – is it normal?

It is quite normal for the blood glucose control to fluctuate during the monthly cycle. Most women find their blood glucose is highest in the pre-menstrual phase and returns to normal during or after their period. Some people need to adjust their dose of insulin during the cycle but rarely by more than a few units. Every woman has to discover for herself the extent of this effect and how much extra insulin, if any, is needed. Your diabetes clinic doctor or diabetes specialist nurse is the best person to turn to for exact advice on how to make these adjustments.

Where is the best place to obtain blood for measuring blood glucose levels?

It is usually easiest to obtain blood from the fingertips. You can use either the pulp, which is the fleshy part of the fingertip, or the sides of the fingertips. Some people like to use the area just below the nail bed. Most people find it easier to use the tip but the sides of the fingertips are less sensitive than the pulp. It may be necessary for some people such as guitarists, pianists or typists to avoid the finger pulp.

The fleshy ear lobes are also suitable areas for obtaining blood and are less sensitive than the fingers but they can be difficult to use as the blood has to be applied to the reagent stick with the use of a mirror. Parents may find that it is easiest to obtain blood from the earlobes of their child with diabetes.

Which is the best finger pricker?

All the currently available blood lancets are very similar and there is very little to choose between any of them. The lancets may either be used on their own or in conjunction with an automatic device. They are obtainable on prescription from your own GP. Alternatively they can be bought from a chemist, or sent for by post from companies such as Owen Mumford (Medical Shop) or D.E.P.T.H. (see Appendix 3 for addresses).

If you have trouble pricking your fingers without an automatic finger pricker there are now a wealth of devices that make the task much easier. The most popular seem to be the Soft Touch (from Roche or D.E.P.T.H.); the Glucolet (from Bayer Diagnostics or D.E.P.T.H.); the Monojector (from D.E.P.T.H.); the Hypolet (from D.E.P.T.H.); and the Autolet Lite and Autolet Mini (from Owen Mumford [Medical Shop] or D.E.P.T.H.). Softclix (from Boehringer Mannheim) has 11 different skin penetration depth settings and uses Softclix lancets. The B-D Lancer (from Becton Dickinson) takes Micro-Fine+ lancets. All these devices are very similar and work on the principle of hiding the lancet from view whilst piercing the skin very quickly and at a controlled depth. They are not available on prescription, but can be purchased from chemists, or by post from the companies named. Contact them direct for details of current prices. The latest products are advertised in *Balance*, the magazine published by Diabetes UK.

Before buying any automatic finger pricker check that you are using the correct lancets with the appropriate finger pricker, as some are not interchangeable. Some manufacturers offer finger prickers as part of the package when you buy a meter.

Should I clean my fingers with spirit or antiseptic before pricking them?

We do not recommend the use of spirit for cleaning your fingers as its constant use will lead to hardening of the skin of your fingertips. It can also interfere with the reagent strips. We suggest that you wash your hands with soap and warm water and dry them thoroughly before pricking your finger.

Will constant finger pricking make my fingers sore?

You may find that your fingers feel sore for the first week or two after starting blood glucose monitoring but this soon disappears. We have seen many people who have been measuring their blood glucose levels regularly three or four times a day for more than 15 years and who have no problems with sore fingers. Don't always use the same finger – instead try to use different fingers in rotation.

Will my fingers take a long time to heal after finger pricking and am I more likely to pick up an infection of the finger?

Your fingertips should heal as quickly as someone without diabetes but make sure that you are using suitable blood lancets. We have seen only one infected finger among many hundreds of thousands of finger pricks. We suggest that you keep your hands socially clean and wash them before collecting your blood sample.

There are a bewildering number of blood glucose sticks and meters on the market. Which are the best to use?

This is purely a matter of preference and may depend on the type of strips or meters used in your local clinic.

Some strips require wiping or blotting and are then compared with a colour chart after careful timing, whilst others do not need wiping or blotting and can only be used with a meter. There is a list of currently available meters in Appendix 1. The magazine *Balance*, produced by Diabetes UK, usually carries advertisements for the latest strips and meters, and their use should be discussed with your diabetes specialist nurse or diabetes physician. Blood glucose testing strips are obtainable on prescription from your GP but the meters have to be purchased.

I have recently started using BM-Test strips but have been told that my results do not compare well with the hospital results. What is the reason for this?

The first thing to do is to make sure that your technique is absolutely correct. Inaccurate results will be obtained if the correct procedures are not followed completely. If your technique is not at fault then it could be that you are not able to interpret the colour chart correctly. If this is so you would be advised to use a meter (see the Plates in the middle of the book) which reads the colour for you.

My blood glucose meter appears to give slightly different results compared with the hospital laboratory. Are the meters accurate enough for daily use?

Most results obtained when you are using a meter will be slightly different from the hospital laboratory results because different chemical methods are used. These slight differences do not matter and the strips and meters are quite accurate enough for home use.

If your results are very different from the laboratory, it could be that your technique is incorrect. The most common fault is not applying a large enough drop of blood to the strip. Other faults are smearing the blood on the strip, or taking too long to apply the blood to the strip. The reaction must also be timed accurately. The insert or carrier of the meter must be kept clean, and you should follow the maker's instructions for cleaning the carrier. Also check that the reagent strips are not used past their expiry date. If all else fails, read the instructions!

I have trouble obtaining enough blood to cover the whole test pad on the strip. Is there anything that I can do to make this easier?

If you are having trouble obtaining enough blood you might find the use of an automatic finger pricker makes it easier. Also try to warm your hands by washing them in warm water before you start, and drying them thoroughly before pricking your finger. Finally, when squeezing the blood out of your finger, try 'milking' the blood out gently, allowing the finger to recover in between each squeeze. Do not squeeze so hard that you end up 'blanching' the finger. The Supreme Test Strips require a very small amount of blood and may be more helpful.

I would like to measure my own blood glucose levels, but as I am now blind I do not know if this is possible. Can it be done?

Unfortunately, this is no longer possible as manufacturers have stopped making 'talking' meters. Maybe you could get a friend to help you.

Urine

I have been told to ignore my urine tests because I have a low renal threshold. Can you tell me what this means?

A low renal threshold means that glucose escapes into the urine at unusually low blood glucose levels. This is particularly common during pregnancy. The presence of a low renal threshold can only be established by careful comparison of simultaneous blood and urine glucose tests. If your renal threshold is low (or indeed if it is high), then urine tests can often be misleading. There is no real way round this problem so it is important to establish where your own renal threshold lies if you are going to rely on urine tests as an indication of your diabetes control.

I do not understand why it is that the glucose from the blood only spills into the urine above a certain level. I gather this level is known as the renal threshold – could you explain it for me in a little more detail?

Urine is formed by filtration of blood in the kidneys. When the glucose concentration in the blood is below about 10 mmol/l, any glucose filtered into the urine is subsequently reabsorbed back into the bloodstream. When the level of glucose exceeds about 10 mmol/l (the renal threshold) more glucose is filtered than the body can reabsorb, and the result is that it is passed in the urine. Once the level has exceeded 10 mmol/l, the amount of glucose in the urine will be proportional to the level of glucose in the blood. Below 10 mmol/l, however, there will be no glucose in the urine and, since the blood glucose level never exceeds 10 mmol/l in people without diabetes, they will not find glucose in the urine, unless they have a particular inherited condition called renal glycosuria.

How do you know if you have ketones in your urine? What are they and are they dangerous?

Ketones are breakdown products of the fat stores in the body. They are present in small amounts even in people without diabetes, particularly when they are dieting or fasting and therefore relying on their body fat stores for energy. In people with diabetes small amounts of ketones in the urine are commonly found. They become dangerous only when they are present in large amounts. This is usually accompanied by thirst, passing large amounts of urine, and nausea. If ketones are present in the urine together with continuous 2% glucose, or blood glucose levels higher than 13 mmol/l, then they are dangerous as this is the condition which precedes the development of ketoacidosis. **Under these circumstances you should seek urgent medical advice**.

You can test your urine for ketones with strips such as BM Ketur-Test (made by Boehringer Mannheim), or Ketostix or KetoDiastix (made by Bayer Diagnostics) which are all available on prescription from your GP.

What does it mean if I have a lot of ketones but no glucose on urine testing?

Testing for ketones in the urine can be rather confusing and, unless there are special reasons for doing it, we do not recommend it for routine use. Some people seem to develop ketones in the urine very readily, especially children, pregnant women and people who are dieting strictly to lose weight.

Usually if glucose and ketones appear together it indicates poor diabetes control, although this may be transient and glucose and ketones which are present in the morning may disappear by noon. If they persist all the time then control almost certainly needs to be improved, probably by increasing the insulin dose.

Ketones do sometimes appear in the urine without glucose, although not very frequently. They are most commonly seen in the first morning specimen and probably occur as the insulin action from the night before is wearing off – in some people the ketone levels increase before the glucose levels. Under these circumstances it is not serious and no particular action is needed.

Finally, ketones without glucose in the urine are very common in people who are trying to lose weight through calorie restriction. Anyone who is on a strict diet and losing weight will burn up body fat which causes ketones to appear in the urine. Provided there is no excess glucose in your urine, these ketones do not mean that your diabetes is out of control.

Why do we not always get a true blood glucose through a urine test (as in my case)?

In most people urine only contains glucose when the glucose concentration in the blood is higher than a certain figure (usually 10 mmol/l), so below this level urine tests give no indication at all to the concentration of glucose in the blood. The level at which glucose spills out into the urine (the renal threshold – discussed earlier in this section) varies from one person to another and you can only assess it in yourself by making many simultaneous blood and urine glucose measurements. If you undertake this exercise you will undoubtedly find, like most other people, that the relationship between the blood and urine concentrations is not very precise. For this reason most people nowadays prefer to do blood tests rather than urine tests, as they find that the increased precision of blood tests outweighs any disadvantage that may stem from having to prick your finger to get a drop of blood.

Which are the best strips to use for urine testing of glucose?

There is little to choose between them. They are all easy to use and can either be dipped into the urine, or urine can be passed directly onto the strip, and they must then be timed accurately. Bayer Diagnostics make a strip called Diastix for testing glucose in urine, and a strip called KetoDiastix for testing glucose and ketones in the urine. Boehringer Mannheim make a strip called Diabur Test 5000 for testing glucose in urine, which has the advantage of retaining its colour for some time after the test has been made, although the timing of the reaction must be for at least two minutes. All these strips are available on prescription.

At what time of day should I test my urine? I am on diet only.

If your first test in the morning before breakfast is continually negative (as it should be if you are on diet only), you can test your urine occasionally before lunch, before your evening meal or at bedtime, and you should find it negative at these times. If these are all negative you should try checking it two to three hours after breakfast which is the most likely time to find glucose in the urine. If this is negative too, then there is nothing further that you can do to monitor your control more accurately by urine tests. You should check that your fasting blood glucose values are 6 mmol/l or less and that your routine haemoglobin A_{1c} is less than 6.5%. If you can achieve these goals, then by all criteria your diabetes is well controlled.

For some time now I have suffered from diabetes. I am always curious to know what type of tests are made on my urine specimens when they are taken off into the laboratory.

Urine specimens are tested for several things but the most common are glucose, ketones and albumin (protein). These tests serve only as a spot check and are meant to complement your own tests performed at home. Clinics like to know the percentage of glucose in samples taken at different times of day as giving some measure of control at home. The detection of ketones is of rather limited value since some people make ketones very easily and others almost not at all, but the presence of large amounts of ketones together with 2% glucose shows that the person is very badly out of control. The presence of protein in the urine can indicate either infection in the urine or the presence of some kidney disease which in people with diabetes is likely to be diabetic nephropathy, one of the long-term complications (see Chapter 9 for more information about this). Another more recent test is for micro-albuminuria – the test detects microscopic amounts of albumin in the urine and can show signs of very early kidney damage.

I have a strong family history of diabetes. My daughter recently tested her urine and found 2% glucose. However, her blood glucose was only 8 mmol/l. She underwent a glucose tolerance test and this was normal. Could she have diabetes or could there be another reason why she is passing glucose in her water?

It is very unlikely that she has diabetes if a glucose tolerance test was normal. If she had glucose in her urine during the glucose tolerance test when all the blood glucose readings were strictly normal, then this would indicate that she has a low renal threshold for glucose (as discussed at the beginning of this section). If this is the correct diagnosis, then it is important to find out whether she passes glucose in her urine first thing in the morning while fasting or only after she has eaten. In people who pass glucose in the urine during the fasting state, there is not known to be any increased incidence of development of diabetes, and the condition (called *renal glycosuria*) is inherited. If on the other hand she only passes glucose in the urine after meals containing starch and sugar, this condition sometimes progresses to diabetes.

A colleague has asked me whether all people with diabetes should be tested for colour blindness in case this might impair their ability to test urine.

You draw attention to a real and not uncommon problem: 20% (one in five) of males are affected by some form of red/green colour blindness and it has been shown that this impairs their ability to read the results of urine sticks. Probably the same problem applies when they are reading sticks used for blood testing.

There is another form of colour blindness that affects both males and females who have diabetic retinopathy, and it has been shown that this form of colour blindness also impairs the ability to read the colours on the urine sticks and probably the blood sticks. We do not recommend the routine testing of all people for colour blindness but, when they are being taught either blood or urine monitoring, their ability to read the colours accurately should be checked by the person (doctor or nurse) who is instructing them.

Haemoglobin A_{1c} and fructosamine

What is haemoglobin A_{1c} and what are the normal values?

Haemoglobin A_{1c} is a component of the red pigment (haemoglobin A; HbA) present in the blood to carry oxygen from the lungs to the various organs in the body. The HbA_{1c} can be measured as a percentage of all the haemoglobin present with a variety of laboratory methods. HbA_{1c} consists of HbA combined with glucose by a chemical link. The amount of HbA_{1c} present is directly proportional to the average blood glucose during the 120-day life span of the HbA-containing red blood corpuscles in the circulating blood.

It is the most successful of all the tests so far developed to give an index of diabetes control. The blood glucose tests which we have used for many years fluctuate too erratically with injections, meals and other events for an isolated sample taken at one clinic visit to provide much information about overall control. HbA_{1c} averages out the peaks and troughs of the blood glucose over the previous two to three months.

Normal values vary a little from one laboratory to another and this can be a source of confusion as results from different clinics cannot be compared directly without the normal range known for each particular laboratory. (Diabetes UK is trying to correct this anomaly.) Normal values usually run between 3% and 5.5%, but you must check the normal range for your own laboratory. In someone with poorly controlled diabetes, or in whom diabetes is recently diagnosed, the value of HbA_{1c} may be as high as 20%, which reflects a consistently raised blood glucose over the preceding two to three months. On the other hand, in someone with perfect control, the HbA_{1c} will be in the normal range of 3–5.5%, while in the occasional person who runs blood glucose levels too low owing to taking too much insulin, the value will be subnormal, i.e. below 3%. Recently HbA_{1c} has replaced HbA_1 as the preferred terminology. It refers to a sub-component of HbA_1 which most closely represents the indicator of average blood glucose level over two months.

What is fructosamine and what are the normal values?

Fructosamine is the name of a test which is similar to that for HbA_{1c} in that it is an indicator of the average level of glucose in the blood over a period of time, in this case the two to three weeks before the test is done (compared with the preceding two to three months for HbA_{1c}). It measures the amount of glucose linked to the proteins in the blood plasma (the straw-coloured fluid in which the red cells are suspended): the higher the blood glucose concentration, the higher will be the fructosamine. Its advantages are that it is usually quicker and cheaper for the laboratory to do and this may mean that it is possible for you to have it done at your hospital clinic visit and have the result ready by the time you see the doctor. The normal values may vary from one laboratory to another depending on the way the analysis is performed; in general, a value of less than 300 micromol/l is a typical laboratory's normal value. In order to make sure you don't get confused we suggest you pay particular attention to what is done in your clinic; please don't hesitate to ask and make quite sure you do know what is going on!

How often should fructosamine tests be done?

Like HbA_{1c}, there is no point in doing them too often; we normally recommend doing one routinely at the time of each clinic visit. If metabolic control is under close scrutiny and treatment is being adjusted, for example in pregnancy, then it may be sensible to do one more often to check that things are going according to plan.

I am 25 years old and have had diabetes since I was 15. I have been attending the clinic regularly every three months and do regular blood glucose tests at home with my own meter. At my last clinic visit the doctor I saw said he did not need to see me again for a whole year because my HbA_{1c} was consistently normal – why did he do this?

It sounds as though your specialist has tremendous confidence in you and your ability to control your diabetes. As long as you can keep it this way he clearly feels that seeing you once a year is sufficient. He can then spend more time with other people who are not as successful as you are.

I am treated only by diet. I find it very difficult to stick to my diet or do the tests between the clinic visits but I am always very strict for the few days before I am seen at the clinic and my blood glucose test is usually normal. At my last clinic visit my blood glucose was 5 mmol/l but the doctor said he was very unhappy about my control because the HbA_{1c} was too high at 10% – what did he mean?

Your experience shows very nicely the usefulness of HbA_{1c} testing, because quite clearly you have been misleading yourself as well as your medical advisers about your ability to cope with your diabetes. The HbA_{1c} has brought this to the surface for the first time. Because the HbA_{1c} reflects what your blood glucose has been doing for as long as two to three months before your clinic visit, your last minute attempts to get your diabetes under control before you went to the clinic were enough to bring the blood glucose down but the HbA_{1c} remained high.

My recent HbA_{1c} was said to be low at 4%. Blood glucose readings look all right, on average about 5 mmol/l. The specialist asked me to set the alarm clock and check them at 3.00 a.m. – why is this?

A low HbA_{1c} suggests that at some stage your blood glucose levels are running unduly low. If you are not having hypoglycaemic attacks during the day, then it is possible that they are occurring at night and you are sleeping through them. By doing 3.00 a.m. blood glucose tests you should be able to determine whether this is so. Incidentally, you will only have to do these middle-of-the-night tests until you have established whether or not you are having hypos at night – they are not going to be a permanent part of your routine!

My diabetes is treated with diet and glibenclamide tablets. By strict dieting I have lost weight down to slightly below my target figure and all my urine tests are negative. My HbA_{1c} test, I am told, is still too high at 9% and does not seem to be falling despite the fact that I am still losing weight. I cannot be any stricter with what I eat. At the last clinic visit the doctor said that I am going to have to go on to insulin injections. I have been dreading these all my life – is he right?

It sounds very much as if you have reached the stage where diet and tablets aren't strong enough to keep your diabetes properly under control. Even in the absence of any glucose in your urine a consistently high HbA_{1c} indicates that your blood glucose is running too high and that you need to move on to the next stronger form of treatment which is insulin injections. You have been given sound advice and we are sure that it will not turn out to be as bad as you imagine. Once you have got over the initial fear of injecting yourself, which most people manage very quickly, you will probably feel a great deal better and it will all have been worthwhile.

Diabetes clinics

They have just appointed a new young consultant at my hospital and I am told they are going to start a special diabetes clinic – will this offer any advantage to me?

Most hospitals these days have at least one senior doctor who specializes in diabetes. By running a special diabetes clinic they can bring together all the specially trained doctors, nurses, dietitians and chiropodists, and this should mean a better service for you and other people attending the clinic. You will have the benefit of seeing people who have special training in diabetes, and most people find this a big advantage.

My GP is starting a diabetes clinic in the local group practice and tells me that I no longer need to attend the hospital clinic. It's much more convenient for me to go to see my GP but will this be all right?

You are very fortunate that your general practitioner clearly has a special interest in diabetes and has gone to the trouble of setting up a special clinic in the practice for this. Quite a number of GPs have had special training in diabetes and these general practice-based 'diabetes mini-clinics' are becoming more common. I am sure that your hospital specialist will know about this, and may even attend the mini-clinic from time to time. If you have any anxieties, why not discuss it with him or her? Many GPs now like to look after their patients with diabetes in general practice without the need to visit hospital. This is usually all right as long as you have uncomplicated diabetes and are well controlled, but you should be aware of the sort of care you should expect – we have reprinted Diabetes UK recommendations on this at the end of this section.

Although they do a blood test every time I go to our local diabetes clinic, they now only test my urine once a year when they look at my eyes and check my blood pressure – why is this?

With the introduction of HbA_{1c} and fructosamine measurement and blood glucose monitoring, the value of urine testing is really for the detection of protein (albumin) in the urine as an indicator of possible kidney damage. This does not need to be done more often than once a year in people who are quite well and free from albumin in their urine. As a general rule everyone with diabetes should have their urine, eyes, feet and blood pressure checked annually.

Why do I have to wait such a long time every time I go to the diabetes clinic?

If you think about it, you probably have quite a lot of tests done when you go to the clinic. It takes time to get the answers back and the results all together before you see the doctor. This is particularly likely to be so if you have had a blood glucose measurement, as the HbA_{1c} or fructosamine levels measured in the clinic take time to process. Although it may be irritating to have to wait for these results, they are very important as they can be used in a two-way discussion between you and the doctor to review your control and progress with diabetes. Many clinics use this waiting time for showing educational films or videos about diabetes and for meeting the dietitian and/or chiropodist, as well as the diabetes specialist nurse. If the clinic appears to be badly organized then you have good grounds for complaint.

What determines whether my next appointment is in one month or six months?

Generally speaking, if your control is consistently good you will not need to be seen very often; on the other hand, if your control is poor it is likely that you will be seen more often. This is not, as you may perhaps think, a subtle form of punishment but it will give you and your medical advisers more opportunity to sort out what is wrong.

At my clinic we have a mixture of people from young children to very old pensioners – why do they not have special clinics for young people?

Young people with diabetes do have special needs which are not usually met by an ordinary diabetes clinic. Growing up and learning to be independent places extra strains on diabetes control and young people prefer a more informal approach from members of the diabetes team. Some hospitals find it difficult to make these changes and there may be extra costs. However, clinics for young people have been set up in many parts of the country and you could ask your GP if you could be referred to one of them.

We have a specialist nurse in diabetes working in the diabetes clinic that I attend. What does she do?

Most clinics in this country now employ specialist nurses who spend their whole time working with people with diabetes. They may work in the community and/or the hospital and have a variety of titles – Diabetic Health Visitor, Diabetic Community Nurse, Diabetic or Diabetes Liaison Nurse, Diabetes Specialist Nurse, Diabetes Sister, Diabetic or Diabetes Care Sister, etc. These senior nurses spend most of their time educating people, giving advice (much of it on the telephone), making decisions about management and teaching other members of the medical and nursing staff about diabetes. They are experts in their field and are very valuable members of the diabetes care team.

As a newly diagnosed person with diabetes what sort of care should I expect?

Targets for improvements in diabetes care have been outlined in a document called the *St Vincent Declaration* which evolved from a meeting of European health officials and diabetes associations in St Vincent, Italy in 1989. In this country, Diabetes UK and the Department of Health set up a task force to put this declaration into practice. The targets are for reduction in disabilities caused by complications of diabetes; improvements in the outcome of pregnancies in women with diabetes; improvements in the care of children with diabetes; provision of effective education in self-care for people with diabetes; and improvements in economic and social conditions for people with diabetes.

Diabetes UK issued a document in June 2000 (from guidelines first produced in 1986) called *What diabetes care to expect*. This document explains clearly what standards of care to expect and as a result we are reprinting the guidelines from it here. If you would like a copy of the complete document, contact Diabetes UK (address in Appendix 3).

When you have just been diagnosed you should have:

- a full medical examination;
- a talk with a registered nurse who has a special interest in diabetes; she will explain what diabetes is and talk to you about your individual treatment;
- a talk with a State Registered dietitian, who will want to know what you are used to eating and will give you basic advice on what to eat in future; a follow-up meeting should be arranged for more detailed advice;
- a discussion on the implications of diabetes on your job, driving, insurance, prescription charges, etc. and whether you need to inform the DVLA and your insurance company, if you are a driver;

- information about Diabetes UK services and details of your local Diabetes UK group;
- ongoing education about your diabetes and the beneficial effects of exercise, and assessments of your control.

You should be able to take a close friend or relative with you to educational sessions if you wish.

PLUS

If you are treated by insulin:

- frequent sessions for basic instruction in injection technique, looking after insulin and syringes or insulin pens, blood glucose and urine ketone testing and what the results mean;
- supplies of relevant equipment;
- discussion about hypoglycaemia (hypos), when and why it may happen and what to do about it.

If you are treated by tablets:

- discussion about the possibility of hypoglycaemia (hypos) and how to deal with it;
- instruction on blood or urine testing and what the results mean, and supplies of relevant equipment.

If you are treated by diet alone:

- instruction on blood or urine testing and what the results mean, and supplies of relevant equipment.

Once your diabetes is reasonably controlled, you should:

- have access to the diabetes team at regular intervals – annually if necessary. These meetings should give time for discussion as well as assessing diabetes control;
- be able to contact any member of the health care team for specialist advice when you need it;
- have more education sessions as you are ready for them;
- have a formal medical review once a year by a doctor experienced in diabetes.

At this review:

- your weight should be recorded;
- your urine should be tested for protein;
- your blood should be tested to measure long-term control;
- you should discuss control, including your home monitoring results;
- your blood pressure should be checked;
- your vision should be checked and the back of your eyes examined with an ophthalmoscope; a photo may be taken of the back of your eyes, and if necessary you should be referred to an ophthalmologist;
- your legs and feet should be examined to check your circulation and nerve supply, and if necessary you should be referred to a State Registered chiropodist;
- if you are on insulin, your injection sites should be examined;
- you should have the opportunity to discuss how you are coping at home and at work.

Your role:

- you are an important member of the care team so it is essential that you understand your own diabetes to enable you to be in control of your condition;
- you should ensure that you receive the described care from your local diabetes clinic, practice or hospital. If these services are not available to you, you should:
  - contact your GP to discuss the diabetes care available in your area;
  - contact your local Community Health Council;
  - contact the BDA or your local branch.

Brittle diabetes

What is brittle diabetes and what treatment does it require?

The term brittle diabetes is applied to someone with type 1 diabetes who oscillates from one extreme to another, i.e. swings from severe hyperglycaemia (blood glucose much too high) to severe hypoglycaemia (blood glucose much too low) with all the problems that are encountered with a hypo. Someone with this problem is frequently admitted to hospital for re-stabilization. The term brittle is not a good one because to some extent the blood glucose of all people taking insulin swings during the 24 hours from high to low and back again. It is therefore restricted to those people in whom the swings of blood glucose are sufficiently serious to cause inconvenience with or without admission to hospital.

It is important to realize that brittle diabetes is *not* a special type of diabetes and only applies when the instability is severe. This normally occurs at a time when perhaps someone may be emotionally unsettled. It is particularly common amongst teenagers, especially girls. It is most encouraging that as emotional stability and maturity are reached so brittle diabetes disappears and most of these people will become reasonably stable and their frequent admissions to hospital will cease. During any particularly difficult period it is well worth remembering that it will not last for ever.

I have 'brittle diabetes' and my doctor has advised me to stop working. Am I entitled to any benefits?

The term brittle diabetes is used rather too loosely. It is usually taken to mean someone whose blood glucose rises or falls very quickly and who may develop unexpected hypos. Many conditions may contribute to this but one of the most common factors is an inappropriate dose of insulin. Other factors which may contribute include irregular meals and lifestyle, poor injection technique, and general ignorance about the problems of balancing food, exercise and insulin. Few people have such difficulty in controlling their diabetes that they have to give up work, but welfare benefits are available to people with diabetes in the same way that they are to anyone else. There are some questions about Social Security benefits in Chapter 5.

5

Life with diabetes

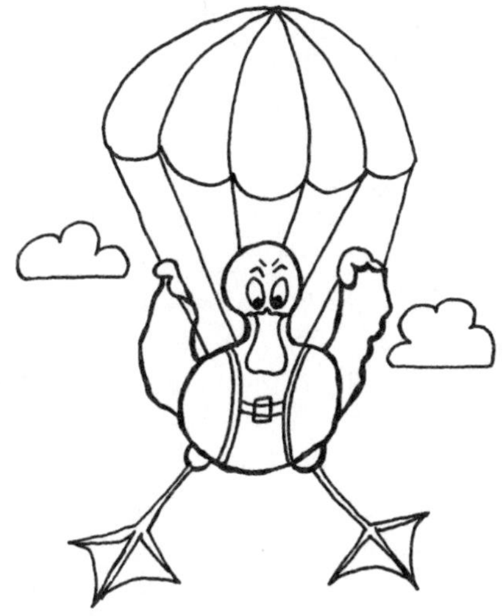

Introduction

This chapter is meant to answer all the questions that affect daily living when you have diabetes. It covers a broad sweep from sport to holidays to surgical operations and illness. The section on ***Other illnesses*** should be read early on, so that you will know how to react if you are struck down by a bad attack of flu. All car drivers should read the section on ***Driving***. At the end of the chapter is a miscellaneous section with questions that we could not find a place for elsewhere (e.g. electrolysis, ear piercing and identity bracelets). After reading this chapter, you will realize that there are very few activities that are barred to people with diabetes. Provided that you understand the condition, you should be able to do almost anything you wish.

Sports

My 13-year-old son is a keen footballer and has just developed diabetes. Will he be able to continue football and other sports? If so, what precautions should he take?

Your son can certainly keep on with his football. There is a very well known professional football player who has type 1 diabetes so, if your son is good enough at the game, diabetes should not stop him becoming another great footballer. People with diabetes have reached the top in other sports, such as rugby, cricket, tennis, sailing, rowing, orienteering and mountaineering. Certainly all normal school sports should be encouraged.

There is, of course, the difficulty that the extra energy used in competitive sports increases the risk of a hypo. Your son should take some extra carbohydrate *before* a match or any other sports period – he could have a couple of sandwiches or biscuits or chocolate wafers. He will probably need another snack at half-time, and he must carry glucose tablets in his pocket.

He also needs to watch what he eats *after* the game has finished. The effect of exercise on the body can last well after the exercise has stopped (the muscles are restocking their energy stores with glycogen) and often blood glucose drops two or more hours after the exercise period. So he may need a snack then or, if he is due a meal or a snack anyway, he may need a slightly larger one than usual. It would also be a good idea for him to have a larger than usual bedtime snack if he has been exercising in the afternoon or evening.

Another way of preventing a hypo during exercise is to reduce the amount of insulin beforehand. So if he is playing football in the morning, he could reduce his morning dose of quick-acting insulin by half. It takes trial and error to discover by exactly how much to reduce insulin for a given amount of exercise.

I used to enjoy swimming, but have been worried about going back to the pool since I have been on insulin. What if I had a hypo?

Whilst a hypo during athletics and most team games can be

inconvenient, a hypo while swimming can be more serious and you are right to be concerned about it. However, don't let your concern stop you swimming, just make sure that you are sensible about it. There are certain simple rules *all* people taking insulin should follow before swimming – by following them you can swim with complete safety.

- Never swim alone.
- Tell your companions (or teacher if you are still at school) to pull you out of the water if you behave oddly or are in difficulties.
- Keep glucose tablets on the side of the pool.
- Get out of the water immediately if you feel the first signs of a hypo.

If you are a keen swimmer and want to take up scuba diving, then the British Sub-Aqua Club does impose some restrictions. They require people taking insulin who wish to scuba dive to have an annual medical review, not to have any long-term complications of diabetes, and insist that they always dive with another person who does not have diabetes. You can contact the Club for more details – the address is in Appendix 3.

Can I take part in all or any forms of sport?

The vast majority of sports are perfectly safe for people with diabetes. The problem lies in those sports where loss of control due to a hypo could be dangerous, not only to you but to your fellow participants or to spectators. Swimming is an example of a potentially dangerous sport but by taking certain precautions (see previous question) it is safe to swim. However, in other sports (e.g. motor racing), the risk of serious injury in the case of a hypo are even greater. For this reason the governing bodies of these high-risk sports discourage people with diabetes from taking part. Discouragement does not necessarily mean a total ban – the restrictions may vary depending on whether you are on diet, diet and tablets, or insulin. You can always contact the appropriate governing body and ask for their advice, and find out what (if any) restrictions they impose. Skiing is discussed in the section on ***Holidays and travel*** later in this chapter.

Are people with diabetes allowed to go parachuting? I want to do a sponsored parachute jump to raise money for charity.

You can probably do your sponsored jump, but it will depend on what your treatment is. If you are on diet alone, or on diet and biguanides, then the restrictions are minimal. If you are on sulphonylureas or insulin the restrictions are much greater – you will need a medical certificate to state that you are well controlled, and you will only be permitted to jump in tandem. The British Parachute Association (address in Appendix 3) can give you more information about this.

As a 30-year-old with type 1 diabetes can I join a keep fit class or do a work-out at home?

Yes, certainly. Keeping fit is important for everybody. Like everyone else, if you are unused to exercise, you should build up the exercises slowly each week so that you do not damage any muscles or tendons. Remember that exercise usually has the effect of lowering blood glucose so you may need to reduce your insulin dose or take extra carbohydrate before exercising.

I take insulin and jog quite a bit. I would like to try running a marathon. Have you any advice on the subject?

Dawn Kenwright who has type 1 diabetes is a long-distance runner at international level. Dawn resumed training within a few weeks of starting insulin and worked hard to discover by trial and error the effect of exercise/food/insulin on her blood glucose levels. Before running, Dawn has found that she needs plenty of 'slow' carbohydrate (in the form of porridge) to maintain her energy levels. During training sessions Dawn wears a bumbag containing glucose tablets and solution, but in competition she cuts back her insulin drastically and just carries glucose tablets. With careful preparation she rarely needs extra glucose. **Dawn warns you to progress gradually from jogging up to a full marathon distance.** She stresses that what is right for her will not necessarily suit everyone and makes the point that each athlete with diabetes has to work out their own solution for their particular sport.

Diabetes UK produces fact sheets on long distance running and some other sports. Once you have reached the required standard, you should think of joining Diabetes UK's team for the London Marathon.

Eating out

My wife and I entertain a great deal and we often go out to meals in a friend's house or in restaurants. I have recently been started on insulin for diabetes. How am I going to cope with eating out?

It is sometimes difficult to know what to do when eating out with friends who have made a special effort to prepare delicious food – which then turns out to be quite unsuitable for people with diabetes. Do you refuse a syrupy pudding and offend your hostess or have a large helping and to hell with your diabetes? You will probably find it less embarrassing to warn your friends in advance that you have diabetes and have to avoid food containing high concentrations of sugar. Restaurants or takeaways should pose less of a problem as you can select suitable dishes from the menu.

People on two or more doses of insulin a day sometimes worry about how they are going to give their injections when they are away from home. Nowadays with insulin pens there should be no difficulty. You can always retire to the lavatory just before sitting down to eat! People who are less shy discreetly give themselves insulin into their abdomen whilst at the table waiting for the first course to arrive. The use of an insulin pen (see the section on ***Insulin pens*** in Chapter 3) can make the injection simpler as bottles of insulin do not need to be carried around. Do not take your evening dose of insulin before leaving home in case the meal is delayed.

Holidays and travel

Do you have any simple rules for people with diabetes going abroad for holidays?

Here is a checklist of things to take with you.

- Insulin (or tablets)
- Syringes or insulin pen and needles
- Test strips (and finger pricker) and/or meter
- Identification bracelet/necklace/card
- Glucose tablets
- Longer-acting carbohydrate in case meals are delayed
- Glucagon
- Medical insurance
- Form E111 (from the DSS) if travelling inside the EU
- Hypostop Gel.

Each year on our summer holidays, our daughter becomes violently sick on the ferry. She recovers quite soon after we get back on dry land but she can keep nothing down during the crossing and it is very worrying.

We presume your daughter is on insulin and, as a general rule, people on insulin need hospital help once they start vomiting. Profuse vomiting leads to dehydration and if this is severe, the only treatment is a 'drip'. The other worry is the risk of a hypo if your daughter has already had her insulin. Don't be tempted to stop her insulin on the grounds that she is not eating.

There is no simple solution (apart from going by the Channel Tunnel) but the following ground rules may help.

- Take a standard anti-sickness tablet (e.g. Sea-Legs) at the recommended time before you sail.
- Try the 'acupuncture' wrist bands for seasickness now on sale at most chemists – they may just work for your daughter!
- Do frequent blood tests during the journey and immediately afterwards.
- If her blood glucose rises alarmingly, try giving her extra small doses of short-acting insulin.

- If her blood glucose values fall too low, give her Lucozade, Coca-Cola or some other non-diet soft drink.

Is it safe for someone with diabetes to take travel sickness tablets?

Travel sickness pills do not upset diabetes, although they may make you sleepy so be careful if you are driving. On the other hand, vomiting can upset diabetes so it is worth trying to avoid travel sickness. If you do become sick the usual rules apply. Continue to take your normal dose of insulin and take carbohydrate in some palatable liquid form, such as a sugary drink. Test your blood or urine regularly.

We are going on holiday and wish to take a supply of insulin and glucagon with us. How should I store them both for the journey and in the hotel?

Insulin is really very stable and will keep for one month at room temperature in our temperate climate. However, it does not like extremes of temperature and can be damaged if kept too long at high temperatures or if frozen. It is best to carry your supplies in more than one piece of luggage in case one suitcase goes astray and you lose everything!

If you are travelling by air you should keep your insulin in your hand luggage – temperatures in the luggage hold of an aircraft usually fall below freezing and insulin left in luggage there could be damaged. Insulin manufacturers say it is stable for one month at 25° C (77° F), so it is perfectly safe to keep insulin with your luggage on the average holiday. Avoid the glove compartment or the boot of your car where very high temperatures can be reached. In tropical conditions your stock of insulin should be kept in the fridge.

Storage of glucagon is no problem as this comes as a powder with a vial of water for dilution. It is very stable and can survive extremes of heat and cold.

Many airports now X-ray baggage for security reasons. Does this affect insulin?

Fortunately not.

I would like to go on a skiing holiday. Is it safe for me to ski, skate and toboggan? Should I take special precautions?

It is as safe for someone with diabetes to ski and enjoy other winter sports as it is for anyone else. Accidents do occur and it is essential to take out adequate insurance to cover all medical expenses. Read the small print in the insurance form carefully to ensure that it does not exclude pre-existing diseases like diabetes, or require them to be declared. In this case you should contact the insurance company and if necessary take out extra medical cover for your diabetes. Physical activity increases the likelihood of hypos so always carry glucose and a snack as you may be delayed, especially if you are injured. Never go without a sensible companion who knows you have diabetes and understands what to do if you have a hypo.

Is sunbathing all right for people with diabetes?

Of course people with diabetes can sunbathe. Lying around doing nothing may put your blood glucose up a little, especially if you overeat as most people do on holiday. So keep up your usual tests and you may need extra insulin. On the other hand, increasing the temperature of the skin may speed up the absorption of the insulin and can precipitate hypos, so be prepared for changes. Remember that sunbathing can increase the risk of skin cancer whether or not you have diabetes, so always take sensible precautions to avoid sunburn by using suncream with a high protection factor.

As I have diabetes should I be vaccinated when going abroad?

People with diabetes should have exactly the same vaccinations as anyone else. You are no more or less likely to contract illnesses abroad but if you do become ill the consequences could be more serious. In addition to the necessary vaccinations it is very important to take protective tablets against malaria if you are going to a tropical area where this disease is found. More cases of this potentially serious disease are being seen in this country, usually in travellers recently returned from Africa or the East.

I am going to work in the Middle East for six months. What can I do if my insulin is not available in the country where I am working?

If you are only working abroad for six months it should be quite easy to take enough insulin with you to last you this length of time. Kept in an ordinary fridge it should keep – but make sure you are not supplied with insulin which is near the end of its shelf life. The expiry date is printed on each box of insulin.

Most types of insulin are available in the Middle East but you may have to make do with a different brand name or even insulin from a different source (pig, cow or human). Strict Muslim countries regard pork and products from the pig as 'unclean' and porcine insulin may be hard to obtain in these countries. We have heard of customs officials in Saudi Arabia confiscating supplies of porcine insulin. To avoid this awkward situation it would be worth changing to human insulin before you try to enter such a country. The change may affect your control, and you should therefore make it in good time to allow yourself to stabilize before travelling. U100 insulin may be difficult to obtain outside the UK, USA, Australia, New Zealand, South Africa and parts of the Far East. Many European countries only stock insulin in 40 units/ml and special syringes for use with U40 insulin will have to be obtained. Diabetes UK can tell you which strength insulin is used in each country.

My husband has just been offered an excellent post in Uruguay which he would love to accept. He is worried about my diabetes there and especially about the availability of my insulin. Can you let me know if my insulin can be sent by post?

It should be possible to obtain an equivalent type of insulin to your own in most parts of the world. If you are keen to keep up your normal supplies, Hypoguard Ltd are prepared to despatch syringes and equipment for testing blood and urine to all parts of the world. Unfortunately Hypoguard are not able to handle insulin. You might be able to make arrangements with a high street chemist who would be prepared to send insulin by post, or John

Bell & Croyden in London will send insulin abroad. The address is in Appendix 3.

My friends and I are going to Spain to work next year. Can you tell me what I should take with me and whether I would have to pay if I needed to see a doctor?

Before you go abroad prepare yourself well – take spares of everything such as syringes, insulin, testing equipment and keep spare supplies separate from the main supply in case your luggage is lost.

Medical attention is free in all European Union countries although you should obtain certificate number E111 (from your local Department of Social Security office) before you go. For longer stays abroad, you should contact the DSS. For countries outside the EU you should insure your health before you go. Diabetes UK Careline can help with this (see Chapter 11 for contact details).

I take insulin and need to fly to the USA. How do I cope with the changing time zones?

Flying from east to west (or vice versa) can be a bit confusing at the best of times and makes it difficult to know which meal you are eating. Here are some typical schedules for travelling from London to the East and West Coasts of the USA plus the return trips. (If you use an insulin pen, the pattern for a basal/bolus regimen is exactly the same as the instructions here, apart from taking short-acting insulin before lunch on the plane. Many people using insulin pens are very used to injecting before each meal whatever time that is!)

1 London – New York

Get up as normal and have your usual dose of insulin and breakfast. The departure for New York is usually around 12.00 noon so have a good snack before boarding the plane. During the flight you will be served lunch and an afternoon snack. You will arrive at about 2.00 p.m. local time but your body thinks it is 7.00 p.m. Eat soon after arrival with your normal evening dose of insulin. If you then go to bed at 10.00 p.m. local time (3.00 a.m. to you) you will need a small dose of long-acting insulin before a well-earned sleep.

2 New York – London

The problem here is that the flights are usually in the evening and the night seems to be very short. Assuming that you are going to try and sleep on the plane, you should reduce your evening dose of insulin by one-third and have this at about 6.00 p.m. New York time followed by a reasonable meal. After take-off at 8.00 p.m. you should be served with a meal and should then sleep. You will arrive at London at about 7.30 a.m. local time although it will feel to you like 2.00 a.m. Most people have another journey followed by a good meal and then a sleep. You should have a dose of long-acting insulin before this sleep and try and get back into phase by the evening (local time).

3 London – Los Angeles

This is an 11 hour flight usually leaving around midday and arriving on the West Coast at 3.30 p.m. local time which feels to you like 11.30 p.m. During this long flight you will have to have an injection of insulin on the plane and this is best if taken before dinner served at 6.00 p.m. London time. It would be safest to give half your normal evening dose as short-acting insulin and then try and sleep. On arrival at the other side you will need to travel to your destination and will probably have an evening meal at what will feel to you like the early hours of the morning. A small dose of long-acting insulin before this meal would cover your subsequent sleep.

4 Los Angeles – London

Leave at 6.30 p.m. and after a 10 hour flight you will arrive in London just after midday local time which will feel to you like 2.00 a.m. Meals on this flight are usually served about an hour after take off and an hour before landing, in the hope that you have a good sleep between these two meals. One way round this arrangement would be to have a dose of insulin immediately before the first meal, giving a normal dose of short-acting insulin and half the normal dose of long-acting insulin. Immediately before the second meal you could have a small dose of short-acting insulin alone. This should last you through until the normal evening meal at your destination which would be preceded by a routine evening insulin dose.

When travelling keep to the following rules.

- Do not aim at perfect control. You have to be flexible especially on international flights. A hypo whilst travelling can be very inconvenient.
- Be prepared to check your blood glucose if you are at all worried and not sure how much insulin you need.
- In general, airlines are prepared to make special allowances for people with diabetes and cabin crew will do their best to help. Airlines say that they like to be warned in advance but in practice this should not be necessary. One of the problems of ordering a 'diabetic' meal is that it is very likely to be carbohydrate-free, so you would be better off eating the standard airline meal.

Work

Can I undertake employment involving shift work?

Yes, certainly. Many people combine shift work with good control of their blood glucose. Shift work does, however, need a little extra care as most insulin regimens are designed round a 24 hour day. Shift workers usually complain that they are just settling into one routine when everything changes and they have to start again. It is hard to generalize about shift work as there are so many different patterns, but if you follow the following rules things should work out all right.

- Aim at an injection of short- and medium-acting insulin every 12–16 hours, or use a basal/bolus regimen.
- Try to eat a good meal after each injection.
- Eat your normal snacks between meals every three hours or so, unless you are asleep.
- If there is a gap of six to eight hours when you are changing

from one shift to another, have some short-acting insulin on its own followed by a meal.

- Because your pattern of insulin and food is constantly changing, you will have to do more blood glucose measurements than normal, as you cannot assume that one day is very much like another.
- If your blood glucose results are not good, be prepared to make changes in your dose of insulin. Soon you will know more about your diabetes than anyone else.

How can I cope with my diabetes if I work irregular hours as a sales rep?

Just as with shift work many people manage to combine an irregular lifestyle with good diabetes control. Many people who lead an erratic lifestyle find that the basal/bolus regimen gives them the freedom they require (there is a section on ***Insulin pens*** in Chapter 3).

If you have had an injection of insulin in the morning and normally have a fairly low blood glucose before lunch, then you will go hypo unless you eat at the right time. So a well controlled person cannot afford the luxury of missing meals completely. However, it is always possible for you to have a few biscuits or even a sweet drink if you are getting past your normal eating time.

The occupational hazard of all sales reps, with diabetes or otherwise, is the mileage they clock up each year on the roads. The dangers of hypoglycaemia while driving cannot be overemphasized and there is really no excuse for this now that instant blood glucose measurement is available. Remember: (i) if driving before a meal, check your blood glucose; (ii) if it is low, eat before driving; (iii) always carry food in your car and have some immediately if you feel warning of a hypo.

Should I warn fellow employees that I might be subject to hypos?

Definitely. Hypos unfortunately can happen, especially when a person first starts using insulin. Warn your workmates that if they find you acting in a peculiar way they must get you to take some sugar. Warn them also that you may not be very co-operative at the time and may even resist their attempts to help you. Some people find it difficult to admit to their colleagues that they have diabetes but, if you keep it a secret, you run the risk of causing a scare by having a bad hypo and being taken to hospital by ambulance for treatment. A needless trip to hospital should be avoided.

My husband's hours of work can be very erratic. Sometimes he only gets three or four hours sleep instead of his normal eight hours. Can you tell me what effect lack of sleep has on diabetes?

Lack of sleep in itself will not affect diabetes although, if your husband is under great pressure and the adrenaline is running very high, his blood glucose may be affected. The real problem with working under a strain is the tendency to ignore diabetes completely and assume that it will look after itself. Unfortunately a few minutes of each day has to be spent checking blood glucose, eating a snack or giving insulin. These minutes are well spent.

I developed diabetes five months ago, one week after I had started a new job. I am coming to the end of my six month probation period and have been given two weeks notice because of my diabetes. They said I could not do shift work because of my diabetes. Could you help?

This is a sad story and a good example of ignorant prejudice against people with diabetes. Of course there are many people on shift work who maintain good control – although it does require a bit of extra thought. You may well have a case under the Disability Discrimination Act and you should seek advice from your local Citizen's Advice Bureau.

I am a public house manager and have had diabetes for the past 19 years but my employers are now making me redundant. Apparently, their insurers cannot accept me for a permanent position owing to my diabetes. Who can help strengthen my case?

We know of several publicans with diabetes who run good pubs and still keep their diabetes under good control. However, people who work in licensed premises are at greater risk of drinking more alcohol than average and heavy drinkers are in danger from hypos (see the section on ***Alcohol*** later in this chapter). We wonder if you have been having a large number of hypos which has made it difficult to continue in your present occupation. Ask your clinic doctor and Diabetes UK to lobby on your behalf, and seek legal advice from your local Citizen's Advice Bureau.

I have been refused a job with a large company because of my diabetes. Have I sufficient grounds to take proceedings against them for discrimination?

The Disability Discrimination Act covers people with diabetes but it can be difficult taking a company to court. We know this sort of discrimination does sometimes happen, especially in large organizations, although, of course, it is very difficult to prove. It may be possible for your case to go to an industrial tribunal to see if there are grounds for unfair dismissal, but as it sounds as if you have been refused a new job rather than dismissed from an exisiting job, then this could be difficult.

It is the responsibility of people with diabetes who are at work to realize that they are, to some extent, on show. If they work well and have no time off for minor complaints, then the next person who applies to the same firm will be looked on kindly and probably be taken on. On the other hand, someone who is constantly having hypos and missing work can give diabetes a bad name.

Diabetes UK has had discussions with medical officers responsible for occupational health in several large organizations. These resulted in an employment handbook which was circulated to diabetes clinics and occupational health doctors.

Other illnesses

I have recently had a severe cough and cold and have been given 'diabetic' cough medicine by the doctor. Since then my blood glucose has been very high. Could this be due to the medicine?

This is a good example of the effect that any infection or serious illness has on diabetes – it nearly always causes a rise in blood glucose. Unfortunately, many people often do not start to feel unwell until the glucose reaches danger level. People on insulin usually need more insulin when they are ill and yet they are sometimes advised to stop insulin completely if they do not feel like eating. This advice can be fatal. The rules when you are ill are as follows:

- Test blood/urine frequently.
- If tests are high take extra doses of short-acting insulin.
- *NEVER* stop insulin.

It is of course possible to get over a bad cold by carrying on with your normal dose of insulin and accepting bad control for a few days. However, this means that your mouth and nose will be slightly dehydrated and it will take a few extra days before you feel back to normal. So you probably get better more quickly if you adjust your insulin and try to keep the blood glucose near normal.

Antibiotic syrup and cough linctus are often blamed for making diabetes worse during an illness such as flu or chest infection. In fact a dose of antibiotic syrup only contains about 5 g of sugar and is not going to make any real difference. It is the illness itself which unbalances the diabetes. In general, medication from your doctor will not upset your diabetes. One antibiotic (Keflex) may cause a muddy colour of the urine which can be confusing.

I have noticed that my son suffers from more colds since developing diabetes. Could this be due to his diabetes?

Many parents make this observation, but there is no real reason why the common cold should be more common in diabetes. However, a relatively minor cold may upset his diabetes control and lead to several days of illness (see previous answer). This may make it a more memorable event. To repeat the previous advice, *never* stop insulin.

My daughter keeps getting infections and has been rushed to hospital on several occasions with high ketones and requiring a drip. How can I prevent these infections? Will vitamins help?

It sounds as though your daughter has so-called 'brittle' diabetes and this must be very alarming for you. There are really two types of people with brittle diabetes. The first type are those who are really very well controlled and can prove this by frequent blood glucose measurements below 7 mmol/l and a normal HbA_{1c}, but who quickly become very ill and 'sugary' at the first sniff of a cold or the beginning of an infection. The other sort are those who are normally poorly controlled with blood glucose results all over the place and who therefore have no leeway when they become ill. In the case of the first type it should be possible to increase the dose of insulin rapidly giving extra doses every few hours depending on the blood glucose. The second type are more of a problem as it is the overall control which needs to be improved and this can be very difficult. Of course if an infection (e.g. cystitis) starts off the trouble then this must be treated immediately with antibiotics.

Provided your daughter has a reasonable diet, vitamins will not help.

My 6-year-old daughter who is on insulin is troubled with frequent vomiting which occurs suddenly. She has ended up in hospital on several occasions as she becomes dehydrated. What can I do to avoid this?

Vomiting in a young child with diabetes has to be taken seriously and the hospital admissions are probably necessary to put fluid back into your daughter by means of a drip.

If the vomiting is associated with high blood glucose levels and ketones then it may be possible to avoid these problems, if extra doses of short-acting insulin are given as soon as the blood glucose levels start to rise before vomiting occurs. As she gets older these attacks of sickness will improve.

What is the best treatment for someone suffering from hay fever? I understand that some products can cause drowsiness which could affect my balance and so be confused with a hypo.

You can have exactly the same treatment for your hay fever as people without diabetes, as it does not affect your control. Antihistamines are often used for hay fever and these may make you feel sleepy, but this should be easy to distinguish from a hypo.

Remember that if you are on antihistamines you should take alcohol with great caution. Hay fever can also be alleviated by sniffing capsules which reduce the sensitivity of the membranes in the nose.

I have just been in hospital with anaphylactic shock from a bee sting. I have diabetes controlled with tablets and wondered if this had anything to do with the severity of my reaction?

There is no connection between diabetes and allergy to bees.

What should I do if my son has an intercurrent illness while on tablets?

This can be a really difficult problem. Of course if your son is ill enough to need hospital admission, he will often be given insulin while his sugars are running high. At home, this is not as simple because there is no way of knowing what dose of insulin he may require and an inadequate dose of insulin may even make matters worse. So, although in a perfect world he would have insulin for the duration of his illness, in reality it is acceptable for him to run high sugars for a day or so, in the expectation that they will soon settle down spontaneously. In a longer lasting illness, there is of course time to adjust the insulin dose in response to the results of blood glucose measurements.

What is the effect of other illnesses on diabetes? Is my son likely to suffer more illness than other children of his age?

Illnesses usually make diabetes worse in the sense that people on insulin need to increase the dose to keep blood glucose controlled. People on tablets or diet alone often find that a bad cold will upset their control. In the case of a prolonged illness or one needing hospital admission, a person with type 2 diabetes may need to have insulin injections for a time.

Diabetes itself does not necessarily make people prone to other illnesses. In fact a survey in a large American company reveals that people with diabetes had no more absences from work than those without. Most children with diabetes grow up without any more illness than their friends.

Since I was diagnosed I have been very depressed. Is there any link between depression and diabetes?

People vary very greatly in their mental response to developing diabetes. Some lucky ones take to their new condition easily, while others, like yourself, find the whole thing very depressing.

The depression seems to take two forms. At first, shock and even anger at the very onset coupled with fear of injections and the unspoken fear of complications. A few weeks later comes the depressing realization that diabetes is for life, and not just a temporary disease that can be 'cured'. This type of depression seems to affect young people who are worried and are insecure about the future.

A few people with diabetes feel that, in some way, they are flawed, especially if they have previously been fitness fanatics. The best way round this feeling of inadequacy is to throw yourself into sporting activities with extra enthusiasm. Exercise is good for us all and people with diabetes have managed to reach the top in most forms of sport from ocean racing to international football.

If you treat your diabetes in a positive way rather than letting the condition control you, the depression will gradually lift.

How does stress and worry affect diabetes? I spend many hours studying and find that, if I study too long, I feel weak and shaky. Are there any side effects to pressure which may affect my diabetes?

In general, stress and worry tend to increase the blood glucose. A Scottish student told us that in the run up to her final examination, she had to double her insulin dose to keep perfect blood glucose control, even though she did not appear to be particularly anxious to her friends. Stress causes a release of adrenaline and other hormones which antagonize the effect of insulin.

During periods of stress it may be difficult to keep to strict meal times, so you could be going hypo. You need to check your blood glucose and, if it is not below normal, then you are simply experiencing the tiredness we all feel after studying hard. Don't blame it on your diabetes but have an evening off from your studies.

Hospital operations

Recently, when I was in hospital to have my appendix removed, I was put on a 'sliding scale'. Please could you explain this, especially as it might save other people in a similar position from worrying?

We agree that the expression 'sliding scale' does sound rather alarming – but it is nothing to worry about. It can be difficult to predict exactly how much insulin someone will need during and after an operation. The way round this is to use a 'sliding scale' so that more insulin is given if the glucose in the blood is high. This is usually monitored every 1–4 hours and the insulin adjusted accordingly. Nowadays, during an operation, insulin is often given straight into a vein using a slow infusion pump. Most surgical wards have machines for measuring blood glucose and by doing this regularly the dose of insulin can be adjusted according to the result. In this way, diabetes control can be carefully regulated throughout the operation and until the person is eating again. At this stage the insulin may be given by three or four injections a day, the dose given at each injection being determined from the amount of insulin according to the 'sliding scale'.

Are there any problems with surgery for a child with diabetes?

Surgical operations on children usually involve a general anaesthetic and it is advisable to have nothing to eat or drink (nil by mouth) for six hours before the anaesthetic is given. Any difficulties caused by this period of fasting can be overcome by a glucose drip into the vein. The normal insulin injection is not given on the day of operation but small regular doses are either injected under the skin or pumped continuously into the vein. The dose of insulin is adjusted according to the blood glucose level. In minor operations where the patient is expected to be eating an hour or so later, these elaborate procedures may not be necessary and insulin may simply be delayed until the next meal is due. If an emergency operation is necessary it is important that the doctors know that the patient has diabetes. This is another good reason for wearing an identification bracelet or necklace.

Must I tell my dentist I have diabetes and will this affect my treatment in any way?

Having diabetes will not affect your dental treatment at all. However, it is important to remove all possibility of a hypo while in the dentist's chair. If you are on insulin, warn your dentist that you cannot run over a snack or mealtime. It is less embarrassing to mention this before the start of a session than to have to munch glucose tablets while the dentist is trying to administer treatment.

Obviously you must warn your dentist if he plans to give you any form of heavy sedation. If someone on insulin is to have dental treatment needing a general anaesthetic, this is usually done in hospital.

Is someone with diabetes more likely to suffer from tooth decay or gum trouble?

There is an increased risk of infection in people who are poorly controlled. The gums may become infected and this in turn may lead to tooth decay. However, someone who is well controlled is not prone to any particular dental problem – in fact, there is a positive advantage to avoiding sweets which cause dental caries (tooth decay).

I have been told that, as I have diabetes, I don't have to pay for dental treatment. Is this true?

No. Dental treatment is not free to people who have diabetes. If you are entitled to benefits such as Income Support, you may be entitled to some help with the cost of treatment.

Driving

I drive a lot in my work and my lunch time varies from day to day. Does this matter? I am on two injections of insulin a day.

Yes, this can be a bit of a problem. The twice-daily insulin regimen is designed to provide a boost of insulin at midday to cope with the lunch time intake of food. Once the early morning injection of insulin has been given, there is no way of delaying the midday surge. It is very common for people who are well controlled on two injections a day to feel a little hypo before lunch. There are two possible solutions to your problem.

- Eat some biscuits or fruit while you are driving – only do this in emergencies as you will not know how much to have for lunch when you do get the chance to eat properly.
- Change your insulin regimen so that you have a small dose of short-acting insulin before each main meal and only have long-acting insulin in the evening to keep your diabetes under control during the night. You may have to eat snacks between meals but the three- or four-injection method should make the timing of meals more flexible. With an insulin pen an extra injection is really no hardship.

If I have diabetes, do I have to declare this when applying for a driving licence? If so am I likely to be required to provide evidence as to fitness to drive?

Anyone whose diabetes is treated by diet alone does not need to inform the DVLA (Driving and Vehicle Licensing Agency). If your diabetes is treated by tablets or insulin, then you must declare this when applying for a driving licence. If you already hold a driving licence, then you must declare your diabetes to the DVLA as soon as you have been diagnosed.

When you have notified the DVLA, they will send you a form asking for details about your diabetes and the names of any doctors you see regularly. They will also ask you to sign a declaration allowing your doctors to disclose medical details about your condition. There is usually no difficulty over someone with diabetes obtaining a licence to drive.

If you are treated by tablets, you will be able to obtain an unrestricted licence, providing you undertake to inform the DVLA of any change in your treatment or if you develop any complications of diabetes.

If you are treated by insulin, the licence will be valid for only three years instead of up to the age of 70, which it is for most people in the UK. It is the risk of sudden and severe hypoglycaemia which makes people liable to this form of discrimination. In general the only people who have difficulty in obtaining a licence are those on insulin with very erratic control and a history of hypos causing unconsciousness. Once their condition has been controlled and severe hypos abolished, they can reapply for a licence with confidence. If you are renewing your licence, you may not be able to drive a minibus (not for hire or reward) or a small lorry over 3–5 tonnes, as legislation has recently changed. For more information, contact Diabetes UK.

People on insulin are no longer allowed to hold PCV or LGV licences.

When I was filling out a form for the DVLA, one of the questions asked whether I had had laser treatment in both eyes. Why do the DVLA need this information?

The DVLA may ask you to have a 'visual fields test' if you have had laser treatment in both eyes, and your licence will be revoked if you cannot pass this test. If you are having a visual fields test, we would recommend that you have the type in which both eyes are tested at the same time. This test which examines both eyes together is the DVLA driving standard.

I have had to have a form signed by my doctor for my insurance company to insure my car. The doctor charged me for this service and pocketed the fee without even giving me a receipt. Is this normal?

Motor insurance is another problem for the driver with diabetes. Failure to inform your insurance company of your diabetes may make your cover invalid, in which case the consequences could be disastrous. The insurance company usually asks your doctor to complete a form. These forms vary but some of them are very long and ask a lot of irritating and irrelevant questions. Unfortunately there is a charge since doctors are not obliged to sign these forms and are therefore entitled to a fee, just as you are entitled to a receipt. You will probably find that doctors at the hospital clinic will fill in the form for nothing.

Unfortunately there may be financial penalties for having

diabetes and some insurance companies will load your premium. Diabetes UK Services has been set up by Diabetes UK to seek a better deal for people with diabetes. This includes a home and motor insurance service which you can contact on 0800 731 7432.

I have heard that a driver who had a motor accident while hypo was successfully prosecuted for driving under the influence of drugs and heavily fined. As someone on insulin I was horrified to hear this verdict.

Several people on insulin have been charged with this offence after a hypo at the wheel when the only 'drug' that they have used is insulin. It may seem very unfair but, for any victim of an accident, it is no consolation that the person responsible was hypo rather than being blind drunk. These cases emphasize the importance of taking driving seriously. Remember the rules.

- Always carry food/glucose in your car.
- If you feel at all hypo, stop your car (as soon as possible), take some glucose and move into the passenger seat.
- Preferably check that your blood glucose is above 5 mmol/l before driving again.
- On a long journey, check blood glucose levels every few hours.

I have been a bus driver for 15 years and was found to have diabetes five years ago. Up till now I have been on tablets but may need to go on to insulin. Does this mean I will lose my job?

As a bus driver you will hold a PCV (Passenger Carrying Vehicle) licence. People on insulin are not allowed to drive a PSV. You are faced with a very difficult choice – either to continue on tablets feeling unwell but holding down your job, or else to start insulin and feel much better, but lose your source of employment. We would have to advise you to go onto insulin as you will come to this eventually.

Any holder of a LGV (Large Goods Vehicle) licence will also lose his licence and thus his livelihood if he has to start insulin treatment. LGV drivers who have been on insulin *since before*

Colour Section

LIST OF PLATES

Plate 1 Using One Touch Profile
Plate 2 Using One Touch Basic
Plate 3 Bayer Esprit
Plate 4 Medisense Sensors
Plate 5 Medisense Precision Q.I.D. Sensor
Plate 6 Blood glucose monitoring: Glucotrend
Plate 7 Drawing up insulin
Plate 8 Mixing insulins
Plate 9 Injection technique
Plate 10 Using a B-D Pen (3 ml)
Plate 11 Using a Novopen 3 Fun and Classic
Plate 12 Using a Humapen Ergo

Plate 1 USING ONE TOUCH PROFILE

Always wash your hands thoroughly and then dry them on a clean towel before starting to test your blood glucose.

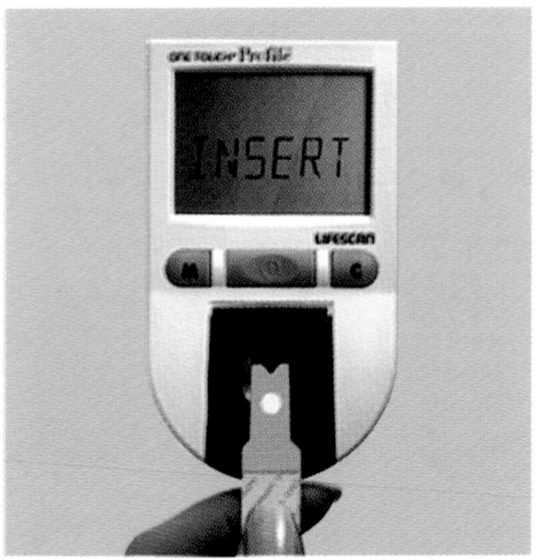

1 **Turn on, Insert strip:** Press middle button to switch on and insert a LifeScan ONE TOUCH test strip, with the notched edge first and the round dot facing upwards.

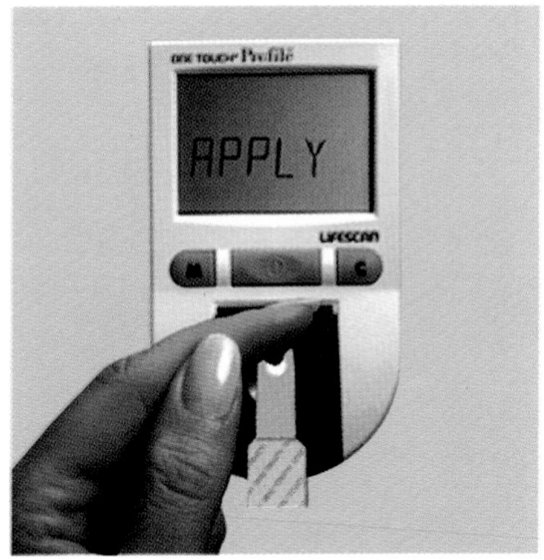

2 **Apply sample:** Apply a small drop of blood on the test spot. No timing, wiping or blotting is required. The Profile automatically starts the test.

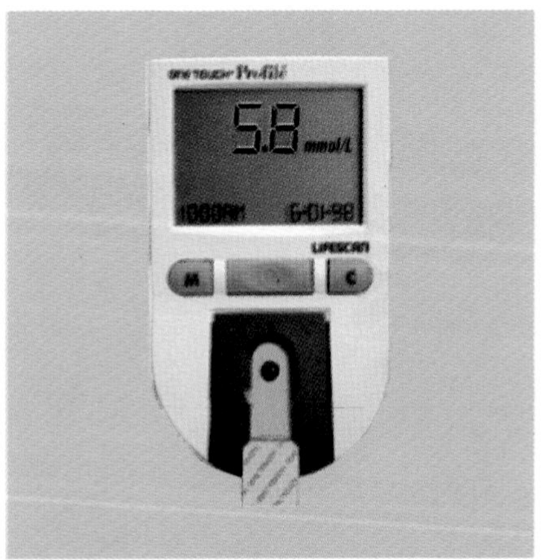

3 **Read result:** An accurate test result is displayed with date and time, in just 45 seconds. If anything has gone wrong that may affect the accuracy of the result, the display will tell you e.g. if not enough blood was applied. The test result is stored in the memory, which holds 250 tests.

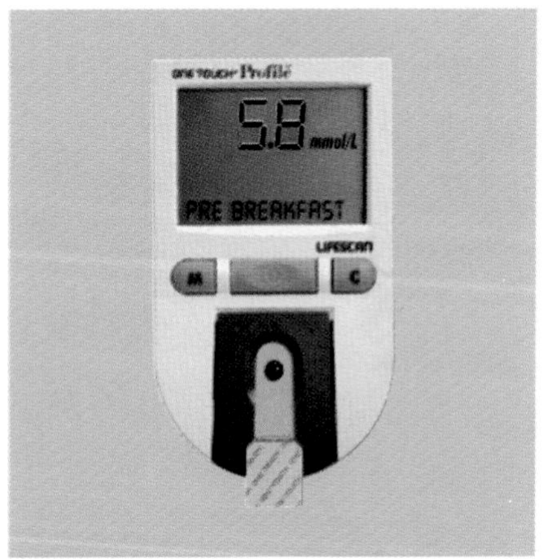

4 **Event label result (optional):** Before removing the test strip, press the button C to select the desired event label, then remove test strip. Averages can then be viewed by a choice of 15 events e.g. pre and post meals, pre and post exercise etc.

Averages and individual results stored, can be viewed by pressing the M button. ***Event labelling results****, entering* ***Insulin doses*** *and* ***Carbohydrate intake*** *are optional features. Data from the Profile can be downloaded to LifeScan's IN TOUCH diabetes management software to produce graphs.*

Plate 2 USING ONE TOUCH BASIC

Always wash your hands thoroughly and then dry them on a clean towel before starting to test your blood glucose.

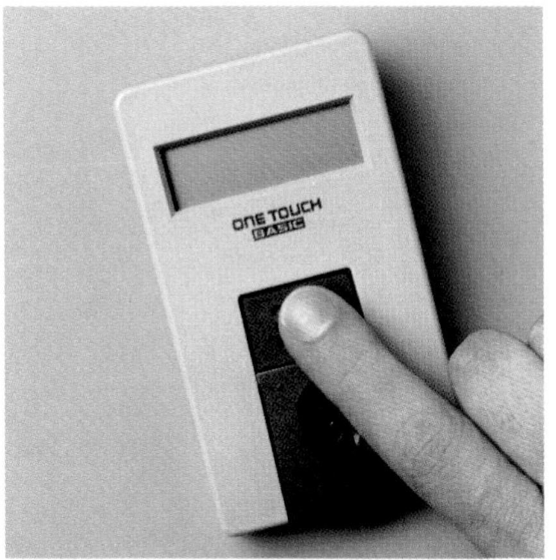

1 **Turn on:** Press the large button on the front to switch the ONE TOUCH BASIC on. Follow the clear instructions on the display that guide you through the test.

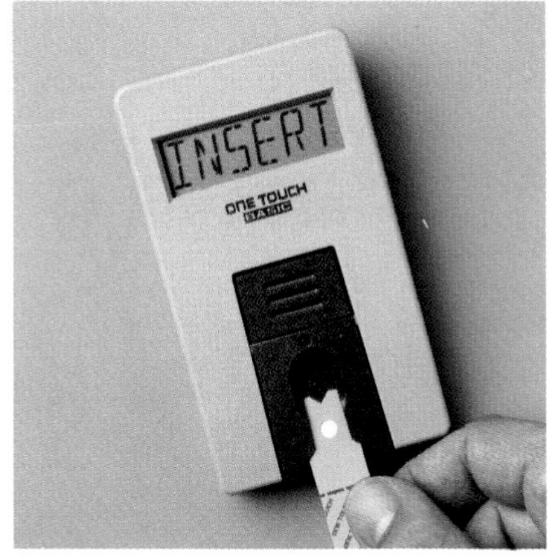

2 **Insert strip:** Insert a Lifescan ONE TOUCH test strip, with the notched edge first and the round dot facing upwards.

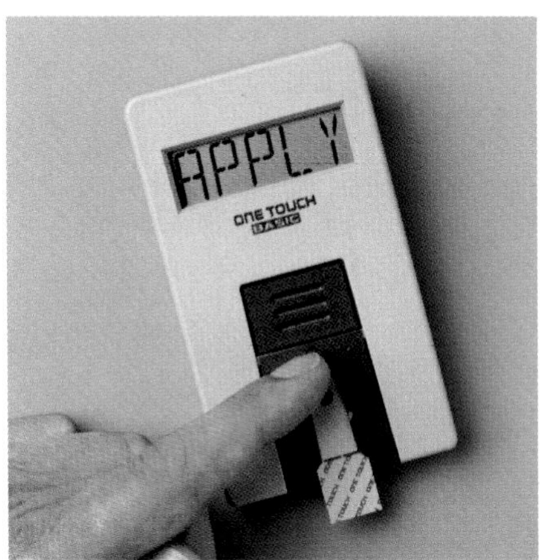

3 **Apply sample:** Apply a small drop of blood on the test spot. No timing, wiping or blotting is required. The ONE TOUCH BASIC automatically starts the test.

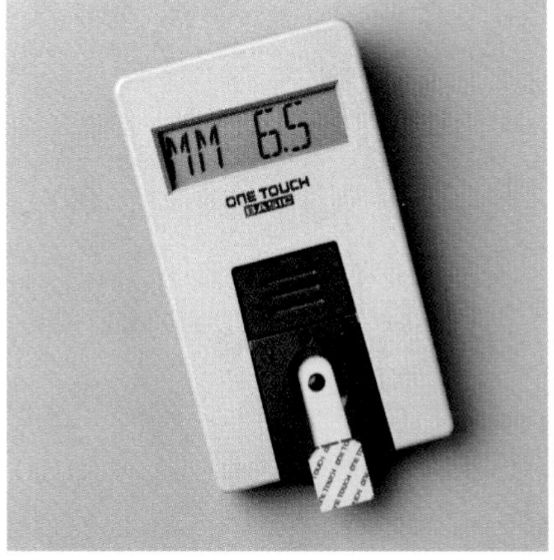

4 **Read result:** An accurate test result is displayed in just 45 seconds. If anything has gone wrong that may affect the accuracy of the result, the display will tell you, e.g. if not enough blood was applied. The test result will be stored in memory until the next test.

Plate 3 BAYER ESPRIT

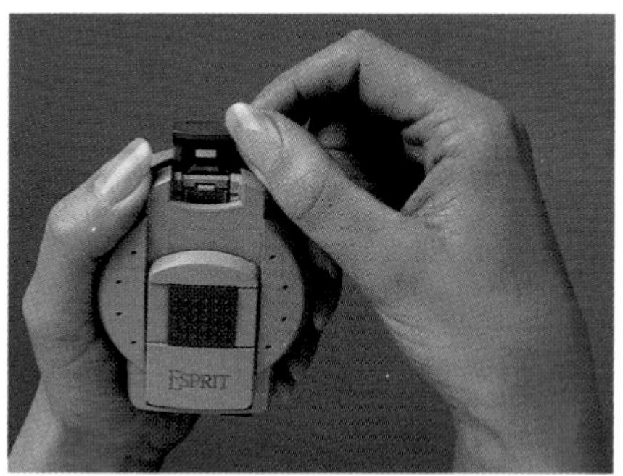

1 Open the meter by releasing the end catch.

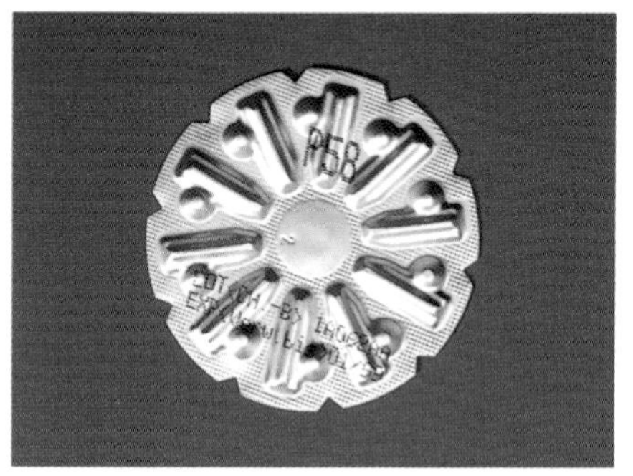

2 Remove the test sensor disc from outer packaging.

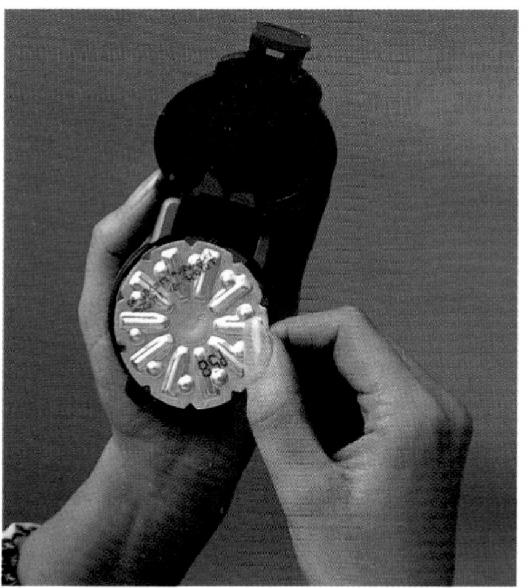

3 Gently press the disc (bump side up) under the two blue corner tabs that hold it in place. Note the programme printed on the disc (Prog. 1–62). Close the Esprit.

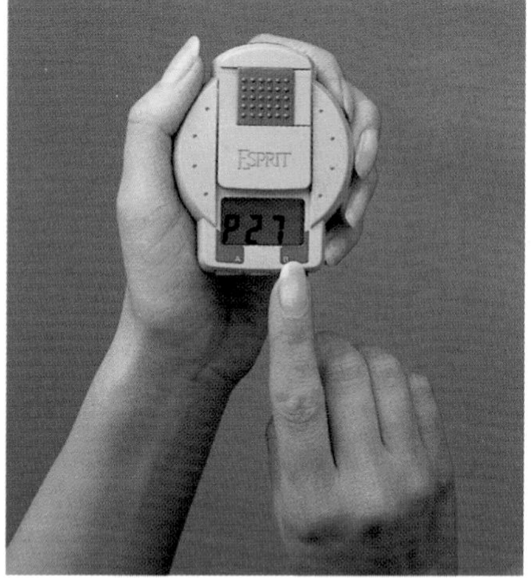

4 To ensure accuracy in test results, programme the meter to correspond with the printed number on the disc. To set the programme number, move the slide forward – the number will flash on the display. Press on B to change, and A to set the number.

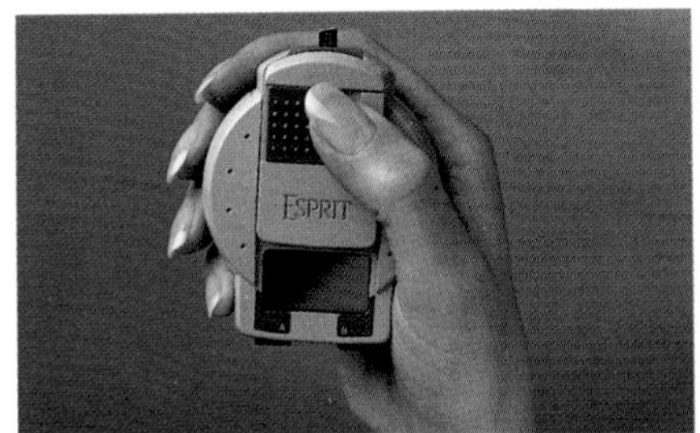

5 To begin test, push slide to the left and move forward. The meter will click and a test strip will appear. The display will show a flashing drop of blood.

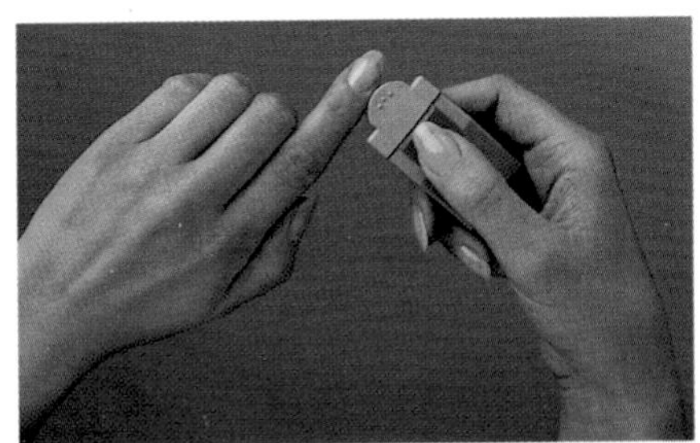

6 Use your finger pricking device as normal to form a rounded drop of blood.

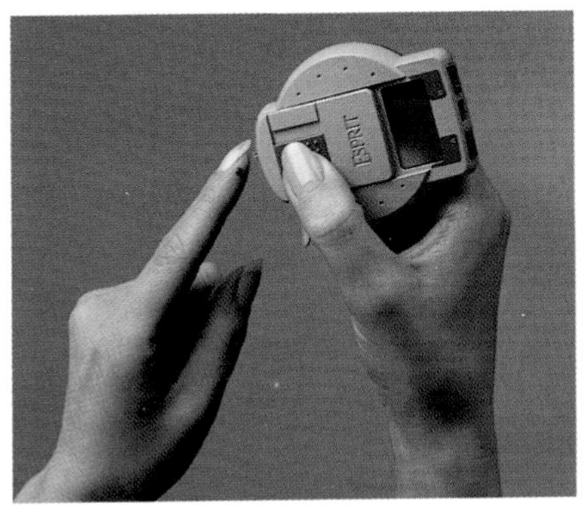

7 Place the entire front edge of the sensor into the droplet. The blood will automatically be drawn into the sensor. Hold in place until beep sounds.

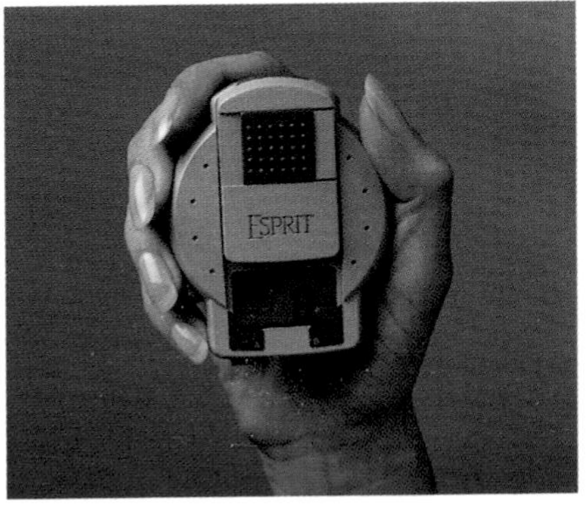

8 Place the Esprit on a flat surface while the display completes its 30-second countdown. The test result will then be displayed followed by a second beep.

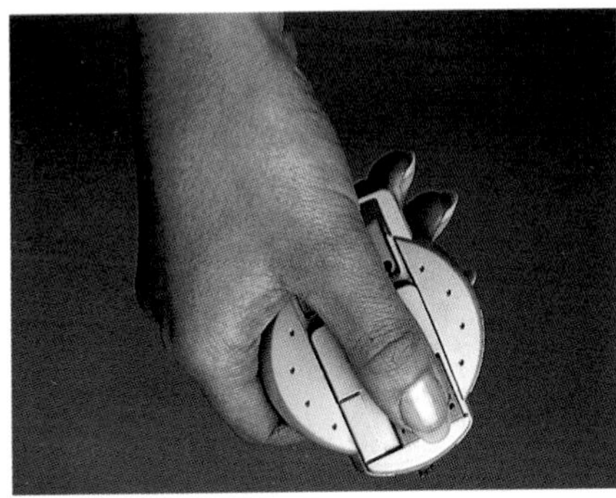

9 Point the meter over a waste container. Move slide back to release and discard used test strip. Results will automatically be stored.

Plate 4 MEDISENSE SENSORS

If you are using the sensor for the first time, refer to the full operating instructions for details on how to calibrate it and for a list of display messages.

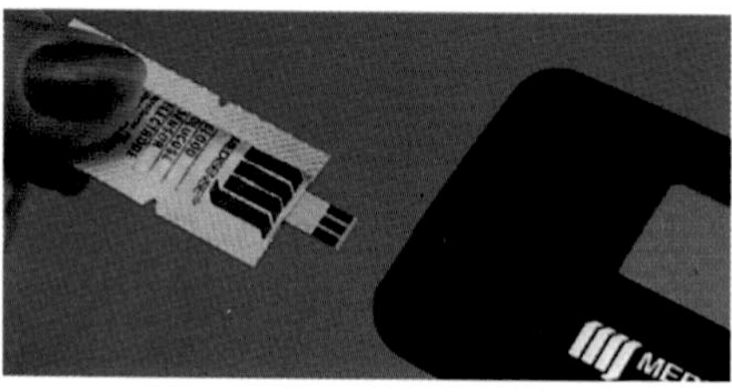

1 Insert the end of the sensor electrode into the sensor (the contact bars should face upwards). The sensor will automatically display 88.8, followed by **CAL**, the calibration code stored in the sensor's memory, and then **rdY**. Remove the remaining foil.

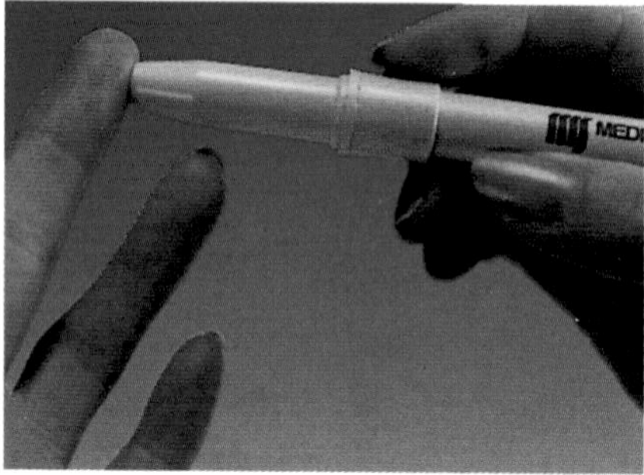

2 Prick the underside of your finger away from your thumb. Wipe away the first drop of blood. Collect a hanging drop of blood.

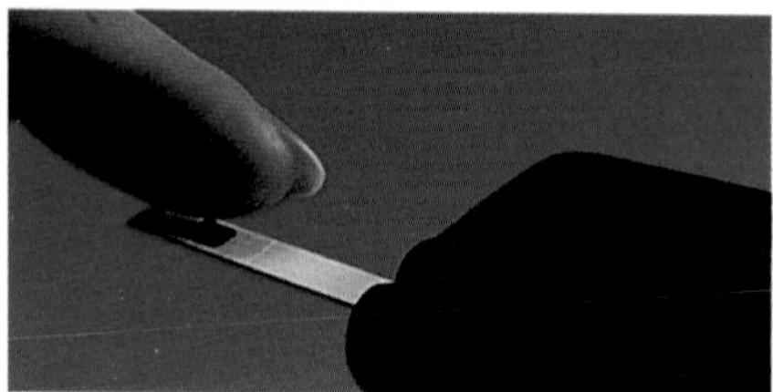

3 Immediately apply the hanging drop of blood to the target area while the display reads **rdY**. The blood will naturally spread over the target area. Make sure that it stays within the target area but completely covers it. Do not touch the sensor electrode with your finger or smear the blood, as this will give you incorrect results.

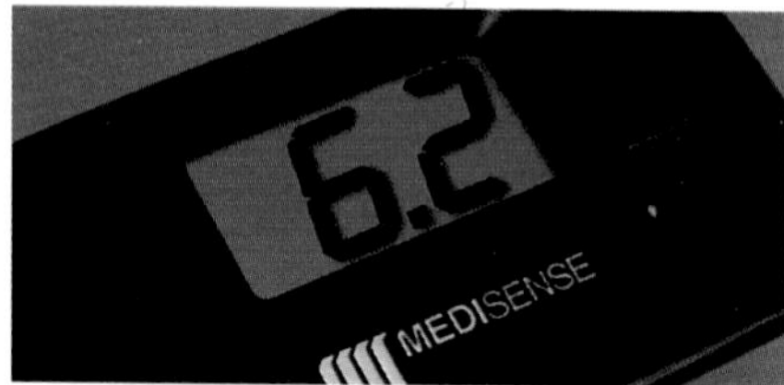

4 Once the drop touches the target area, the display will show ---, --, -, and then **ctd**. The sensor will start automatically and count down from 20 to 1. The blood glucose result will then be displayed. Record this result.

Plate 5 MEDISENSE PRECISION Q.I.D. SENSOR

If you are using the sensor for the first time, refer to the full operating instructions for details on how to calibrate it and for a list of display messages.

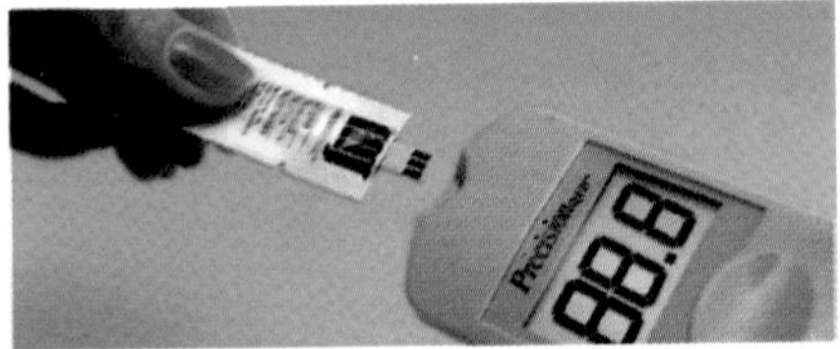

1 Insert the end of the sensor electrode into the sensor (the contact bars should face upwards). The sensor will automatically display 88.8, followed by **CAL**, the calibration code stored in the sensor's memory, and then **rdY**. Remove the remaining foil.

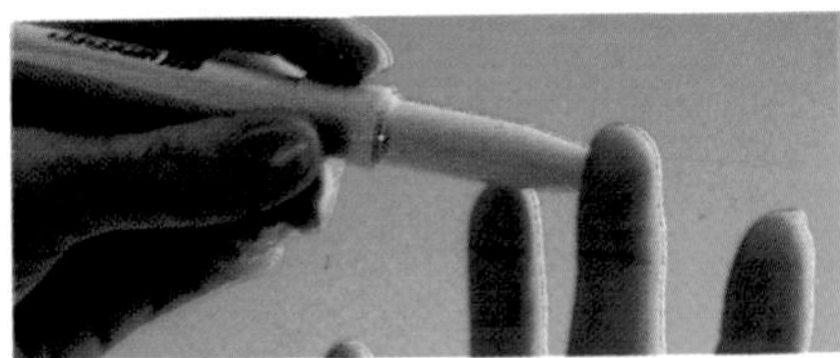

2 Prick the underside of your finger away from your thumb. Wipe away the first drop of blood. Collect a hanging drop of blood.

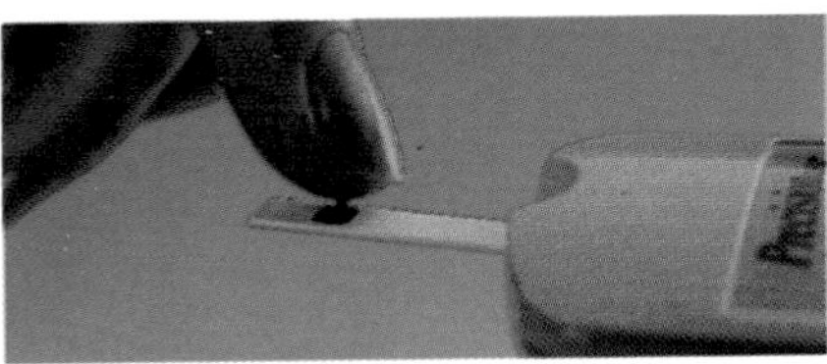

3 Immediately apply the hanging drop of blood to the target area while the display reads **rdY**. The blood will naturally form a dome and spread over the target area. Make sure that it stays within the target area but completely covers it. Do not touch the sensor electrode with your finger or smear the blood, as this will give you incorrect results.

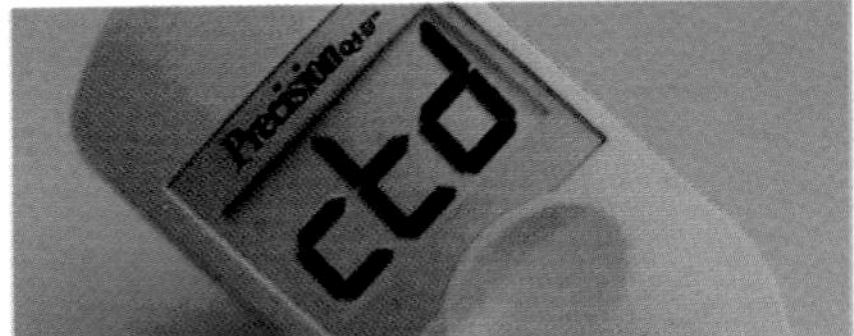

4 Once the drop touches the target area, the display will show ---, --, -, and then **ctd**. The sensor will start automatically and count down from 20 to 1. The blood glucose result will then be displayed. Record this result.

Plate 6 BLOOD GLUCOSE MONITORING: GLUCOTREND

If you are using the meter for the first time refer to the full operating instructions for details on how to calibrate it and for further hints.

Wash and dry your hands thoroughly. Take a test strip from the Glucotrend Glucose test strip vial and replace the cap immediately.

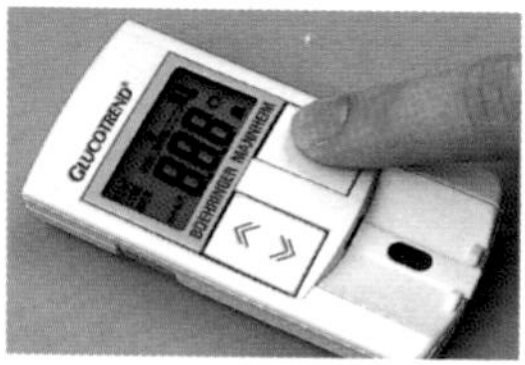

1 Switch on the meter by pressing the on/off button marked ⏻. When the screen displays [888] check that all parts of the digits appear in full. A three digit code will then appear. **Check that the number is the same as the one printed on the Glucotrend Glucose test strip vial. If it differs, recalibrate the meter before proceeding with the test.**

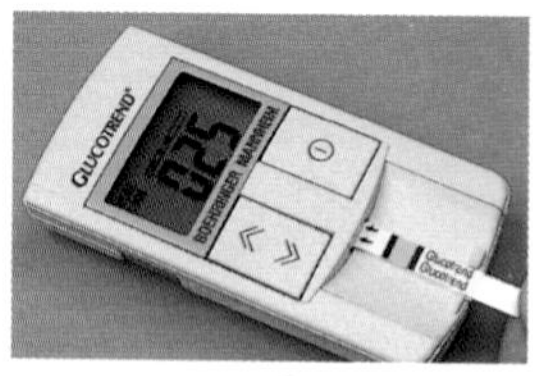

2 When the test strip symbol on the screen is displayed and the red light flashes in the measuring window, insert the test strip into the slot in the direction of the arrows. **Push in firmly until the strip locks into place.** The symbols showing a drop of blood and the sample application zone begin flashing, confirming that blood can now be applied.

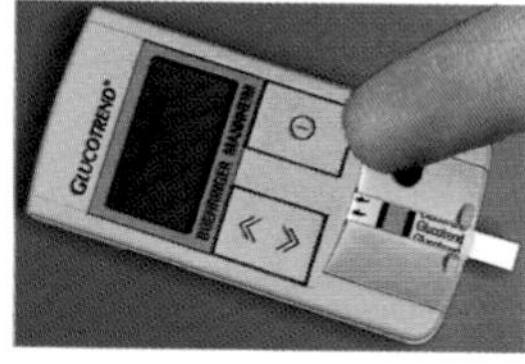

3 Using a sterile lancet, prick the side of your fingertip and squeeze gently to form a **hanging drop of blood** and cover the yellow pad in one application. If the blood does not cover the whole pad, repeat the process using a fresh test strip and a larger drop of blood.

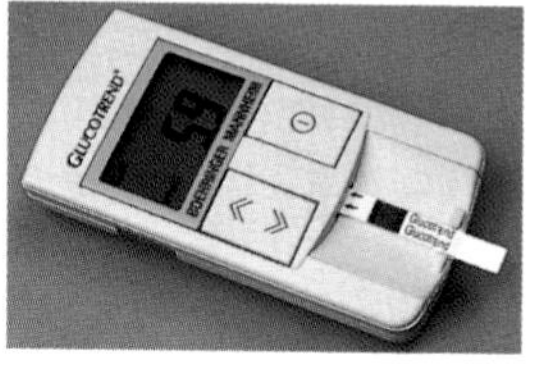

4 After 30 seconds, the meter automatically displays and stores the result. Switch off the meter and remove the test strip. If the meter switches itself off during the test, it means that no key has been pressed during the last 90 seconds.

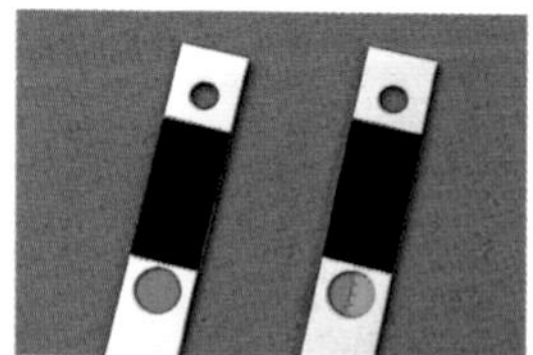

5 Turn the test strip over and check that the circular window is fully and uniformly coloured **(a)**. If the window is partially coloured **(b)** there was not enough blood on the pad to ensure an accurate result. Repeat the process using a fresh test strip and a larger drop of blood. **It is important that you perform this check after every test.**

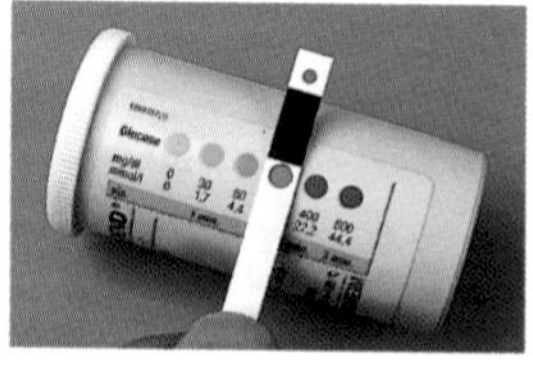

6 As a rough check of the meter's accuracy, compare the colour in the circular window on the back of the strip with the colour chart on the Glucotrend Glucose test strip vial.

To recall any of the last 10 automatically stored results, press the ⏻ button to switch on the meter. The lower part of the rocker key on the left ∨ displays the most recent result, and the upper part ∧ displays results 2–10. Press the ⇕ button up or down repeatedly to display places 1–10.

Plate 7 DRAWING UP INSULIN

Thoroughly wash and dry your hands.
Check the label on the insulin bottle for any special instructions and make sure that the expiry date has not passed. Check that the top of the bottle is undamaged and that the insulin is clear, if it should be.

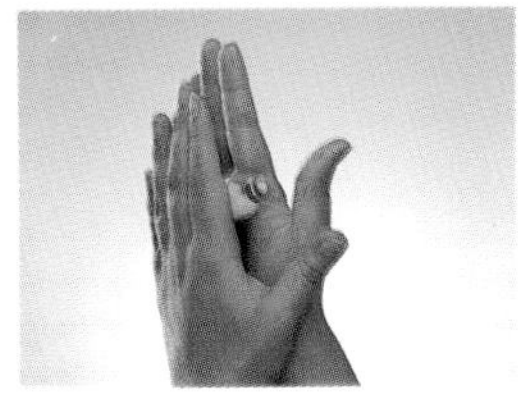

1 Gently rotate the bottle to make sure that the insulin is properly mixed (never shake the bottle). This is especially important when using cloudy insulin.

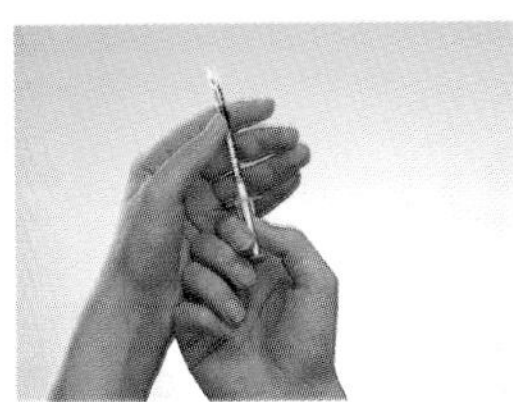

2 Remove the white plunger cap, then carefully remove the orange needle cap by gently twisting and pulling. Pull back the plunger of the syringe to measure the amount of air equivalent to the amount of insulin you require.

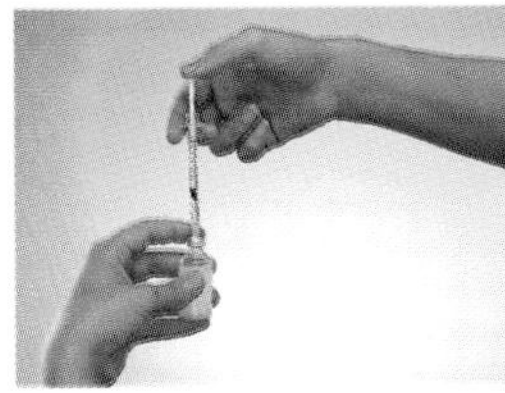

3 With the bottle standing upright, insert the needle straight through the centre of the rubber cap of the insulin bottle and push the plunger down. This pushes air into the bottle, making it easier for you to draw the insulin out of the bottle.

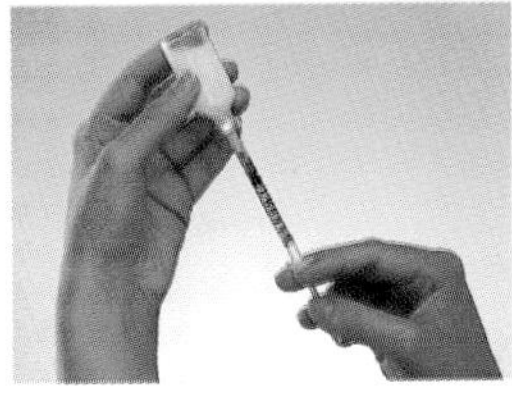

4 Turn the bottle upside down. Make certain that the point of the needle inside the bottle is well beneath the surface level of the insulin. Pull back the plunger until you have measured slightly more than your correct dose of insulin.

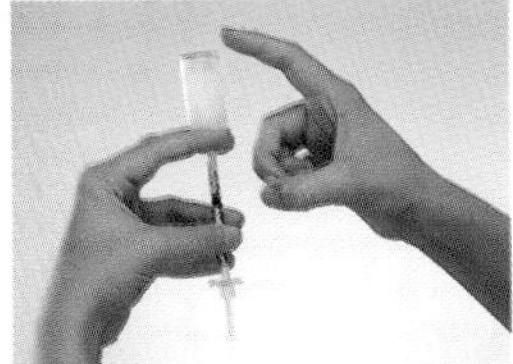

5 If there are air bubbles in your syringe, remove them. Flick or tap the syringe at the bubble with your finger. When the air bubble goes to the top of the syringe, push the plunger up to expel the bubble back into the bottle.

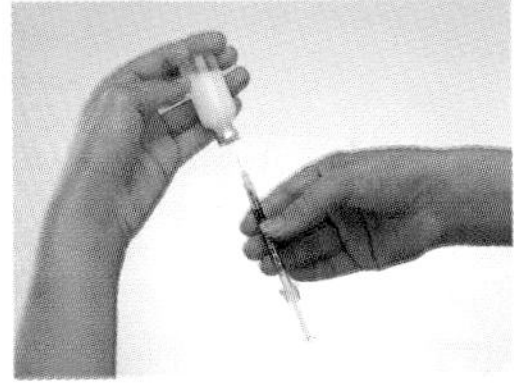

6 Remove the syringe from the bottle. You are now ready to inject.

Note: Although air bubbles are not dangerous if injected, it is important to get the air bubbles out of the syringe so that you have an accurate dose of insulin. If air bubbles persist, expel all of the insulin back into the bottle and start again.

Plate 8 MIXING INSULINS

A combination of two types of insulin can be prescribed by your doctor to provide the benefits of both a fast acting insulin and a longer acting insulin in one injection.

Before you start:

- Thoroughly wash and dry your hands.
- **Always** inspect both insulin bottles before using them to make sure the tops are not damaged and that the expiry dates have not passed.

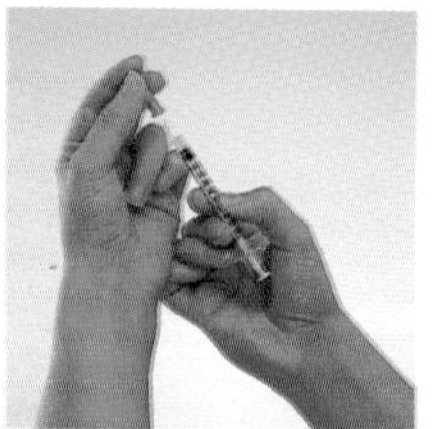

1 Remove the white plunger cap, then carefully remove the orange needle cap by gently twisting and pulling.

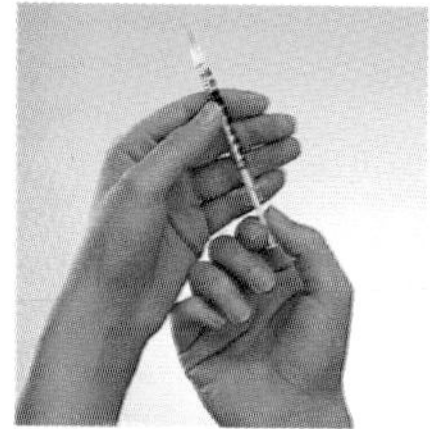

2 Pull back the plunger of the syringe to measure the amount of air equivalent to the amount of **cloudy** insulin you require.

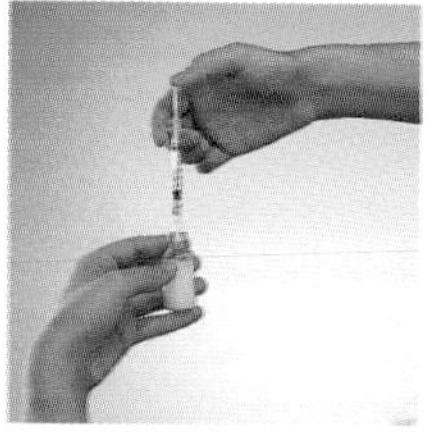

3 With the bottle standing upright, insert the needle straight through the centre of the rubber cap on the **cloudy** insulin bottle and push the plunger down. (This injects air which will make it easier to draw up the insulin later.) You are not going to draw up any cloudy insulin yet. Remove the needle **without** drawing up the insulin.

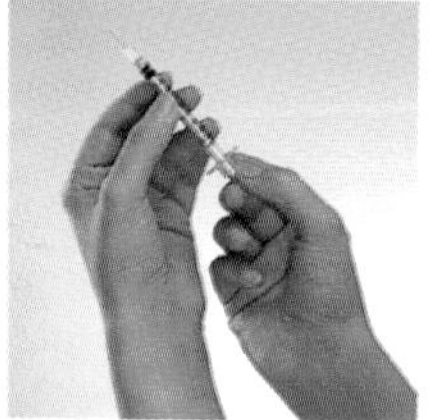

4 Pull back the plunger of the syringe again to measure the amount of air equivalent to the amount of **clear** insulin you require.

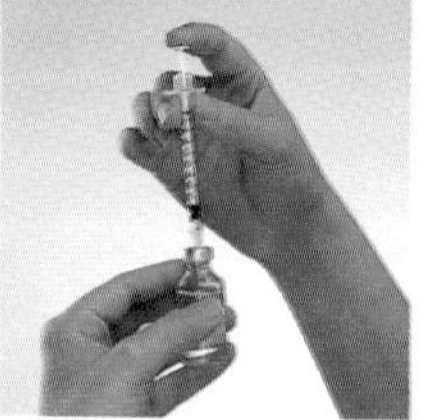

5 With the bottle standing upright, insert the needle straight through the centre of the rubber cap on the **clear** insulin bottle and push the plunger down. This time leave the needle in the bottle.

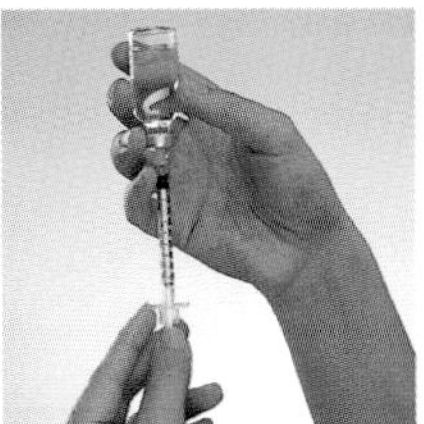

6 Turn the bottle upside down and support to avoid bending the needle. Ensure that the needle point is beneath the surface level of the insulin. Pull back the plunger to measure slightly more than your correct dose of insulin.

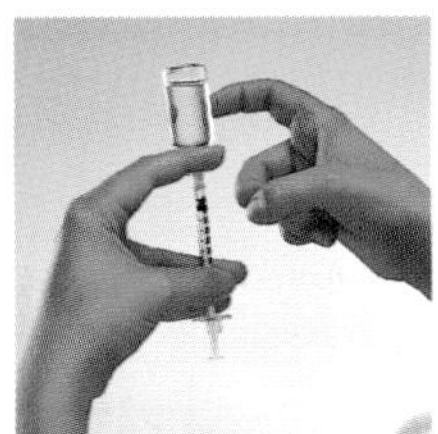

7 If any air bubbles are in your syringe, flick or tap the syringe at the bubble with your finger. Then push the plunger up to the correct dose to expel bubbles and excess insulin back into the bottle.

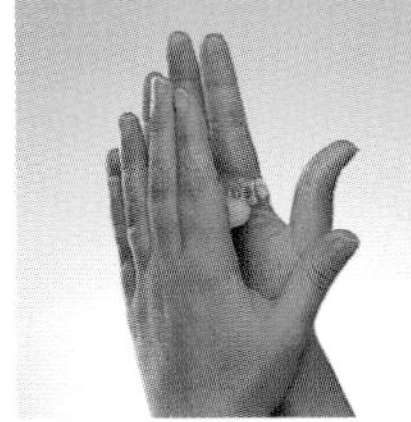

8 Gentle rotate the **cloudy** bottle to make sure the insulin is properly mixed. (Never shake the bottle.)

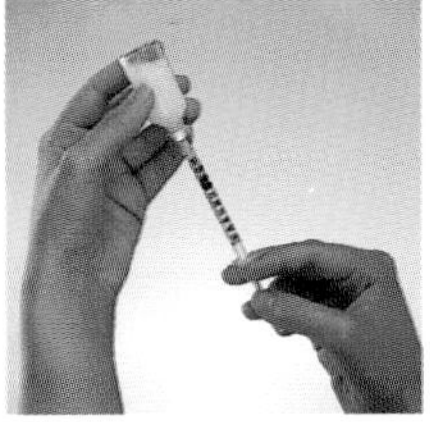

9 Holding the bottle of **cloudy** insulin upside down, push the needle through the rubber cap. Ensure that the needle point is beneath the surface level of the insulin. Pull back the plunger until you have measured the exact dose of **cloudy** insulin.

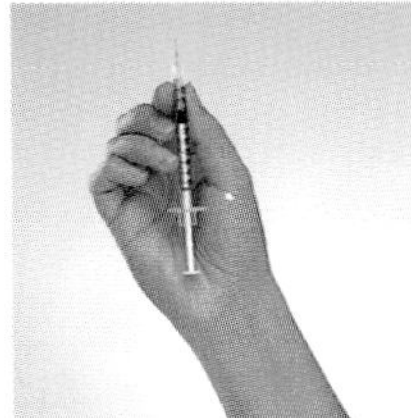

10 Withdraw the needle from the **cloudy** bottle. Check again for air bubbles. It is rare to see them at this step, but if you do, discard all of the measured insulin into the sink and start again. If there are no bubbles, you are ready to inject.

VERY IMPORTANT

Clear insulin should always be drawn into the syringe before **cloudy**. If you accidentally measure too much **cloudy** insulin, do not press the plunger to return the excess into the bottle because some **clear** insulin will also be injected into the **cloudy** insulin bottle. Remove the needle from the bottle and discard all of the insulin from the syringe into the sink and start again.

Plate 9 INJECTION TECHNIQUE

Your doctor or the nursing staff at the hospital are the final authorities regarding precisely how you should inject and where you should give your injection. Follow their advice carefully.

It is important to remember the following tips when using insulin syringes:

- Carefully twist and pull off the orange needle cap making sure not to touch the exposed sterile needle.
- NEVER attempt to re-straighten a bent or damaged needle – simply clip it off with a B-D Safe-Clip and use a new syringe.
- Do not clean or flush out sterile disposable syringes.
- For comfort and safety, Becton Dickinson recommends that disposable insulin syringes be used once only.

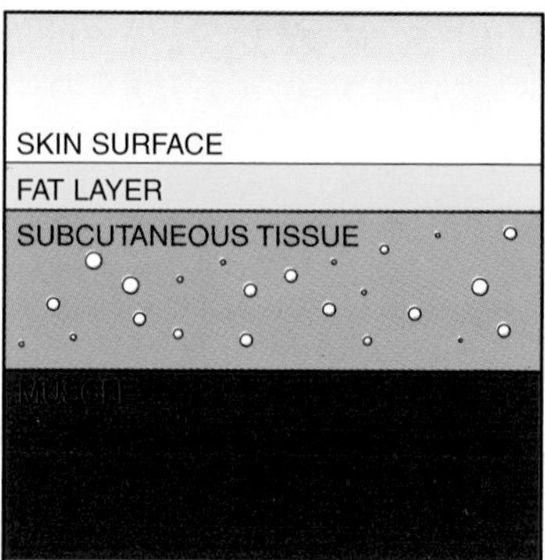

1 Choose an injection site where there is subcutaneous tissue. This type of tissue is located between the fat layer under the skin and the muscles which are below that.

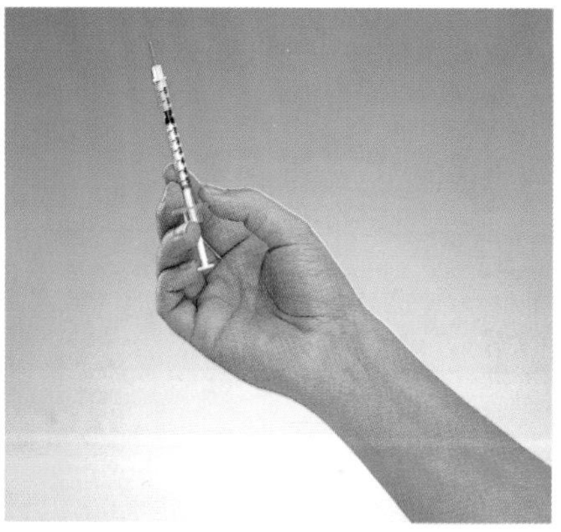

2 Make absolutely certain once again that you have measured your insulin dose correctly.

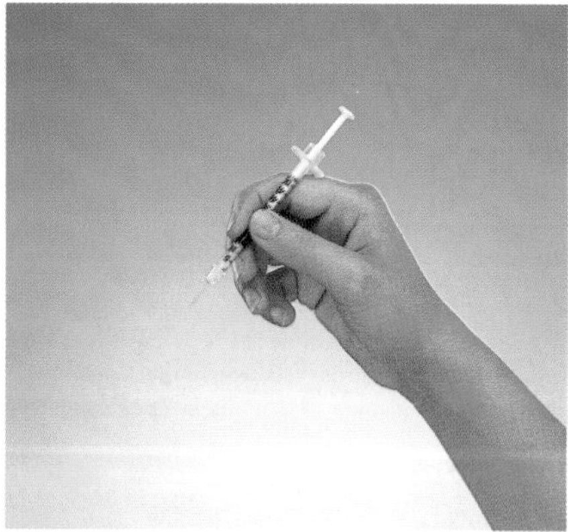

3 Taking care not to touch the sterile needle, hold the syringe firmly near the top, as if you were going to write with it like a pencil.

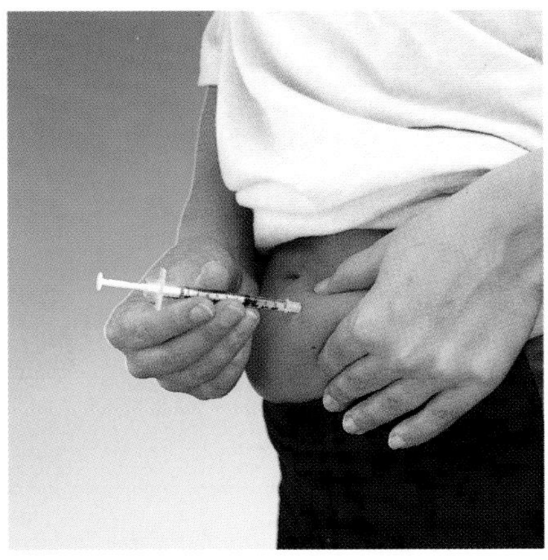

4 Using the other hand, pinch a mound of clean skin between your thumb and index finger and quickly push the needle straight into the mound as far as it will go.

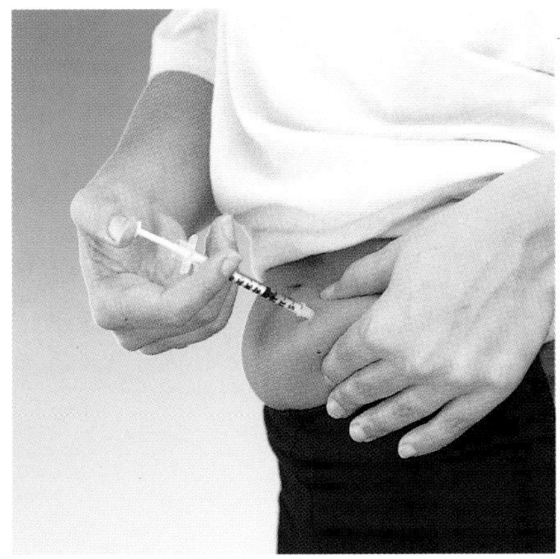

5 Holding the pinched mound through the injection, with your thumb on top of the plunger, quickly and smoothly inject all of the insulin from the syringe. **After the plunger is pushed in leave the syringe in the skin for 5 seconds.**

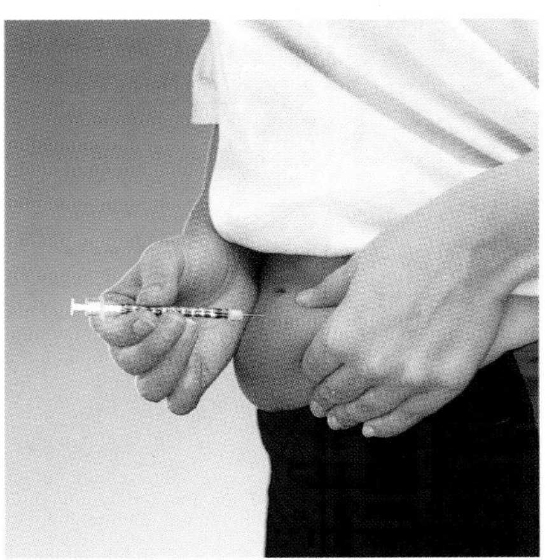

6 Withdraw the needle slowly straight out of the mound of skin, then release the mound and, if necessary, gently wipe the site with a clean piece of tissue or cotton wool. Your injection is now completed.

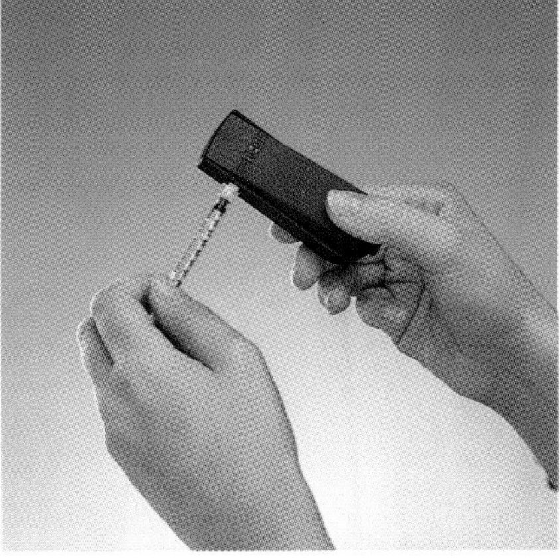

7 Dispose of syringes carefully. Clip the needle off the syringe body using a B-D Safe-Clip. Place the unusable syringe into a sealable container, such as a bleach bottle – keep out of the reach of children. When full, seal the lid securely and place in the refuse.

Plate 10 USING A B-D PEN 3 ml

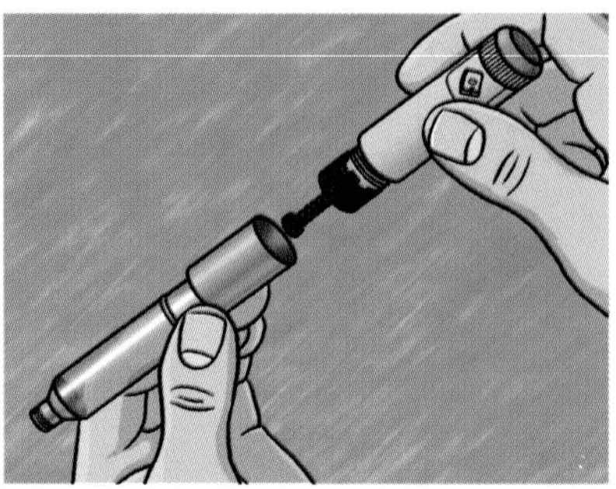

1 Remove the cap. Unscrew the two parts of the B-D Pen 3 ml.

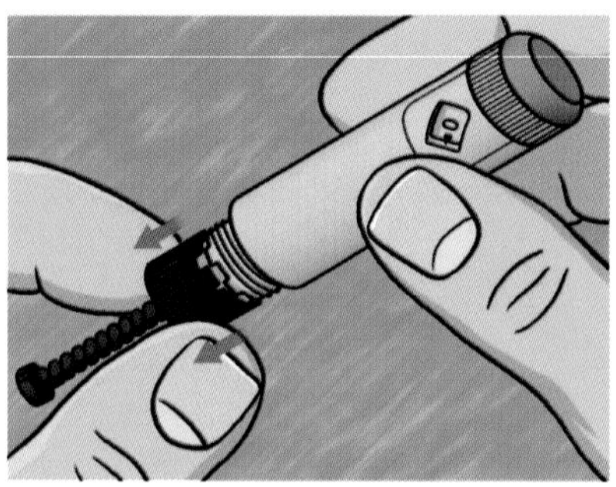

2 Disengage the black ring lock.

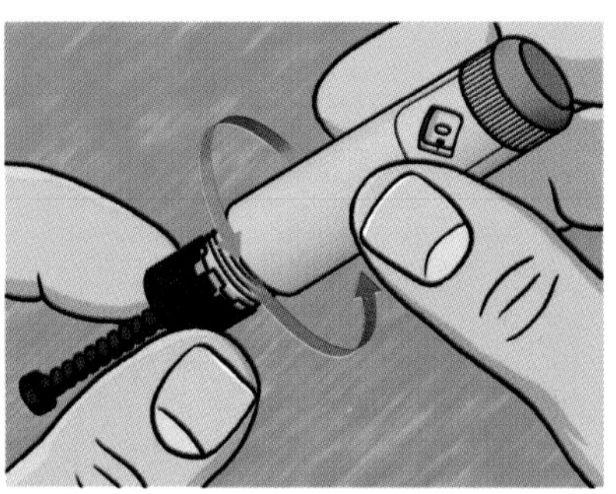

3 Rewind the black plunger screw until flush with black ring lock.

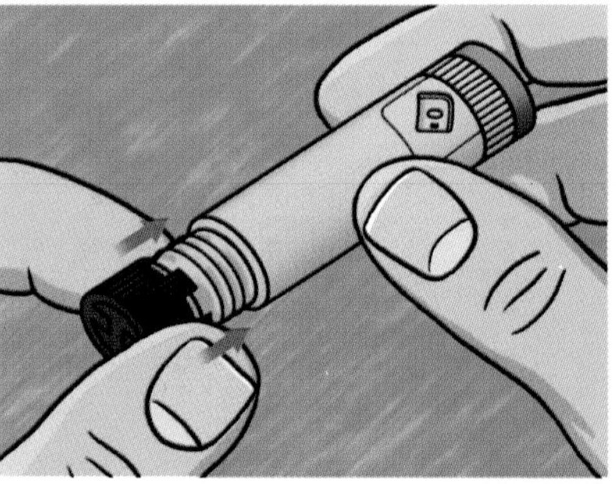

4 Return the black ring lock to original locked position.

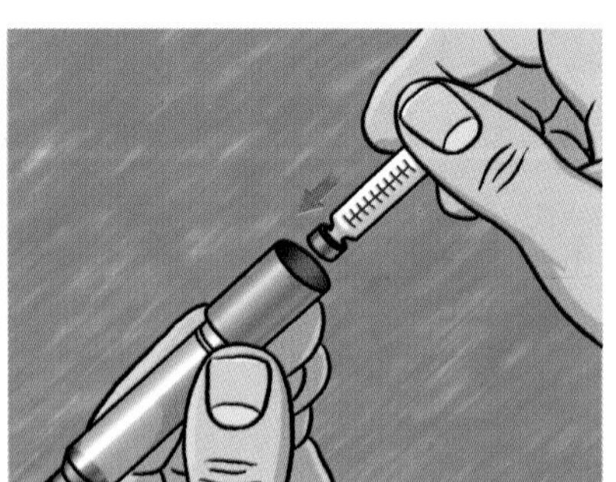

5 Put the 3 ml U-100 Eli Lilly insulin cartridge into the transparent housing.

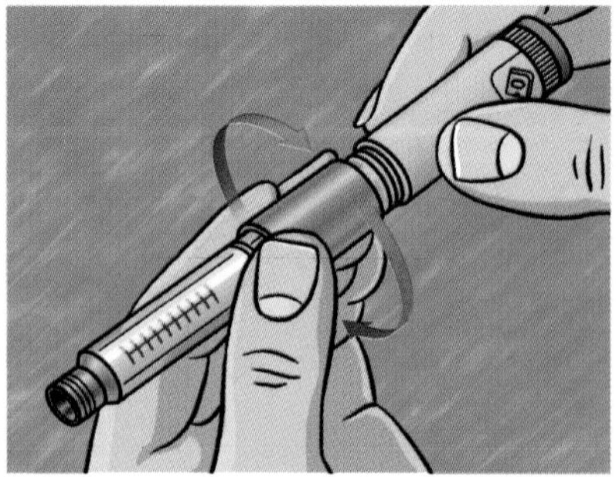

6 Screw together the two parts of the B-D Pen 3 ml. Resuspend the insulin. Attach a B-D MICRO-FINE + pen needle. Remove the needle cover and shield.

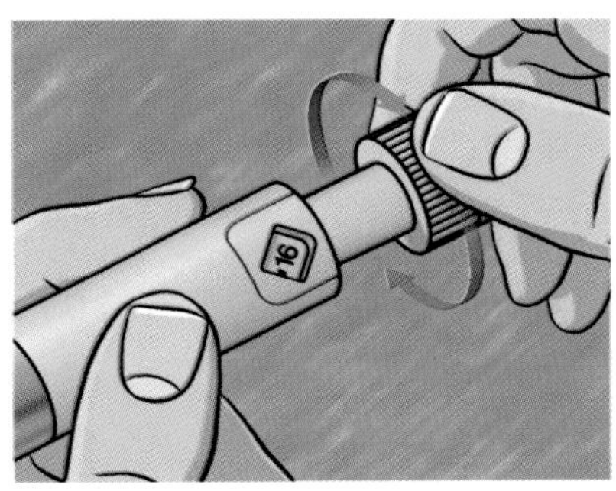

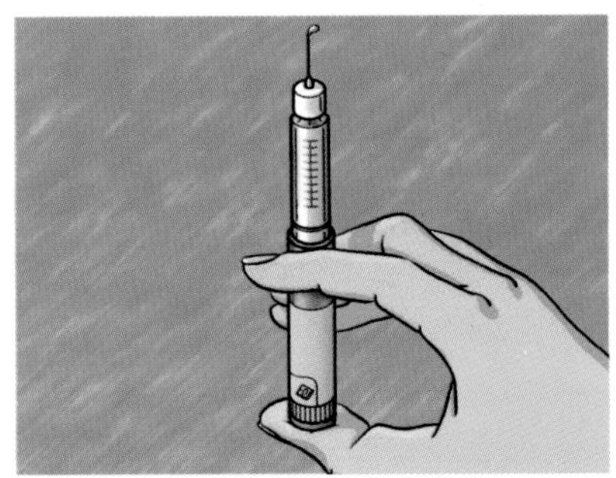

7 Prime by setting 16 units and holding the pen vertically, push the injection button fully, maintaining the pressure for 5 seconds.
If no insulin appears at the needle tip, dial another 2 units and repeat the procedure until insulin appears.

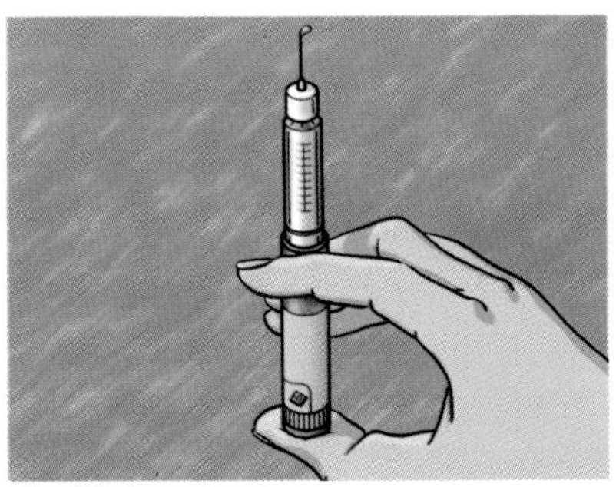

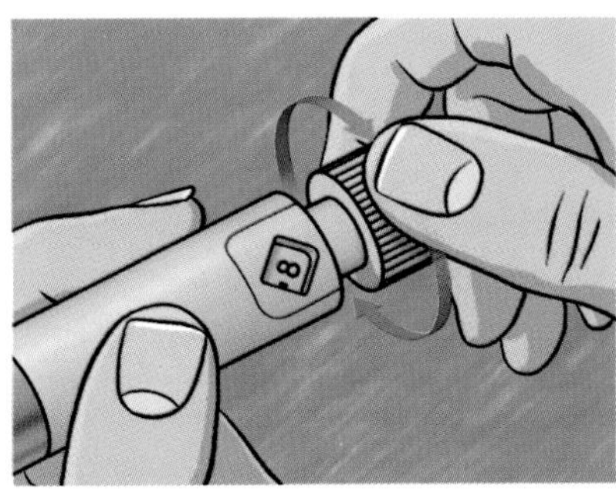

8 Check the insulin flow by dialling 2 units and pushing the injection button fully (maintaining the pressure for 5 seconds).

9 Select the insulin dose required.

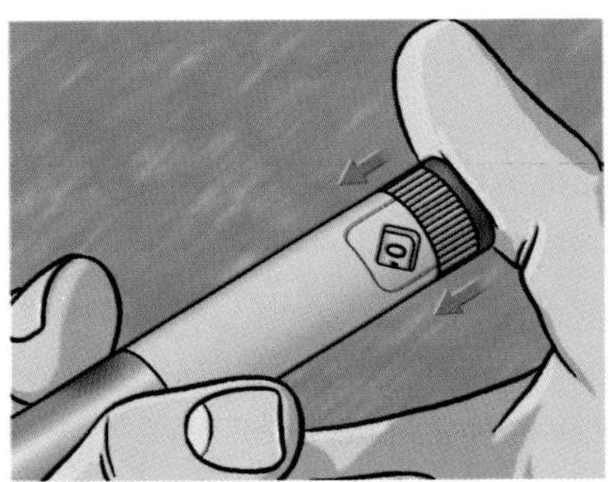

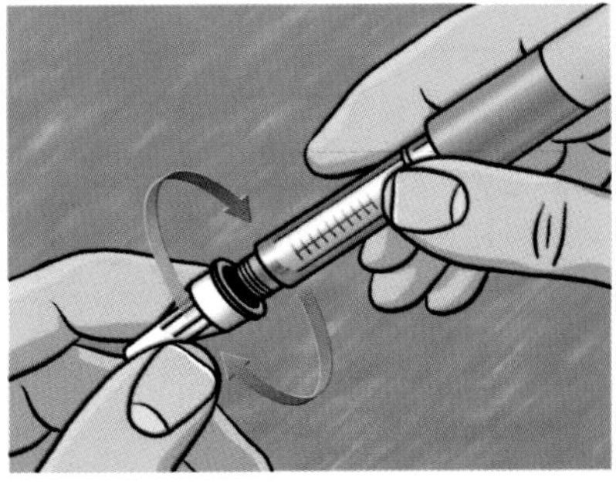

10 Insert the needle in the skin and push injection in fully. Maintain pressure on the injection button for 5 seconds. Remove the needle from the skin.

11 Clip the needle off using a B-D Safe-Clip. Using the needle cover, unscrew the needle hub from the B-D Pen 3 ml and dispose of according to local guidelines.

Plate 11 USING A NOVOPEN 3 FUN AND CLASSIC

INSTRUCTIONS FOR USE

1 Remove the pen cap and unscrew the cartridge holder. Dial the return mechanism clockwise to ensure the piston rod is in its starting position. NEVER PUSH THE PISTON ROD BACK AS THIS MAY DAMAGE THE PEN.

2 Insert the cartridge into the holder - the coloured cap goes in first.

3 Screw both halves of the pen together firmly.

4 Cloudy insulins must be evenly mixed before injecting. Do not try to inject cloudy insulins if you can see the rubber piston in the small inspection window.

5 Screw a needle onto the end of the pen and remove the outer and inner caps. Remember to do an 'air-shot' before each injection.

6 Check the push button is fully depressed then dial the number of units you need to inject. Up to 70 units may be delivered as one dose.

7 Inject the insulin into your chosen injection site by pressing the push button fully home.

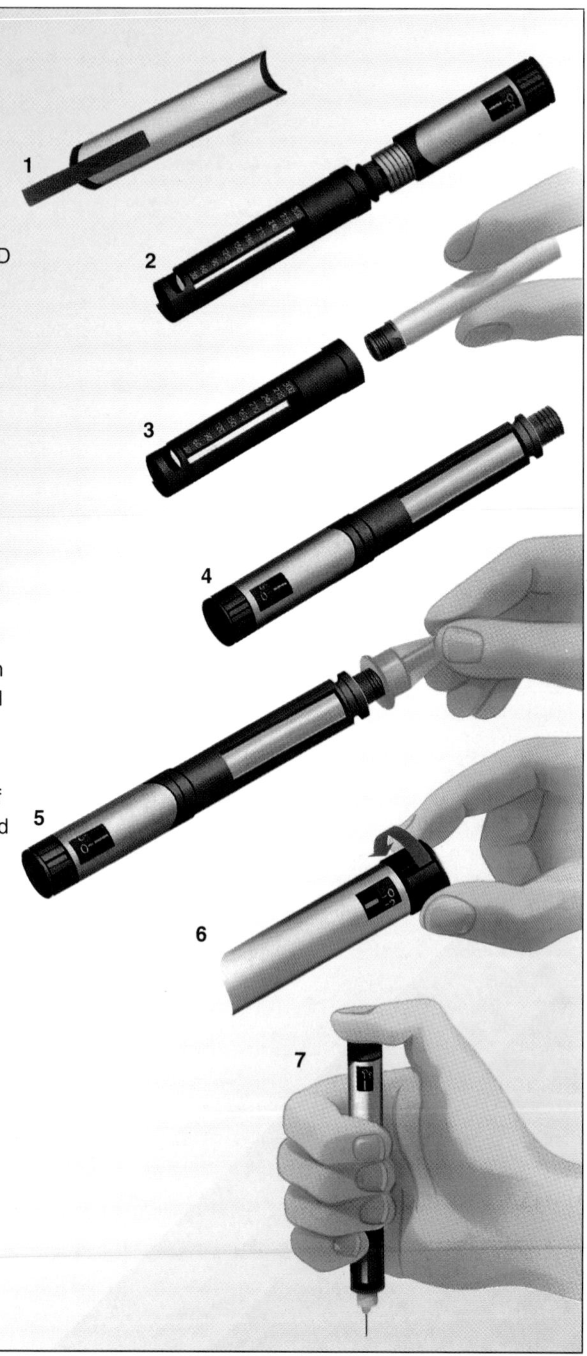

HELPFUL HINTS

A Air-shot: check that the dosage selector is set at zero, then dial 2 units. Hold the pen so that the needle points upwards, tap the cartridge holder gently and press the push button fully. A small drop of insulin should appear at the needle tip. If not, repeat this procedure until a drop of insulin appears.

B If you have dialled too large a dose by mistake, simply pull the spring-loaded mechanical section and the cartridge holder slightly apart, grip firmly and press the push button back to zero. Upon releasing your grip, the cartridge holder will slide back into place.

C NovoPen 3 Fun and Classic allow you to select a dosage larger than the number of units remaining in the cartridge; therefore you should always check the scale on the cartridge holder to see if there is enough insulin for your requirements. If you do inject an insufficient number of units, the remaining number to be injected is displayed in the indicator window. Simply change the cartridge and, after an 'air-shot', dial the appropriate remaining dose and inject as usual.

NovoPen 3 Fun and Classic are supplied free to people with diabetes, when recommended by a doctor or nurse.

Plate 12 USING A HUMAPEN ERGO

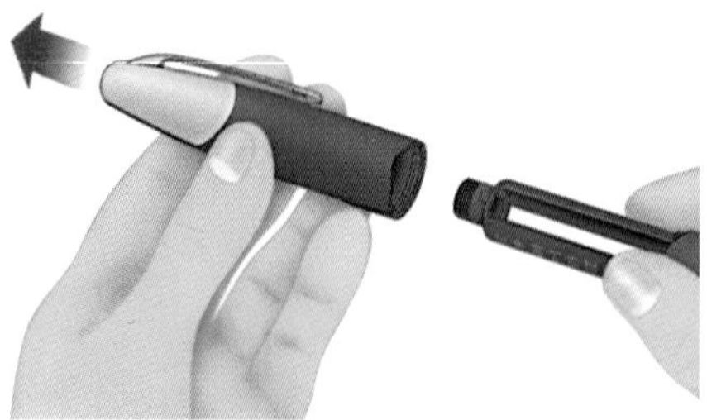

1 Remove the cap.

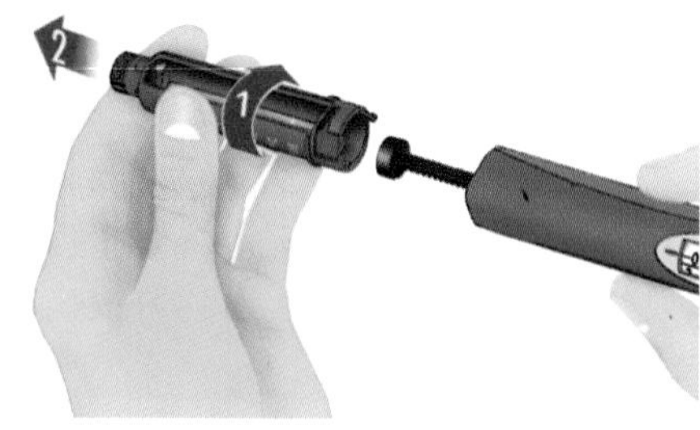

2 Remove the cartridge holder.

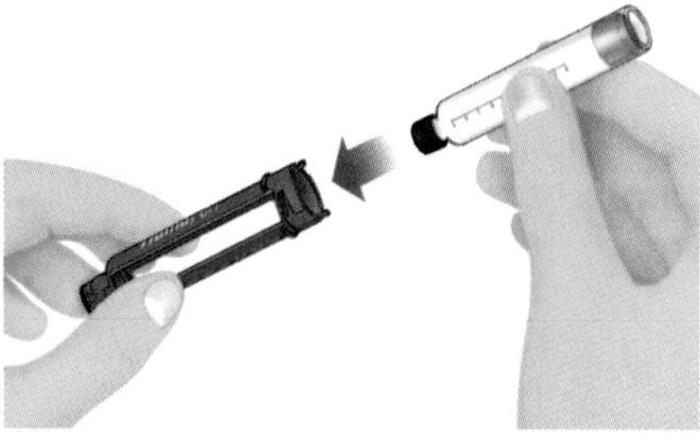

3 Load the cartridge.

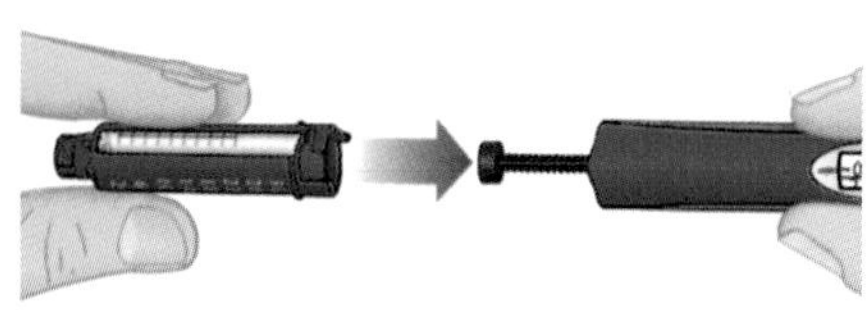

4 Reset the lead screw. The cartridge plunger pushes the lead screw back.

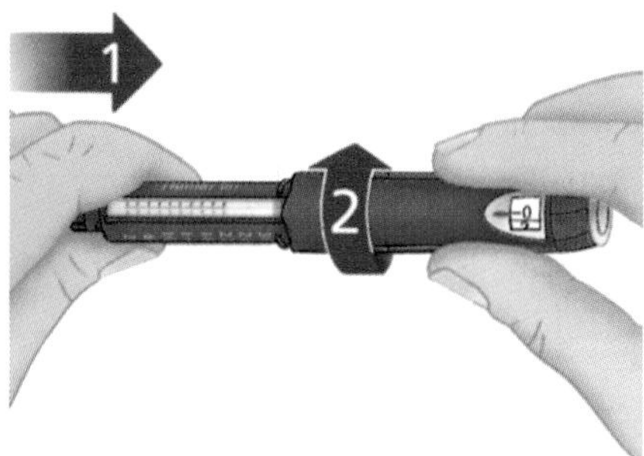

5 Attach the cartridge holder by pushing together and partially turning until it stops.

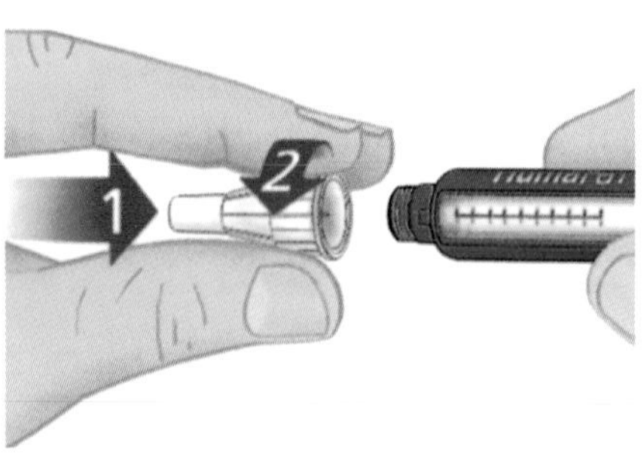

6 Attach the needle.

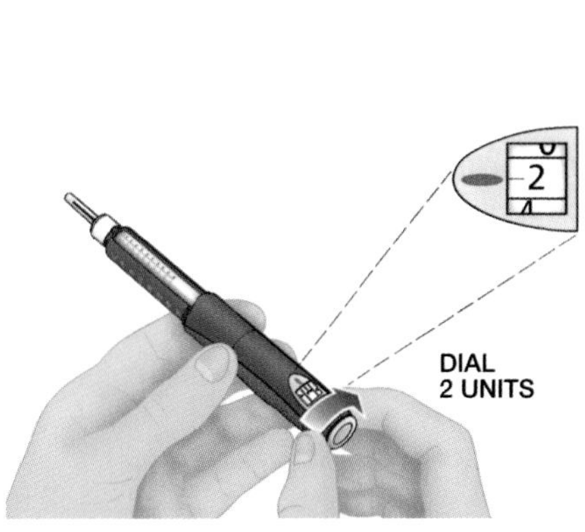

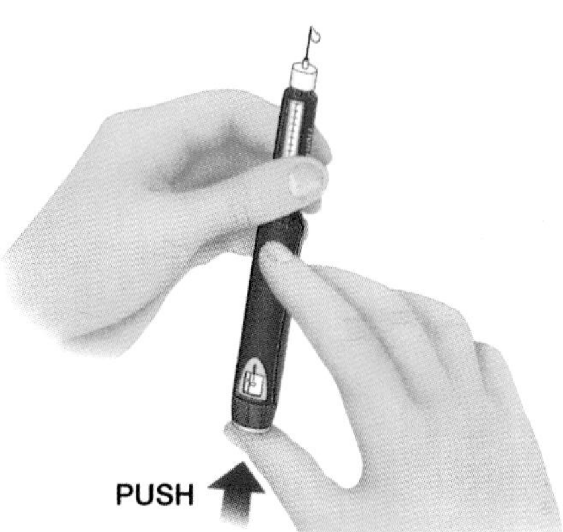

7 Check the insulin flow before each injection to make sure that the pen is ready for use. For cloudy insulin, roll the pen and mix 10 times by turning it up and down. Dial 2 units. Take the top off the needle and push up from the bottom. If the insulin does not come out, repeat the flow check until the insulin is seen.

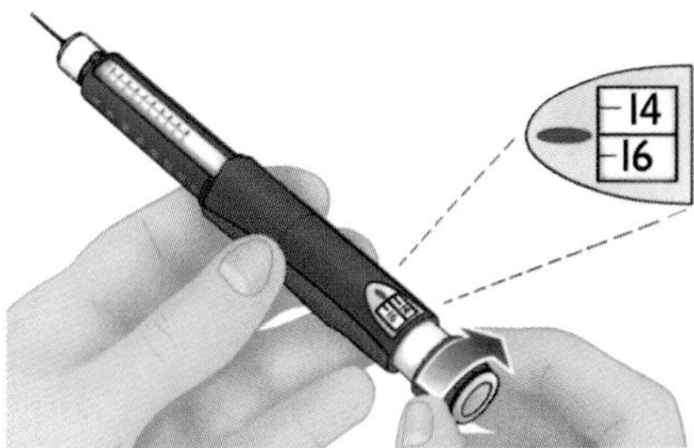

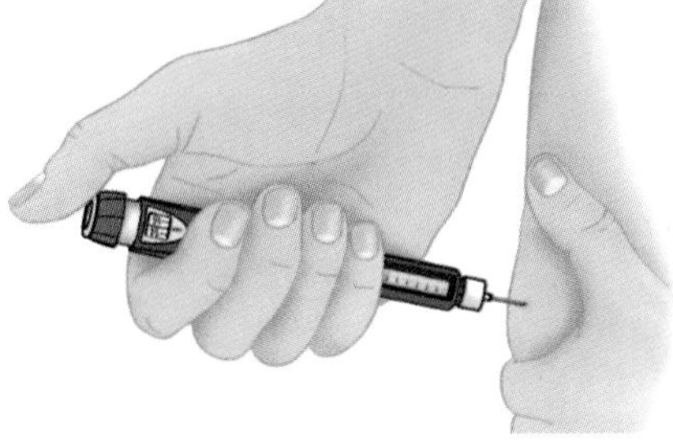

8 Dial **your** dose. You can dial backwards if you dial too many (be careful not to push on the injection button).

9 Inject your dose, pushing until the injection button stops. Count to 5 slowly and then remove the needle from the skin. The pen should read zero after the injection. If not, the number in the window is the amount you did not receive. Change the cartridge, check the insulin flow; dial and inject your remaining dose.

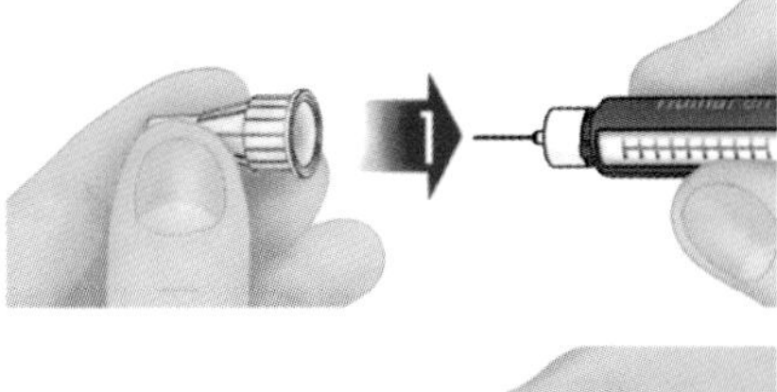

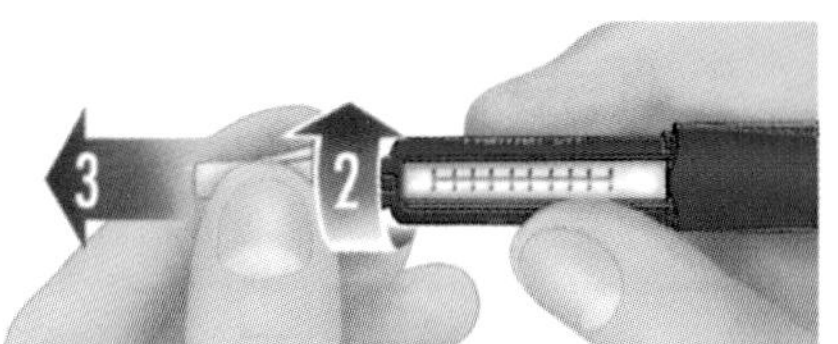

10 Remove and dispose the needle carefully. Replace the cap. Do not store the pen with the needle attached.

1991 and held their HGV licence then may keep their licences provided that they can prove that their control of their diabetes is good and they are not subject to hypos.

I recently read a newspaper article which implied that people with diabetes who are breathalyzed can produce a positive reading even though they have not been drinking alcohol. What does this mean?

Diabetes has no effect on breathalyzer tests for alcohol even if acetone is present on the breath. However, the Lion Alcolmeter widely used by the police does also measure ketones, though this does not interfere with the alcohol measurement. Anyone breathalyzed by the police may also be told that they have ketones and that they should consult their own doctor. These ketones may be caused either by diabetes which is out of control or by a long period of fasting.

Alcohol

My husband likes a pint of beer in the evening. He has now been found to have diabetes and has to stick to a diet. Does this mean he will have to give up drinking beer?

No. He can still drink beer but if he is trying to lose weight he will need to reduce his overall calorie intake and unfortunately all alcohol contains calories. There are about 180 calories in a pint of beer and this is equivalent to a large bread roll. Special 'diabetic' lager contains less carbohydrate but more alcohol so in the end it contains the same number of calories, with the drawback of being more expensive and more potent. He should probably also avoid the 'strong' brews which are often labelled as being low in carbohydrate, as these are higher in alcohol and calories than the ordinary types of beer and lager. Low-alcohol and alcohol-free beers and lagers often contain a lot of sugar, so if he decides to change to these he should look for the ones which are also labelled as being low in sugar.

So overall your husband is probably better off drinking ordinary beer, but if he is on the fat side he will have to restrict the amount he drinks.

My teenage son has had diabetes since the age of seven. He is now beginning to show interest in going out with his friends in the evening. What advice can you give him about alcohol?

Most people with diabetes drink alcohol and it is perfectly safe for them to do so. However, if your son is on insulin he must be aware of certain problems that alcohol can cause – in particular alcohol can make hypos more serious. When someone goes hypo a number of hormones are produced which make the liver release glucose into the blood stream. If that person has drunk some alcohol, even as little as two pints of beer or a double measure of spirits, the liver will not be able to release glucose and hypos will be more sudden and more severe.

In practice most alcoholic drinks also contain some carbohydrate which tends to increase the glucose in the blood. So the overall effect of a particular alcoholic drink depends on the proportions of alcohol to carbohydrate. For instance lemonade shandy (high carbohydrate/low alcohol) will have a different effect on blood glucose from vodka and slimline tonic (low carbohydrate/high alcohol). Your son may notice that 'diabetic' lager is more likely than ordinary beer to cause a hypo because it contains less carbohydrate but more alcohol.

If your son has been drinking in the evening then his blood glucose may drop in the early hours of the morning. To counteract this it would be sensible for him to eat a sandwich or some similar long-acting carbohydrate before going to bed.

The best way for your son to discover how a certain alcoholic drink affects him is to do an experiment. He could stay at home one evening with a supply of his favourite drink and by measuring his blood glucose every hour he would actually discover how different quantities of drink affected him. Someone else could also stay at home to do the blood tests for him. The experiment would provide useful information and could prevent an awkward experience later on. People are sometimes accused of being drunk when really they have become hypo after a modest amount of alcohol.

I am 18 and go out a lot with my friends. I am careful never to drink and drive but when it is not my turn to drive I do drink quite a lot. I am careful not to miss any meals and I am not increasing my insulin as I used to when I first started drinking but I have had quite a few bad hypos recently. Why should this happen?

Briefly, because alcohol blocks the release of glucose from the liver (see the previous question for more information about this). If your blood glucose is dropping because it is a while since you have eaten or because you have been out and active longer than usual, then your body cannot come to the rescue as it normally does. Ideally it would be better if you could try not to have more than three or four units of alcohol in any one session. One unit of alcohol is half a pint of beer or lager or cider OR one glass of wine OR one single pub measure of spirits OR one measure of sherry or aperitif.

If you are going to have more than three or four units in one go, then make sure you have your usual meal before you go out, have a snack while out and, very importantly, have a sandwich or a take-away meal before you go to bed. Following this plan will help prevent your hypos.

I believe it is dangerous to drink alcohol when taking certain tablets. Does this apply to tablets used in diabetes?

In general the answer is no. Some people on chlorpropamide (Diabenese) experience an odd flushing sensation when they drink alcohol but those people can easily be changed on to an equivalent tablet (e.g. glibenclamide) which does not cause this problem.

The other consideration is that alcohol may alter the response to a hypo (this has been discussed in an earlier question in this section) and most tablets used for diabetes can cause hypos. If you are on tablets and are going to drink any alcohol then you must be extra careful not to go hypo.

Drugs

Could the toxic affect of diazepam, Parstelin or Lentizol cause damage to the pancreas and, as a result, cause diabetes?

You mention examples from the three main groups of drugs used to treat depression and anxiety. None of these is known to have any affect on the pancreas or to be related in any way to diabetes.

My son was told that people with diabetes should not use Betnovate cream because it contains steroids. Is this true and why?

Most skin specialists avoid using powerful steroid creams such as Betnovate unless there is a serious skin condition. Very often a weak steroid preparation or some bland ointment is just as effective in clearing up mild patches of eczema and other rashes. Unfortunately too often the very strong steroids are often used first, instead of as a last resort. These strong steroids can be absorbed into the body through the skin and lead to a number of unwanted side effects. This advice applies to all people with skin problems and not just people with diabetes. One of the side effects of steroids is to cause a rise in the blood glucose level. Thus, someone without diabetes may develop it while taking steroids and a person treated with diet may need to go onto tablets or insulin.

If there are good medical reasons for your son to take steroids, in whatever form, he should be prepared to test their blood for signs of poor control. If he is already taking insulin, the dose may need to be increased.

Can you tell me if any vaccinations including BCG are dangerous for people with diabetes?

There is no reason why a child should not have full immunization against the usual diseases. Sometimes the inoculation is followed by a mild flu-like illness which may lead to a slight upset of diabetes control. This is no reason to avoid protecting your child against measles, whooping cough and the rest. In some areas school children are given BCG as a protection against tuberculosis.

Children should also have the normal immunization procedures if they are travelling to exotic places.

I understand that aspirin lowers the blood glucose. Should I avoid taking it?

You may take aspirin or any other painkiller in the same way as someone without diabetes. Large doses of aspirin given to people not taking insulin may have a small effect in lowering blood glucose but in practice this does not cause any problem from hypoglycaemia. It has no effect on the blood glucose of people taking insulin. Aspirin can also cause indigestion and irritation of the stomach lining but this is not a particular risk for people with diabetes.

My wife suffers from bad indigestion. She is afraid to take indigestion tablets in case they upset her diabetes. Can you advise her what to do?

Indigestion tablets and medicines do not upset diabetes.

Is it safe to take water tablets (diuretics) if one has diabetes?

Diuretics are given to people who are retaining too much fluid in the body. This fluid retention may happen in heart failure and cause swelling of the ankles or shortness of breath. Diuretics are usually very effective but, as a side effect, they may cause a slight increase in the blood glucose. This is especially true of the milder diuretics such as Navidrex, which belong to the thiazide group. The increase in glucose is only slight but can sometimes mean that someone controlled on diet alone may need to take tablets. People already on insulin are not affected by diuretics. The thiazide group of tablets is also used in the treatment of raised blood pressure.

Is there any special cough mixture for people with diabetes?

Yes, there are various sugar-free cough mixtures that can be bought from your chemist. However, there are only a few grams of sugar in a dose of ordinary cough mixture and this amount is not going to have any appreciable effect on the level of blood glucose.

I have been on insulin for diabetes for seven years. I was recently found to have raised blood pressure and was given tablets, called beta-blockers, by my doctor. Since then I have had a bad hypo in which I collapsed without the normal warning signs of sweating, shaking, etc. Could the blood pressure tablets have caused this severe hypo?

Beta-blockers are widely used for the treatment of high blood pressure and certain heart conditions. They have an 'anti-adrenaline' effect which sometimes damps down the normal 'adrenaline' response to a hypo (there is a section on ***Hypos*** in Chapter 3). Thus the low blood glucose may prevent someone thinking clearly without the normal sweating and shaking that warns of an impending hypo. Some beta-blockers have been designed to have their effect only in the heart without blocking the general adrenaline reaction of the body. These are theoretically much safer for people taking insulin.

Someone who is already taking beta-blockers and having no unexpected problems from hypos should carry on taking them without worry. Anyone taking beta-blockers for the first time should be warned by their doctor that their reaction to a hypo may be blunted. Where a problem has already occurred, as in your case, then your doctor should either try a different beta-blocker or some other type of treatment for your blood pressure.

Please could you give me a list of tablets or medicines which may interfere with my diabetes?

The important medicines which affect diabetes have already been discussed in this section. There are no medicines which must never be used but the following may increase the blood glucose and upset your control.

- Steroids (e.g. prednisolone, Betnovate ointment). Steroid inhalers (e.g. Becotide) should not have any ill effect.
- Thiazide diuretics (e.g. Navidrex, Neo-Naclex).
- The contraceptive pill.

- Hormone replacement therapy (e.g. Harmogen, Prempac, Trisequens, Progynova).
- Certain bronchodilators (e.g. Ventolin) may have a slight effect on raising the blood glucose.
- Aspirin in large doses may lower blood glucose.
- Beta-blockers (e.g. Inderal, Tenormin) may prevent people on insulin from recognizing a hypo.
- Growth hormone treatment.

Smoking

I am a 16-year-old on insulin. I would like to know whether smoking low tar cigarettes could interfere with my diabetes? Would it cause any restriction in my diet?

Smoking is unhealthy not only because it causes cancer of the lung but because it leads to hardening of the arteries – affecting chiefly the heart, brain and legs. The proper advice to all people, especially teenagers, is not to smoke. Smoking will not directly affect your diabetes except, perhaps, by reducing your appetite.

When my doctor diagnosed diabetes, he told me to stop smoking. Could you tell me if there is a particular health hazard associated with smoking and diabetes? The problem is made worse for me by the fact that I have to lose weight and if I stop smoking I will do just the opposite.

Smoking is a danger, not only to the lungs but because of the risk of increased arterial disease affecting any smoker. Someone who has long-standing diabetes is also at risk of problems with poor blood circulation. It is foolish to double this risk by continuing to smoke. If the discovery that you have diabetes has come as an unpleasant surprise, this is a good time to turn over a new leaf and alter your lifestyle, by eating less and giving up cigarettes. It may be a lot to ask, but many people manage to carry out this 'double'. It will not kill you – on the contrary, you may live longer.

There is a lot of support available now for people who want to give up smoking, and your GP or practice nurse should be able to offer you advice on whom to contact. You may even find that they run an anti-smoking group or clinic. Some people find nicotine gum or patches useful, and we deal with these in a later question in this section.

Since my husband, who has had diabetes for 23 years, has stopped smoking, he has had high blood glucose tests for a while. Why?

Your husband should be congratulated for giving up smoking. Most people who give up smoking do put on weight, on average 4 kg (9 lb). Presumably this is because cigarettes suppress the appetite and people feel the need of another form of oral gratification when they stop smoking. If your husband has put on weight this explains why his diabetes has gone out of control. If so, then he must reduce weight and his diabetes should improve. If he is already thin and his blood glucoses are high then he will have to take tablets or insulin to get things under control.

My doctor has stongly advised me to give up smoking and suggested that I try nicotine patches. I was surprised to find that the information leaflet enclosed with the patches advised people with diabetes not to use the patches. Is this true?

It sounds as though the company are being over-cautious. The main reason for giving up smoking is the effect it has on the blood supply to the heart and legs. Each time someone has a cigarette, the nicotine they inhale narrows the small blood vessels. This narrowing eventually becomes permanent which explains why smoking increases the risk of such problems as heart attacks and gangrene. Nicotine patches have been shown to be one of the most effective ways of helping people to stop smoking.

Nicotine has the same effect on the blood vessels whether from patches or from cigarettes. However, patches are no worse than cigarettes and, if they help you to give up smoking, the overall benefit will be enormous, especially with regard to your circulation. Don't be afraid to try nicotine patches in the recommended dose. The same advice applies to nicotine chewing gum and the newer nicotine inhaler.

Prescription charges and Social Security benefits

I believe that people with diabetes are entitled to free prescriptions. Please could you tell me how to apply?

One of the few definite advantages of having diabetes is exemption from payment on all prescription charges – even for treatment which is not connected to the diabetes itself. This does *not* apply to people who are treated on diet alone and who are *not* exempt from prescription charges.

You must obtain a form called *NHS Prescriptions – How to get them free* from a chemist, hospital pharmacy or a Post Office. Having filled in the form yourself, it must be signed by your family doctor or clinic doctor and sent to the local Family Practitioner Committee. The chemist should be able to give you the address. You will, in due course, receive an exemption certificate. Please remember to carry this certificate wherever you are likely to need a prescription, for example when coming to the clinic or going on holiday in the UK. The certificate currently lasts for five years, and you will need to renew it at the end of that time by filling in the form again.

To what Social Security benefits am I now entitled now that I have diabetes?

There are no special benefits given automatically to people with diabetes. You may claim disability living allowance if you have a child with diabetes who is under the age of 12, and it may be possible to obtain this allowance for a child up to the age of 16 if you can prove that the child needs extra supervision and care. Diabetes UK Careline can provide you with information to help you complete the necessary forms.

The benefits system is currently under review, but it may be possible to obtain benefits if you receive renal dialysis, or are visually handicapped, or are of working age and needing to care for someone over the age of 65.

For more information about benefits, we suggest that you contact either Diabetes UK Careline, or the Disability Alliance (addresses in Appendix 3), or the Benefits Agency. The Benefits Agency is the organization which deals with Social Security benefits on behalf of the Department of Social Security, and you can make enquiries either at their offices or by phone. You will find their addresses and telephone numbers (they have several freephone enquiry lines) in your local phone book under 'Benefits Agency'.

Since developing diabetes I have found that my food bills have risen alarmingly. Are there any special allowances I can claim to offset the very high cost of the food?

Most people with diabetes are not entitled to any special allowance and, indeed, there is no real need for them to eat different food from others. Special diabetic products are not necessary and, if eaten at all, should be treated as luxuries. Now that people are encouraged to eat food that is high rather than low in carbohydrate, they do not have to fall back on expensive protein as a source of calories. There is a question in the section on ***Diet*** in Chapter 2 which offers some suggestions on keeping food costs down.

My mother has had diabetes for 12 years and is subject to crashing hypos for no reason. She needs someone to be with her all the time. Would we be eligible for an attendance allowance as she needs watching 24 hours a day?

If you have to provide a continuous watch over your mother then you would be able to apply for an attendance allowance. Before admitting defeat, however, it would be better to try every means to prevent the hypos. Presumably your mother is having insulin, though you do not mention the dose or type of insulin she takes. At a guess, she is having a large dose of lente insulin every morning. This method of giving insulin sometimes leads to severe hypos at unexpected times of the day or night. Changing to more frequent but smaller doses of insulin might solve the problem. You may have to spend a lot of time and energy getting to grips with your mother's diabetes. It would do more for her self-confidence to abolish the hypos than to get an attendance allowance.

Miscellaneous

Is there any objection to my donating blood? I am on two injections of soluble insulin a day and my general health is fine.

There is no obvious reason why a fit person with diabetes should not be a blood donor. However, the blood transfusion authorities do not accept blood from people on insulin. They suggest that the antibodies to insulin found in all people having injections may, in some mysterious way, harm the recipient of the blood.

My local youth group is holding a sponsored fast over a weekend. I have type 1 diabetes – can I take part?

It would be very difficult and perhaps dangerous for you to go without food and, even more important, drink for 48 hours. The problem is that even in the fasting state you need small amounts of insulin to prevent the blood glucose rising. Having taken insulin, you would then need food to prevent an over-shoot leading to a hypo. Anyone who goes without food for long periods produces ketones which could be another hazard.

Is it true that someone with diabetes should not use an electric blanket?

It is perfectly safe for you to use an electric blanket although most underblankets should only be used to warm up the bed in advance. The manufacturers usually recommend that underblankets should be switched off before you get into bed – tempting though it is to lie there toasting yourself. However, there are now a few underblankets which can be left on all night on a very low heat and these would be safe to use, providing that you follow the manufacturer's instructions. Overblankets can be left on all night, but again you should always check the manufacturer's instructions.

Hot-water bottles are rather more dangerous as their temperature is not controlled. People with a slight degree of nerve damage can fail to realize that a bottle full of very hot water may be burning the skin of their feet. This is a common cause of foot ulcers. It is better to be safe than sorry and avoid the comfort of a hot water bottle. Bedsocks are a possible alternative for cold feet, or you could perhaps try one of the small electric heating pads now on the market. Again you need to be careful how you use these and follow the manufacturer's instructions – not all of them are suitable for use in bed.

My 10-year-old daughter has had diabetes for three months. She has started to lose a lot of hair and now has a bald patch. Is this connected with her diabetes?

Yes, it could be. There are three ways in which diabetes and hair loss may be connected.

- If your child was very ill with ketoacidosis at the time of her diagnosis, this could lead to a heavy loss of hair. If this is the case, her hair will regrow over the next few months.
- Alopecia areata is a skin condition which is slightly more common in people with diabetes. This is the likely diagnosis if your daughter has a well-defined bald patch with the rest of her hair remaining a normal thickness. If the patch is on the top of her head there is every chance that her hair will regrow over the next six months. There is no way of encouraging growth and steroid ointments may even cause permanent skin changes and make matters worse.
- Myxoedema or lack of thyroid hormones may occur with diabetes. If this is the cause of your daughter's hair loss you will notice other symptoms such as mental slowing, weight increase and an inability to keep warm. All these symptoms can be corrected by taking thyroid tablets.

Shortage of body iron may also cause hair loss although this is not connected with diabetes.

I recently enquired about having electrolysis treatment for excess hair. I was told that, as I had diabetes, I would need a letter from my doctor stating that my diabetes did not encourage hair growth. Could I use wax hair removers instead?

There is no objection to you having electrolysis. Diabetes does not cause excessive hair growth. It sounds as though the firm doing the electrolysis is keen to turn away customers.

Many women find wax hair removers useful for the less sensitive parts of the body. Make sure that the wax is not too hot.

Is it safe for people with diabetes to use sunbeds and saunas?

As safe as for those without diabetes. Exposure to ultraviolet radiation is known to increase the risk of skin cancer. Make sure you can recognize a hypo when you are hot and sweaty. Keep some means of treating a hypo with you – not with your clothes in the changing room.

I would dearly love to have my ears pierced but when I asked my doctor about this, he said there was a chance that my ears would swell. Please could you advise me if there is a great risk of this happening?

Anyone who has their ears pierced runs a small risk of infection until the wound heals completely. The risk in a well controlled person is no higher than normal. If your ears do become red, swollen and painful, you may need an antibiotic.

Is there any connection between vertigo and diabetes? I have had diabetes for just over two years controlled on diet alone.

Vertigo, in the strict medical sense, describes that awful feeling when the whole world seems to be spinning round. It is usually due to disease of the inner ear or of the part of the brain which controls balance. This is not connected with diabetes in any way. However, simple dizzy spells are a common problem with many possible causes which may be difficult to diagnose. If dizziness occurs when you move from sitting down to the standing position, it may be the result of a sudden fall in blood pressure. This can sometimes be due to a loss of reflexes from diabetic neuropathy (see Chapter 9 on ***Long-term complications*** for more information about neuropathy). There are no other connections between diabetes and vertigo.

My husband's grandmother is 84 and has diabetes. Although she is fiercely independent, she cannot look after herself properly and will have to go into a home. Can you let me know of any homes which cater especially for people with diabetes?

Because diabetes becomes increasingly common in the elderly, most homes for the elderly are well experienced in looking after diabetes. The staff of the home will probably be happy to do urine tests, ensure that diet is satisfactory and make sure she gets her tablets and, if necessary, insulin injections. If your grandmother-in-law is too fit and independent to accept an old people's home, she may be a suitable candidate for a warden-controlled flat.

My wife, who developed diabetes a few weeks ago, is about to return to work. I feel that she should wear some sort of identity disc or bracelet showing she has diabetes but she is reluctant to wear anything too eye-catching. Have you any suggestions?

It is very important that all people with diabetes, especially those on insulin, should wear some form of identification. Accidents can and do happen and it may be vital that any medical emergency team knows that your wife has diabetes.

Medic-Alert provide stainless steel bracelets or necklets which are functional if not very beautiful. They can also be obtained in silver, gold plate, and 9 carat gold. Medic-Alert's address is in Appendix 3.

SOS/Talisman produce a medallion which can be unscrewed to reveal identification and medical details. These can be bought in most jewellers and come in a wide range of styles and prices, including some in 9 carat gold. They are also obtainable from The Golden Key Co., whose address is also in Appendix 3.

Could you tell me what ointment to use for skin irritation?

The most common cause of skin irritation in people with diabetes is itching around the genital region (*pruritus vulvae*). The most important treatment is to eliminate glucose from the urine by controlling diabetes. However, the itching can be relieved temporarily by cream containing a fungicide (e.g. Nystatin).

I have recently been given a foot spa and was surprised to see a caution on the side of the box that it was not suitable for people with diabetes. Is this true?

If you have neuropathy (nerve damage) you should check with your diabetes team before using the spa. If you don't have neuropathy, make sure that you check the temperature of the water carefully and don't soak your feet for too long!

6

Sex, contraception and HRT

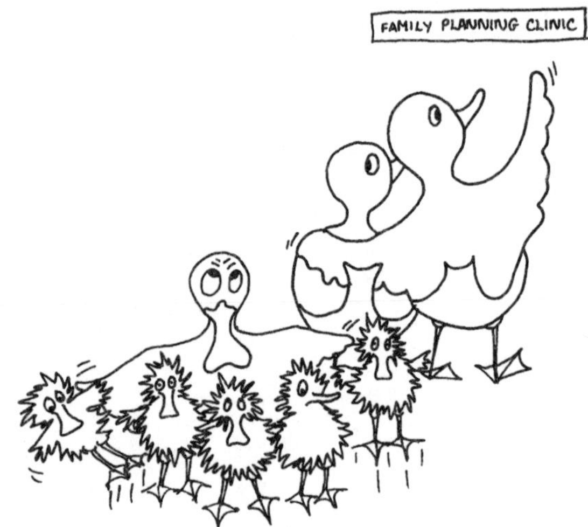

Introduction

Although modern society has removed many of the taboos and inhibitions surrounding sex and contraception, many people still find it a difficult subject on which to ask personal questions. There are very many old wives' tales about diabetes and sex and most of these are rubbish. Basically, people with diabetes are no different from people without diabetes in any aspect of sex, sexuality, fertility, infertility and contraception. There are, however, a few exceptions, such as the undoubted risk of impotence in men who have had diabetes for many years with evidence of extensive neuropathy. Even this has to be considered in relationship to the fact that impotence is a common problem in people without diabetes. There is certainly good evidence that women with diabetes are totally without risk of developing any problem analogous to impotence. Frigidity, on the other hand, is not uncommon in women with and without diabetes, just as impotence is not uncommon in men who do not have diabetes as well as in those who do.

Various contraceptive devices have at times been claimed to be less effective in women with diabetes – the evidence to support this is poor and, in our opinion, people with diabetes should consider themselves entirely normal as far as contraceptive practice is concerned.

There was, in the 1960s and 70s, much emphasis on the potential risk of precipitating diabetes when taking oral contraceptives. It is now felt that the risks were grossly exaggerated in the press.

Impotence

Will diabetes affect my sex life (especially as I am male)?

No. The vast majority of people, both male and female, are able to lead completely full and normal sex lives. This does not mean that problems do not occur but that most of these problems have nothing to do with diabetes. If, for any reason, diabetes control is lost with severe hyperglycaemia (high blood glucose), then this can affect sex life. In a minority of people who have either severe nerve damage or arterial disease, a loss of sexual potency can be directly attributed to diabetes but this is uncommon. The majority of people, both male and female, can look forward to a completely normal sex life.

Is it normal for people with diabetes to suddenly find themselves totally uninterested in sexual intercourse?

No more so than in people without diabetes. The feeling you describe is more common in females than males but no more common in those with diabetes than those without.

Does a low blood glucose affect the ability to achieve or maintain an erection and more importantly, the ability to ejaculate?

No, unless the blood glucose is very low (less than 2 mmol/l), in which case many aspects of nerve function are impaired and this can affect both potency and ejaculation. These return to normal when the blood glucose is back to normal.

Is there some drug or hormone which will help cure impotence?

It is extremely rare that impotence is due to a hormonal abnormality. Most cases of impotence are due to psychological causes and often respond to appropriate advice and occasionally drug treatment. If there is a hormonal defect, treatment with replacement hormones (testosterone) will cure that particular form of impotence. It is essential to get a correct diagnosis in order to ensure appropriate therapy. Recently it has been shown that the injection of a drug called papaverine directly into the penis can sometimes be helpful. It leads to an erection and, in people who have become impotent, the result is often good enough to make this an acceptable and effective form of therapy.

Am I likely to become impotent? I have had diabetes for five years.

There is no doubt that many people with diabetes worry about possible complications which may lie ahead of them at some stage in the future, and many men have loss of potency at the top of their worry list. Our advice is to worry more about keeping your diabetes under control and balanced and less about what future skeletons there might be in the cupboard. By ensuring that you have good control of your diabetes you are doing everything that you possibly can to avoid trouble in the future and the chances are that you will steer clear of difficulties throughout your life.

My wife left me because I was impotent and the doctors say that there is nothing they can do for me – why was I not told about this?

We are surprised that the doctors said that there is nothing they can do for you, because even for those who are completely impotent there are now several treatments that can be tried. There is a question about treatments for impotence later in this section.

It must be very upsetting to think that your marriage broke up on account of your impotence. In our experience, most wives are sympathetic and understanding about impotence (whatever the cause) provided both partners can talk about the matter in an open manner. We have known frank discussions lead to an increase of affection within marriage. Keeping things bottled up leads to the aggression and resentment that emerges from your question.

I have had trouble keeping an erection for the last few months – has this anything to do with my diabetes? I also had a vasectomy a few years ago.

This is difficult to answer without knowing more about you and your medical history. Certainly it is unlikely that the vasectomy had anything to do with your current problem. Failure to maintain an adequate erection may occasionally be an early symptom of diabetic neuropathy. However, and at least as commonly, it is often a symptom of overwork or simply growing older and you would need detailed tests to be sure of the cause.

I suffered a stroke affecting the right side of my body 12 months ago at the age of 40 and now suffer from partial impotence. The onset seemed to coincide not with the stroke but with taking anticoagulants. Are these known to cause impotence? I have heard that blood pressure tablets can cause impotence and I have been taking these for three months and wonder whether this is a factor?

A severe stroke can sometimes be associated with impotence. A stroke is often due to narrowing of the arteries inside the head: the arteries elsewhere may also be narrowed and if those supplying blood to the penis are affected, it could contribute to your impotence. You are also quite right about the question of drugs. Some blood pressure lowering drugs may cause impotence and can interfere with ejaculation. It may be possible to try other drugs which may help the problem. It would be unwise to stop taking the drugs since this would lead to loss of control of your blood pressure. We suggest you ask your doctor to try different tablets for your high blood pressure to see if this helps. Anticoagulant tablets are not known to cause impotence.

My husband, who is middle-aged with type 1 diabetes, has been impotent for the past two years. Please will you explain his condition as I am worried that my teenage son, who also has diabetes, may also discover that he is impotent.

Impotence (or the fear of it) worries many people and is certainly not so rare that we can ignore it. It has been claimed that as many as 20% of males with diabetes (though the figure is probably not as high as this) may at some stage become impotent. Most impotent men are not suffering from diabetes: anxiety, depression, overwork, tiredness, stress, guilt, alcohol excess and grief can contribute to impotence. Any man may find that he is temporarily impotent and there is no reason why men with diabetes should not also experience this. Fear of failure can perpetuate the condition. Overwork or worry is frequently the cause of lack of interest in sex and even of impotence. Excess alcohol can cause prolonged lack of potency.

Some men with diabetes do become impotent, due to problems with the blood supply or the nerve supply to the penis. This usually develops slowly and in the younger person we believe it can be prevented by strict blood glucose control. In the older person (who does not require insulin) the condition does not usually respond well to treatment. In this age group impotence is more commonly due to other factors and not to diabetes. We hope you will be encouraged to discuss the matter further with your own doctor or with the doctor at the diabetes clinic which your husband and son attend.

Is there any treatment for impotence?

Yes. Depending on the cause, there are several effective forms of therapy. Counselling by a therapist trained in this subject can be helpful, particularly in cases where the stresses and conflicts of life are the root cause. Testosterone is effective in those with a hormone deficiency. Vacuum therapy, with a device that looks like a rigid condom, is also a harmless (if expensive) form of therapy which has been useful in many cases. Injections of papaverine or alprostadil into the penis, and penile implants (which require an operation) are more invasive but also effective. The best choice for an individual requires a considerable amount of thought and discussion with your doctor. Many diabetes clinics hold special clinics for treatment of impotence.

After sexual intercourse I recently suffered quite a bad hypo. Is this likely to happen again and if so, what can be done to prevent it?

This form of physical activity can, like any other, lower the blood glucose level and lead to hypoglycaemia. When this happens, and it is not at all uncommon, then the usual remedies need to be taken – more food or sugar beforehand or immediately afterwards. You may find it useful to keep some quick-acting carbohydrate close at hand, perhaps on a bedside table.

The pill, IUD and vasectomy

Are there any extra risks that women with diabetes run in using the contraceptive pill?

Use of the oral contraceptive pill is the same in both women with diabetes and women without diabetes. It is now well known that the pill carries with it small risks of rare conditions such as venous thrombosis and pulmonary embolus, as well as occasionally leading to high blood pressure, although these risks are obviously less than those of pregnancy itself. This is why all women should be examined and questioned before starting the pill because there are a few conditions in which it is best avoided and other methods of contraception used. The same arguments apply equally to women with and without diabetes. Healthy women with diabetes who have been checked the same way as those without diabetes may certainly use the pill and there are no additional risks.

When women with diabetes start using the pill there is sometimes a slight deterioration of control. This is rarely a problem and is usually easily dealt with by a small increase in treatment, which in those taking insulin may mean a small increase in insulin dose. It is a simple matter to monitor the blood or urine level and make appropriate adjustments.

There is nothing to suggest that the pill causes diabetes. It is all right for the relatives of people with diabetes to use the pill but of course they, like others, should attend for regular checks by their general practitioner or family planning clinic.

My doctor prescribed the pill for me but on the packet it states that they are unsuitable for people with diabetes. As my doctor knows that I have diabetes is it safe enough for me?

Yes. There used to be some confusion about whether the pill was suitable for women with diabetes but there is now general agreement that they may use the pill for contraceptive purposes without any increased risks compared with those who do not have diabetes.

Is the progesterone-only pill suitable for women with diabetes?

Yes, although recently these have become less popular for all women.

I have just started the menopause and wondered if I have to wait two years after my last period before doing away with contraception?

Although the periods may become irregular and infrequent at the start of the menopause it is still possible to be fertile and this advice is a precaution against unwanted pregnancy. It applies equally to women with diabetes as with those who do not have diabetes.

I have diabetes and I am marrying a man with diabetes in eight weeks time. Please could you advise me on how to stop becoming pregnant?

We are not quite clear whether you wish to be sterilized and not have children at all or whether you are just seeking contraceptive advice. If it is that you and your fiancé have decided that you do not want to have the anxiety of your children inheriting diabetes and that you have made a clear decision not to have children, then you have the option of your fiancé having a vasectomy or being sterilized yourself.

These are both very fundamental decisions and will require careful thought because they are probably best considered as irreversible procedures. If you are quite certain about this plan, then they are probably the best procedures to consider. We would advise you both to discuss this with your GP and seek referral either to a surgeon for vasectomy for your fiancé or to a gynaecologist for sterilization. Whichever referral you get, you must both attend since no surgeon is going to undertake this procedure unless he is absolutely clear that you have thought about it carefully and have come to a clear, informed decision.

If our interpretation of your question has not been right and you are merely looking for contraceptive advice, then the best source of this is either your GP or the local family planning clinic. All the usual forms of contraceptives are suitable for women with diabetes, so it is just a question of discovering which best suits you and your partner.

Can you please give me any information regarding vasectomy and any side-effects it may have for men with diabetes?

Vasectomy is a relatively minor surgical procedure which involves cutting and tying off the vas deferens, which is the tube that conveys the sperm from the testis to the penis. Vasectomy may be carried out under either local or general anaesthesia usually, but not always, as a day case. You may be advised that it would be simpler to have it under local anaesthesia since in this way your eating should not be affected and the balance of your diabetes not disturbed. The side effects of the operation are primarily discomfort although infections and complications do rarely occur.

There are a few medical reasons for avoiding this operation but they apply equally to men without diabetes as they do to men with diabetes.

I have been warned that IUDs are more unreliable in women with diabetes. Is this really true?

IUDs (intrauterine contraceptive devices) are generally regarded as slightly less reliable contraceptives than the pill and there has been one report suggesting they may be even less reliable when used by women with diabetes. Not all experts agree about this, as there are no other reports confirming this observation. There has also been a report suggesting that women with diabetes may be slightly more susceptible to pelvic infections when using an IUD. On balance, our recommendation is that IUDs should be considered as effective and useful in women with diabetes as in those who do not have diabetes.

Thrush

I keep getting recurrence of vaginal thrush and my doctor says that as I have diabetes there is nothing that I can do about this – is this correct?

Thrush is due to an infection with a yeast that thrives in the presence of a lot of glucose. If your diabetes is badly controlled and you are passing a lot of glucose in your urine then you will be very susceptible to vaginal thrush and, however much ointment and cream you use, it is likely to recur. The best line of treatment is to control your diabetes so well that there is no glucose in your urine and then the thrush will disappear, probably without the need for any antifungal treatments, although these will speed the healing process. As long as you keep your urine free from glucose you should be free from any recurrence of the thrush.

I suffer with thrush. My diabetes has been well controlled for 10 years now. I do regular blood tests and most of them are less than 10 mmol/l and whenever I check a urine test it is always negative. I have been taking the oral contraceptive pill for three years and I understand that both diabetes and the pill can lead to thrush. Can you advise me what to do?

Since your diabetes is well controlled and your urine consistently free from glucose, diabetes can probably be excluded as a cause of the thrush. One has to presume that in your case you are either being reinfected by your partner or that it is a relatively rare side effect of the pill and you would be best advised to seek alternative forms of contraception.

Hormone replacement therapy (HRT)

Can you tell me if hormone replacement therapy for the menopause is suitable for people with diabetes?

Hormone replacement therapy is given to women who are suffering unpleasant symptoms, usually hot flushes, around the time of the menopause. Hormone replacement therapy is not usually given to people with certain conditions such as stroke, thrombosis, high blood pressure, liver disease or gallstones. This form of treatment may have a slight worsening effect on diabetes similar to the contraceptive pill (as we have discussed earlier in this chapter). Some doctors are reluctant to use these hormones in any patient and may use diabetes as an excuse for not prescribing them. However, small doses of female hormones can cause dramatic relief of severe menopausal symptoms and there is no reason why you should not benefit from them provided you have no history of stroke, thrombosis, etc.

I have read in a magazine that the pill can now be taken by women with diabetes. Does this mean that hormone replacement therapy can also be used for women with diabetes?

Hormone replacement therapy (HRT) for the menopause consists of small doses of oestrogens and progesterone which are given to replace the hormones normally produced by the ovaries. Oestrogen levels in the blood at this time begin to decline, and if they decline rapidly can cause unpleasant symptoms. Replacement therapy is thus designed to allow a more gradual decline in circulating hormones. There is now very good evidence that HRT reduces both osteoporosis and vascular disease in post-menopausal women. The benefits of HRT outweigh any risk.

Are the patch forms of HRT suitable for women with diabetes?

Yes.

Are women with diabetes able to take HRT to prevent osteoporosis?

Yes.

During the past five years I have had trouble with my periods being very heavy and on several occasions I have become very anaemic. I have tried hormone replacement therapy (HRT) which interferes with my control of my diabetes and it has been suggested that I have a hysterectomy. I have heard that depression is common after this operation and that HRT is often given to alleviate this feeling but if this treatment makes my control more difficult, how will I cope?

Many people do have the impression that depression is common following hysterectomy. There is no reason for this. Anyone might get a little bit depressed after an operation in the same way that they would after any illness. A few women may feel that if they have their womb removed they have lost some of their femininity and therefore will become depressed. However, the womb is merely a muscle and has no effect at all on feminine characteristics apart from its relationship with menstruation. Unless the ovaries are taken out at the same time there is no reason why you should require HRT. If the ovaries are removed then HRT should not then upset your diabetes as you will be taking it to replace the hormones you were producing yourself before the operation. The best person to discuss this with is your doctor.

Termination of pregnancy

Is diabetes grounds for termination of pregnancy?

Not unless your doctor considers that pregnancy would be detrimental to your health which may occasionally be the case. All the reasons for termination of pregnancy apply equally to people without diabetes as to people with diabetes.

Is it safe for a woman with diabetes to have an abortion?

There is no added hazard for women with diabetes who undergo termination of pregnancy, and care of the diabetes during this operation does not raise any special difficulties.

Infertility

Are people with diabetes more likely to be infertile than those who do not have diabetes?

There is nothing to suggest that men with diabetes are any less fertile than men who do not have diabetes and this is generally true also for women. In the case of women, however, extremely poor diabetes control with consistently high blood glucose readings is associated with reduced fertility. This is probably just as well as there is good evidence to show that the outcome of pregnancy is much worse in women who conceive when their control is poor.

Can people with diabetes expect the same treatment for infertility as people without?

Yes. As mentioned in the previous question, diabetes is rarely the cause of infertility. If control is anything other than excellent, then improving control should be the first goal. If that is not successful than expert opinion on management from a specialist is the next step.

7

Pregnancy

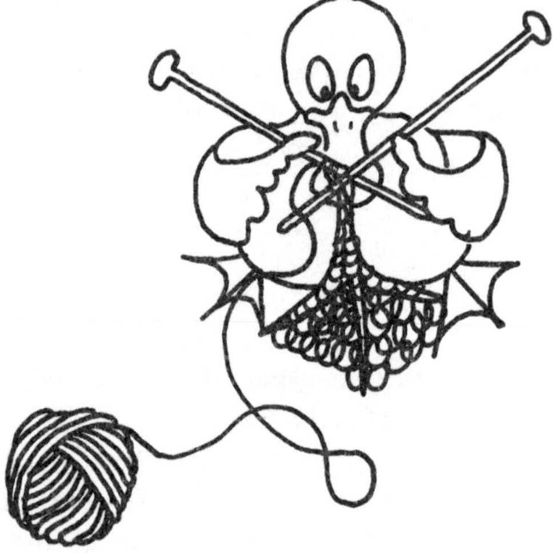

Introduction

Pregnancy was the first aspect of life with diabetes where it was shown without any doubt that poor blood glucose control was associated with many complications for both mother and child, and that these complications were avoidable by strict control. The outcome for women with diabetes who are pregnant and for the babies that they carry is directly related to how successful these mothers are in controlling blood glucose concentration. If control is perfect from the moment of conception to delivery, then the risks of pregnancy to mother and baby are little greater than in women without diabetes.

We now know that poor control at the time the egg is fertilized (conception) can affect the way in which the egg divides and changes into the fetus (in which all organs and limbs are present but very small) in such a way as to cause congenital abnormalities (such as harelip, absence of the bone at the base of the spine, and holes in the heart). The risk of this happening can be reduced to a minimum, and possibly even eliminated, by ensuring perfect control (normal HbA_{1c}) before getting pregnant.

For women who become pregnant when their control is poor, there will be an increased risk of congenital abnormalities in their babies – some of which may be detectable by ultrasound very early in pregnancy, when termination is possible, if a major defect is found. When no defect is detected the outcome of the pregnancy will still be dictated by the mother's degree of control during her 40 weeks of pregnancy and during labour and delivery. Modern antenatal care is usually shared between the diabetes specialist and the obstetrician, often at a joint clinic. So long as control remains perfect (normal HbA_{1c}) and pregnancy progresses normally, there is no need for hospital admission. With the excellent control that is now possible, the baby will develop normally and we believe that the pregnancy can be allowed to go to its natural term (40 weeks). If spontaneous labour begins, the procedure is no different from that for a woman without diabetes, other than the continued need to keep the mother's blood glucose normal to prevent hypoglycaemia in the infant shortly after birth.

Women with diabetes are not immune to obstetric and antenatal complications and these will be treated in the same way as they would be in women without diabetes. If a woman cannot achieve satisfactory control of her diabetes at home, then her admission to hospital becomes essential, but there are very few mothers who cannot achieve and maintain normal blood glucose values as an out-patient, at least while they are pregnant. It is a remarkable example of the importance of motivation in the struggle for good diabetes control. The single-mindedness of a pregnant woman makes her able to cope with almost anything to protect her growing baby from harm. Sadly this motivation is often lost once the pregnancy is over and control slips back to where it was before.

A very comprehensive pregnancy magazine is available from Diabetes UK.

Prepregnancy

The man I am going to marry has diabetes. Will there be any risk in having children?

If you do not have diabetes yourself and there is no diabetes in your family then the risk of your children developing diabetes in childhood or adolescence, if their father has diabetes, is probably about 1 in 20. Provided you are both in good health it is certainly all right to have a family. If you and your fiancé both had type 1 diabetes, then there would be an even greater risk of your children developing diabetes.

There is a rare form of type 2 diabetes in which there is a strong hereditary tendency. This is called maturity onset diabetes of the young, commonly known as MODY. Were you or your fiancé to have this, the risk of your children getting diabetes of this unusual kind would then be rather high. It is often a relatively mild form of diabetes and runs true to type throughout the generations.

The study of inheritance of diabetes is a complicated subject and you would be well advised to discuss this further with your specialist or a professional genetic counsellor.

I am worried that if I become pregnant whilst my husband's diabetes is uncontrolled the child will suffer – am I right?

No. There is no known way in which poor control of your husband's diabetes can affect the development of your child.

I am 25 years old and have type 1 diabetes. My husband and I plan to start a family but first I would like to complete a three year degree course at university. By the time this course finishes I will be 29. Can you tell me if this will be too old to have a baby?

You pose a difficult question as to the ideal age at which someone with diabetes should have a baby. The age of 29 is not too old to start a family but there are certain advantages in starting younger, particularly if you have diabetes and if you plan more than one pregnancy. Starting a family may be hard work whether you have diabetes or not. If you add increasing age to the difficulties, we are sure you will understand why one normally recommends starting earlier rather than later. It is difficult to give exact personal advice to individual people and the right person to talk to is your clinic doctor who knows both you and your diabetes.

I have diabetes treated by tablets which I chose rather than insulin and I want to become pregnant again. As I have had a previous miscarriage I am worried about the chance of this recurring. Both my husband and I smoke a lot. How can I make sure that this pregnancy is successful?

Your control of your diabetes will certainly affect the outcome of your pregnancy – better control leads to more successful pregnancies. As you are planning your pregnancy, you can make sure that you establish good control before conception. Your control is probably best maintained by either diet alone or if this fails, by diet with insulin. We do not advise women to take tablets throughout pregnancy although they do not harm the baby if they are taken inadvertently in the early part of pregnancy. The tablets can cross into the baby's circulation and stimulate insulin secretion from the pancreas causing hypoglycaemia in the baby shortly after birth.

It should also be said here that most women of childbearing age are already being treated with insulin, so that they are not normally faced with your decisions.

You obviously know already that smoking affects the baby and that heavy smoking is associated with more miscarriages and smaller babies. In asking the question we suspect that you already know the answer – take insulin and give up smoking.

There is also more recent evidence to link even modest regular alcohol intake in pregnancy with an unfavourable outcome as far as the baby is concerned, so we suggest that you should stop drinking alcohol until the pregnancy is over.

Why must I ensure that my diabetes control is perfect during pregnancy?

To ensure that you reduce the risks to yourself and your baby to an absolute minimum. If you are able to achieve this degree of control from before the time of conception through to the time of delivery, you can reduce the risks to your baby to those which are virtually indistinguishable from babies born to women without diabetes. On the other hand, if you do not control your diabetes properly and pay no attention to it then the risk to your baby increases dramatically.

Management

When seven months pregnant I developed diabetes. I had 8 units of insulin a day. After my baby was born, the tests were normal so I stopped taking insulin. I would now like another baby. My GP says I could develop permanent diabetes. Another doctor, however, says this is very unlikely – please could you advise me?

You have had what we call gestational diabetes (i.e. diabetes that occurs during pregnancy and then goes away again when you are not pregnant). The chances are that this will recur in all your subsequent pregnancies. You may well find that at some stage it does not get better at the end of the pregnancy and that you then have permanent diabetes. Even if you do not have further pregnancies, you are a 'high risk' (greater than 1 in 2) case for developing diabetes at some stage in the future. Your pancreas produces enough insulin to cope with everyday life but the extra demands of pregnancy are more than it can manage, hence the need for extra insulin. You should pay particular attention to your diet and fitness, and keep your weight at even slightly below your ideal weight for your height. The decision about further pregnancies with the greater risk of developing permanent diabetes is one that you and your partner must make after you understand the facts.

When I had my first baby, I was in hospital for the last two months and I was given a caesarian section after 36 weeks of pregnancy. My baby weighed 3.7 kg (8 lb 4 oz) even though it was four weeks early. During my most recent pregnancy I was allowed to go into labour which occurred at 39 weeks and the baby weighed 3.2 kg (7 lb) and I spent absolutely no time at all in hospital other than going into hospital as I went into labour. Why was there such a big change in treatment?

The last 15 years have seen a dramatic change in our attitudes to the care of pregnancy in women with diabetes. Good blood glucose control is the most important goal and with home blood glucose monitoring this can be achieved in the majority of women without the need for admission to hospital at any stage. It sounds as if your control was worse during your first pregnancy than your second. Early delivery by caesarian section was decided on because the baby had already grown to 3.7 kg by 36 weeks and they were worried that it would become even bigger if left to 38 or 39 weeks. The heavier baby in the first pregnancy was because the high blood glucose you were running resulted in more fat being laid down on the baby to increase its weight. However, during your second pregnancy, when your control was clearly a good deal better, the baby grew at a more normal rate so that it was at the correct weight when you went into labour at the end of pregnancy.

During my last labour I was given a drip and had an insulin pump up all day. Why was this necessary?

Strict blood glucose control during labour is very important to ensure that you do not put your baby at risk from hypoglycaemia in the first few hours of life. If there is any possibility that your labour may end up with an anaesthetic (e.g. for forceps delivery or possible caesarian section) then the simplest way to keep your diabetes well controlled is with glucose being run into your circulation and matched with an appropriate dose of insulin. With the pump this means that – should an emergency arise – you will be immediately ready.

During my pregnancy I found attending the antenatal clinic a nuisance and I did not like to keep my diabetes too well controlled because if I did I had many hypos. Labour and delivery seemed to go quite normally but my baby was rather heavy. He was 4.2 kg (9 lb 4 oz), and had to spend a long time in the Special Care Baby Unit because they said he was hypoglycaemic – how do I avoid all this trouble in my next pregnancy?

If you want to go ahead and have further babies then it is essential that you change your attitude to the antenatal clinic and to controlling your diabetes throughout the pregnancy. The trouble your baby had from hypoglycaemia was a reflection of the fact that it had been exposed to a very high glucose concentration throughout pregnancy and had had to produce a lot of insulin from its own pancreas to cope with this extra load of glucose from you. Immediately after birth it no longer had the glucose coming from you but still had too much insulin of its own, hence the hypoglycaemia.

You can prevent this risk in future pregnancies by ensuring that your control is immaculate. This will require you to attend the antenatal clinic on a regular basis and to do frequent blood glucose monitoring to ensure that your control is excellent. If you can do this you should be able to eliminate any risk of hypoglycaemia in your baby.

Is it all right for me to breast-feed my baby if my blood glucose is too high?

Breast-feeding is generally encouraged these days for all women. There are no special difficulties for women with diabetes and the presence of a slightly raised blood glucose need not worry you too much provided that your control of your diabetes is not too bad. For the best results with breast-feeding, keep up a high fluid intake and keep an eye on your diabetes, making appropriate adjustments to your insulin dose if necessary. If you find this all too much, it is perfectly all right to bottle-feed. Do not breast-feed whilst having a hypo – feed yourself first, so that you and your baby will both be satisfied!

My diabetes was fairly easy to control during my pregnancy, but since the birth of my baby it has been more difficult to control, and I am needing much less insulin. I am breast-feeding – could this have anything to do with it?

Various hormones are produced during pregnancy and these lead to an increase in your insulin requirements and alter your body's metabolism in such a way that obtaining good control is usually easier. After the birth these hormones decrease which means that you need much less insulin, and in many people this dose is even lower than was required *before* pregnancy. When breast-feeding the dose usually drops even more and you should be prepared to lower your dose of insulin should hypos occur.

I am married to a man who takes insulin to control his diabetes. I have just fallen pregnant, so what special things do I need to do during pregnancy to ensure that it goes smoothly and without complications?

You need take no special precautions other than those taken by all pregnant women, as the fact that your husband has diabetes does not put your pregnancy at any particular risk. It is only when the mother has diabetes that strict control and careful monitoring of blood glucose become essential.

I have been told that I must keep my blood glucose levels as low as possible during pregnancy. Please can you tell me what they should be?

Your blood glucose before meals should be 4–6 mmol/l and two hours after meals no higher than 10 mmol/l.

I am frightened of having hypoglycaemic attacks especially as I have been told to keep my blood glucose much lower during pregnancy. What should I do?

All people treated with insulin should be prepared for a hypo whether or not they are pregnant (there is a section on ***Hypos*** in Chapter 3). Carry glucose or dextrose or something like a mini Mars bar on you at all times. Most convenient are Dextro-energy tablets – one of these raises the blood glucose by about 0.5 mmol/l, so you should take two to four for a hypo.

Do hypoglycaemic attacks during pregnancy harm the baby?

No. There is no evidence to suggest that a very low blood glucose in the mother can harm the baby.

Complications

My second son was born with multiple defects and has subsequently died. I have been on insulin for 14 years (since the age of 10). Are women with diabetes more likely to have an abnormal baby?

The secret to a successful pregnancy is perfect blood glucose control starting before conception and continuing throughout pregnancy. There is good scientific evidence to suggest that multiple developmental defects are caused by poor control in the first few weeks of pregnancy and that the risk of this can be avoided by ensuring immaculate control at the time that the baby is conceived. The risks in terms of multiple congenital defects seem to be confined to the very early stages of the pregnancy. This is hardly surprising because this is the stage when the various components of the baby's body are beginning to develop and is the stage where other illnesses such as German measles (rubella) also affect development.

Good control is also needed for the rest of the pregnancy because the gradual development and growth of the baby can be disturbed by poor control. In particular, with poor control, the baby grows rather faster than normal and is large in size, although the development of the organs remains relatively immature in terms of their function. This does not happen with well controlled diabetes. Because the baby is large, the mother has to be delivered early and, because the baby is immature, it is susceptible to a number of added risks immediately after birth.

I had three hypoglycaemic comas when expecting my son nearly 12 years ago and I wondered whether this could have caused brain damage? Although he is bright and is in the A stream at school he doesn't seem to be able to keep his work reasonable and presentable.

We are sure that we can reassure you that your son has not got brain damage. This rarely happens even to women with diabetes themselves and if you have managed to survive the comas without brain damage then there was no risk to your child. Untidy work is certainly not a sign of brain damage!

I have read that the babies of mothers with diabetes tend to be fat and have lung trouble shortly after birth and also be susceptible to hypoglycaemia. Is this true, and if so why does it happen?

We know that if the mother runs a high blood glucose throughout pregnancy, glucose gets across the placenta into the baby's circulation and causes the baby to become fat. This is because the baby's pancreas is still capable of producing insulin even though the mother's cannot. As a result of this the baby grows bigger during pregnancy and delivery has to be carried out earlier to avoid obstruction of labour by the large baby. This used to be carried out most commonly by caesarian section at about 36 weeks of pregnancy. One of the complications of this method of delivery was lung trouble in these babies, known as the Respiratory Distress Syndrome (RDS), caused by the fact that the babies were born before their lungs were properly developed.

If the mother's blood glucose levels are kept strictly within normal limits during pregnancy, babies do not grow faster than they should and pregnancy can be allowed to continue for the normal period of 40 weeks. This avoids the risk of caesarian section in the majority of women and RDS is rarely seen because the babies are fully mature when they are born.

Low blood glucose (hypoglycaemia) during the first few hours after birth is a result of the fact that the baby's pancreas has been producing a lot of insulin during the pregnancy to cover its mother's high blood glucose, which was passed across the placenta to the baby. If the mother's blood glucose is strictly controlled during pregnancy and delivery, hypoglycaemia in the baby is much less of a problem.

Are babies of mothers with diabetes more likely to have jaundice?

Babies born to mothers with diabetes are more likely to be jaundiced. This is partly because they tend to be born early. We do not know the other reasons why the mature babies are jaundiced. The jaundice is usually mild and clears without treatment.

I developed toxaemia during my last pregnancy and had to spend several weeks in hospital even though my control of my diabetes was immaculate. Luckily everything turned out all right and I now have a beautiful healthy son. Was the toxaemia related to me having diabetes? And is it likely to recur in future pregnancies?

Women with diabetes are a little more prone to toxaemia. You are not more likely to get toxaemia in your future pregnancies – indeed the risk is less.

During my last pregnancy I had hydramnios and my obstetrician said that this was because I had diabetes. Is this true? And is there anything that I can do to avoid it happening in future pregnancies?

Hydramnios is an excessive amount of fluid surrounding the fetus and it is, unfortunately, more common in mothers with diabetes. It does appear to be related to how strictly you control your diabetes throughout your pregnancy. Our advice is that in future pregnancies you can reduce the risk to an absolute minimum by aiming to keep your HbA_{1c} and blood glucose levels completely normal from the day of conception.

During the recent delivery of my fourth child (which went quite smoothly) I had an insulin pump into a vein during labour. I had not had this in my previous three pregnancies, despite having diabetes. Why did I need the pump this time?

We now know that it is very important to keep your blood glucose within normal limits during labour to minimize the risk of your baby developing a low blood glucose (hypoglycaemia) in the first few hours after birth. This is most effectively and easily done using an intravenous insulin infusion combined with some glucose given as an intravenous drip. This means that your blood glucose can be kept strictly regulated at the normal level until your baby has been delivered. It also ensures that should any complications arise and something like a caesarian section be required, you are all ready immediately for an anaesthetic and operation.

I have had a previous child that was delivered by caesarian section. Do I have to have a caesarian section with my next pregnancy ?

It all depends on why you had the caesarian section. If it was performed for an obstetric reason which is likely to be present in this pregnancy, then the answer is yes. If it was performed because the first baby was large or just because you have diabetes, the answer could be no.

Some doctors do consider it safer to deliver a woman by caesarian section if she has had a caesarian section before. Others would allow you a 'trial of labour'. In other words, you would start labour and, if everything was satisfactory, you would be able to deliver your baby vaginally in the normal way.

My doctor tells me that I will have to have a caesarian section because my baby is in a bad position and a little large. What sort of anaesthetic is best?

Nowadays approximately 50% of women who have caesarian sections have them under epidural anaesthetic rather than under general anaesthetic. If you have an epidural anaesthetic your legs and abdomen are made completely numb by injecting local anaesthetic solution through a needle into the epidural space in your spine. You remain awake for the birth of your baby and therefore remember this event. In most cases an epidural is preferred because your baby receives none of the anaesthetic and therefore is not sleepy.

If you are interested in having your baby this way, you should discuss it with your obstetrician.

My baby had difficulty in breathing in his first few days in the Special Care Unit. They said this was because my control of my diabetes was poor – why was this?

It sounds as if your baby had what is called Respiratory Distress Syndrome (RDS) which occurs most commonly in premature babies. It occurs in babies of mothers with diabetes where the baby has grown too quickly because of the mother's poor blood glucose control, and so the baby is born before it has become fully mature. It used to be a relatively common cause of death in the babies of mothers with diabetes but now, because of stricter control and supervision, the mother does not have to be delivered early, so the baby is fully mature when it is born. It is now uncommon and indeed can probably be completely prevented if women control their blood glucose throughout pregnancy, thus allowing the pregnancy to proceed for the normal 40 weeks.

8

Diabetes in the young

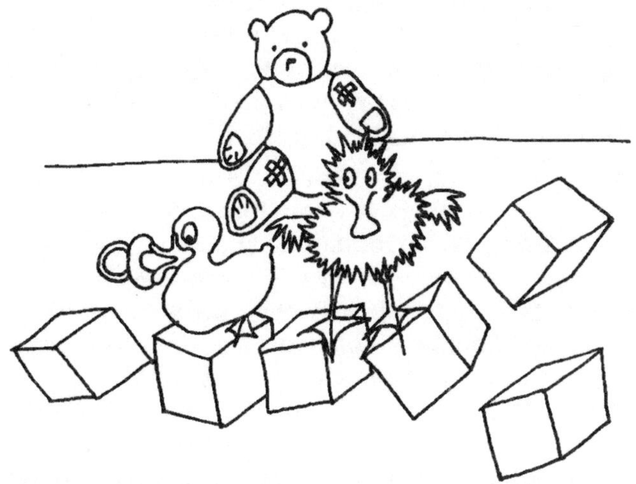

Introduction

This chapter about diabetes in young people divides naturally into three main age groups: babies, children and adolescents. The sections on babies and children consist of questions asked by parents and the answers are naturally directed at them. The section on adolescents is for both young people and their parents.

Apart from the experience of Diabetes UK camps, none of the authors has actually lived with the daily problems of bringing up a child with diabetes. However, we have listened to hundreds of parents who have felt the despair of finding that their child has diabetes and then overcome their fears to allow their child to develop to the full. Mothers and fathers usually end up by being especially proud of children who have diabetes. We hope to pass on some of this experience to those parents who are still at the frightened stage.

The baby with diabetes

My baby developed diabetes when she was four weeks old. She is now six weeks old and looks very healthy but I would like emergency advice in order to protect her life. What food and treatment should I give her?

You must be relieved that your baby is better now that she has started treatment, but worried about the difficulties of bringing up a child with diabetes from infancy. Diabetes is very rare in infants less than 12 months old, so you will not find many doctors with experience of this condition. However, the general principles are the same for all infants with diabetes and there is no reason why she should not grow into a healthy young woman.

Diabetes UK has produced a special youth pack for children less than five years old, which contains many useful documents including a booklet about babies with diabetes. Diabetes UK might also be able to put you in touch with other people who have had the same problem. Practical advice and reassurance from these people would be more use than any theoretical advice.

Like all babies, your daughter will be fed on breast or bottle milk. For the first four months frequent feeds are best – 3-hourly by day and 4-hourly by night. Bottle-fed babies usually need 2½ ounces of milk per pound of body weight each day (168 g per kg). Some babies grow very rapidly and need more milk than this, while others may need solids earlier than four months. This may be a help in babies with diabetes as the solids will slow down the absorption of milk. It is important to wake young babies for a night feed to avoid night-time insulin reactions. If there is any doubt about this, do a blood glucose check while your baby is asleep. If her blood glucose is low an additional 5–10 g carbohydrate (100–200 ml milk) should be given.

My little boy is nearly 12 months old and has been ill for a month, losing weight and always crying. Diabetes has just been diagnosed. Does this mean injections for life?

Yes. We are afraid it does literally mean injections for life. The thought of having to stick needles into a young child quite naturally horrifies parents. But with loving care, explanations and playing games like injecting yourself (without insulin) and a teddy bear (using a different needle) and perhaps some bribery, most children accept injections as part of their normal day. Young children grow up knowing no other way of life and they often accept this treatment better than their parents. Encourage your child to help at injection time by getting the equipment ready or perhaps by pushing in the plunger and pulling out the needle.

How can I collect urine for testing from my 18-month-old son? I have been given lots of different suggestions but none of them seem to work.

It is not easy to get clean samples of urine from babies in nappies. Many infants will produce a specimen by reflex into a small potty when undressed. You can also squeeze a wet nappy directly onto a urine testing stick. But be warned – washing powders or fabric softeners in the nappies alter the urine test result.

Diastix or Diabur-Test 5000 can be used for testing for glucose, whilst Ketostix or Ketur Test are used to test for ketones. Keto-Diastix tests for glucose and ketones. Infants are much more likely than older people to have ketones in the urine. This is because they rapidly switch to burning up fat stores in the fasting state. It is important to check on ketones and try to keep his urine ketone-free, although you should not worry if ketones appear for a short time.

You will also have to do blood tests on your son. Parents expect children to find these painful but blood tests taken from a finger, heel or ear lobe are surprisingly well accepted by young people. They enable you to check accurately what is happening if your son feels unwell or looks ill. Urine tests only provide a guide about the state of his diabetes since his last urine specimen. The blood test confirms what is happening at that very instant. It is the only reliable way of deciding whether your son is hypo or just tired and hungry. Blood glucose measurements are also necessary to check your overall control of his diabetes and to help you decide on the dose of insulin if his blood glucose rises during an illness. Blood samples should be obtained with an automatic finger pricker – the Autolet (Owen Mumford Medical Shop) has a special platform for children, but the Soft Touch and Softclix (Roche), the Glucolet (Bayer Diagnostics), the B-D Lancer (Becton Dickinson) and the Monoject (Mariner Medical) are all suitable. Addresses for all these suppliers are given in Appendix 3.

My 2-year-old daughter has diabetes and makes an awful fuss about food. Meals are turning into a regular struggle. Have you any suggestions?

Food is of great emotional significance to all children. If meals are eaten without complaint, then both mother and child will be satisfied. All children go through phases of food refusal because of a need to show their growing independence, their ability to provoke worry or anger in parents and their attempts to manipulate the situation. Food leads to the well-known breakfast battleground which occurs in all families at some stage. The only way for you to win is to remain in control of the weapon. Usually when young children begin this phase (at 10–18 months), they dislike being told to leave the table and go away. They often return and eat rather than remain alone and hungry.

The battle is even more difficult for parents like you where the child has diabetes – your daughter has some explosive weapons! However, you must stay in control: try distracting her attention away from food by toys, music, talk or your own relaxed approach to eating. You may have to send your daughter away from the table if she is refusing to eat properly. Hypoglycaemia often provokes hunger and, anyway, a couple of mild hypos due to food refusal are a small price to pay for better behaviour next time. Be prepared to modify the type of carbohydrate within reason if she consistently refuses the diet recommended by the hospital. Bread, potatoes, biscuits, fruit juices and even ice-cream can be offered as alternatives.

The child with diabetes

My 5-year-old son has had diabetes since he was 18 months and he is only 3′ 2″ (96 cm) tall. I have been told that he is very short for his age. The doctor says that poorly controlled diabetes could be slowing his growth. Is this true?

The average height for a five year old boy is 3′ 6″ (108 cm), so your son is certainly short for his age. Having high glucose levels for several years could be the cause of this. If you now keep his diabetes under control and make sure that he has plenty to eat, he should grow rapidly and may even catch up with his normal height. However, his short stature may be due to a growth disorder and may need further investigation.

My 6-year-old daughter has had diabetes for four years. She is on 12 units of Monotard insulin, once a day. Her urine test in the morning is always 2% and the teatime test 1/4%. My own doctor is satisfied with her tests and says that negative tests in a child of this age means a risk of hypos. However, the school doctor says her diabetes is out of control and she should have two injections a day. What do you advise?

Until a few years ago most doctors did not try to achieve close control of diabetes in children. It was considered good enough if the child felt well and was not having a lot of hypos. The feeling nowadays is that good control is important to allow normal growth and prevent long-term complications.

In the first place, you should start measuring your daughter's blood glucose. This will tell you how serious her early morning high glucose actually is, and also whether she is running the risk of a hypo at any other time of the day. It is likely that she will need an evening injection to control her morning blood glucose.

It is true that keeping her blood glucose down towards normal may make a hypo more likely. Mild hypos do not cause any harm and even severe reactions do no damage, except to the parent's confidence! You must not worry about a few days or weeks of poor control and you will never achieve perfection in a little girl whose activities and lifestyle are changing daily.

I have been told not to expect my daughter to be as tall as she would have been if she had not had diabetes. Is this true? If so, what can I do to help her reach her maximum height?

Unless your daughter's diabetes control has been very poor, there is no reason why she should not reach her proper height without any special encouragement. We know of one 16-year-old boy who is 6′ 2″ (165.8 cm) tall and has had diabetes for 15 years. Diabetes does not have to stunt your growth.

My son, aged 10, started insulin last year and his dose has gradually dropped until recently he has come off insulin completely and is on diet alone. Will he now be off insulin permanently?

No. There is a 99.9% chance that he will have to go back on insulin. This so-called 'honeymoon period' (there is more about this in the section on ***Insulin*** in Chapter 3) can be very trying as it raises hopes that the diabetes has cleared up. Unfortunately, this never happens in young people.

Are there any special schools for children with diabetes?

There are no special schools for children with diabetes and they would not be a good idea. It is most important that a young person with diabetes grows up in normal surroundings and is not encouraged to regard himself or herself as 'different'. These children should go to normal schools and grow up in a normal family atmosphere.

I think my newly diagnosed son is using his insulin injections as a way of avoiding school. I can't send him to school unless he has his insulin but it sometimes takes ages before I can get him to have his injection. I have two younger children and a husband whom I also have to help to get to school and work. How should I cope with my temperamental son?

You raise several related points. Firstly, you assume that he is using his insulin injections to avoid school. You may be right if he resisted going to school before developing diabetes. In this case you should try the same tactics you used before. Alternatively, his dislike of school could be related to the diabetes, for example an overprotective attitude by sports instructors, frequent hypos or embarrassment about eating snacks between meals. If you suspect such difficulties, a talk to your son and his form teacher might clear the air.

He may in fact be happy about school but actually frightened of his insulin injections so that things get off to a slow start in the morning. Problems with injections have been reduced with the introduction of insulin pens, but some children focus their dislike for diabetes as a whole on the unnatural process of injecting themselves.

Diabetes UK has produced an Information for Schools and Youth Organizations Pack to help parents communicate with the school. It contains information to be given to teachers and those responsible for children with diabetes. You can contact Diabetes UK (the address is in Appendix 3) for a copy of this publication.

When my son starts school, would it be better for him to return home for lunch or let him eat school dinners?

It depends largely on your son's temperament and attitude to school. Some 4-year-olds skip happily off to their first day at school without a backward glance (much to their mother's chagrin), while other perfectly normal children make a fuss and have tummy aches at the start of school. Diabetes will tend to add to these problems. You will have to talk to his teachers and it would be worth asking their advice and making sure that someone will take the responsibility of choosing suitable food for your son – you can't leave that to a 4- or 5-year-old child.

My 10-year-old son has recently been diagnosed with diabetes. What is the best age for him to start doing his own injections?

The fear of injections may loom large in a child's view of his own diabetes. Many children actually make less fuss if they do their own injections and most diabetes specialist nurses would encourage a 10-year-old to do his own injections right from day one. We know a girl who developed diabetes at the age of six and who gave herself her own first injection without any fuss – and has been doing so ever since. Insulin pens take a lot of the horror out of injections.

If you do have an injection problem or if you want your son to have a good summer holiday, encourage him to go on a Diabetes UK holiday – you will find details in *Balance* or contact the care interventions team of Diabetes UK (address in Appendix 3).

When I heard that I was to have a child with diabetes in my class (I am a junior school teacher), I read up all I could about diabetes. Most of my questions were answered but I cannot discover what to do if the child eats too much sugar. Will he go into a coma? If so, what do I do then?

Eating sugar or sweets may make his blood glucose rise in which case he may feel thirsty and generally off-colour. Coma from a high blood glucose takes some time to develop and there is only cause for concern if he becomes very drowsy or starts vomiting. If this does happen, you should contact his parents. A child who is vomiting with poor diabetes control may need to go to hospital.

The most common sort of coma, which may occur over a matter of 10 minutes, is due to a hypo. In this case the blood glucose level is too low and he needs to be given sugar at once. The causes of hypo are delayed meals, missed snacks or extra exercise.

Can I apply for an allowance to look after my son who has frequent hypos and needs a lot of extra care?

Yes, as the parent of a child with unstable diabetes you can apply for a disability living allowance which is a non-means-tested benefit. Many people in your position have successfully applied and feel that it provides some recognition of the burden of being responsible for a child with diabetes, especially if hypos are a major problem. There is more information about Social Security benefits in Chapter 5.

There is an opposing view that diabetes should not be regarded as a disability and that applying for an allowance fosters a feeling that the child is an invalid.

My little boy has diabetes and is always having coughs and colds. These make him very ill and he always becomes very sugary during each illness despite antibiotics from my doctor. Could you please give me some guidelines for coping with his diabetes during these infections?

Yes, of course. The main guidelines are as follows.

Insulin

Never stop the insulin even if your son is vomiting. During feverish illnesses the body often needs more insulin, not less. During an illness it may be useful to use only clear (short-acting) insulin. You may have to give three or four injections a day as this is much more flexible and so you can respond more quickly to changes in the situation. Give one third of the total daily insulin dose in the morning, as clear insulin only.

Food

Stop solid food but give him sugary drinks, e.g. Lucozade 60 ml (10 g) or orange squash with two teaspoons of sugar (10 g). Milk drinks and yogurt are an acceptable alternative for ill children. Aim to give 10–20 g of carbohydrate every hour.

Blood tests

At midday, check his blood glucose and if it is 13 mmol/l or more, give the same dose of clear insulin as in the morning plus an extra 2 units. Repeat this process every four to six hours, increasing the dose of insulin if the blood glucose remains high. Once he is better, cut the insulin back to the original dose.

Ketones

Check his urine for ketones twice daily. If these are +++, either your son needs more food or his diabetes is going badly out of control.

Vomiting

Young children who vomit more than two or three times should always be seen by a doctor or specialist nurse to help supervise the illness. They can become dehydrated in the space of a few hours and if vomiting continues they will need fluid dripped into a vein. Unfortunately this means a hospital admission.

I am headmaster of a school for deaf children and one of my pupils developed diabetes two years ago. Since then his learning ability has deteriorated and I wondered if this had any connection with his diabetes?

No. Diabetes in itself has no effect on learning ability and there are plenty of children with diabetes who excel academically. Poorly controlled diabetes with a very high blood glucose could reduce his powers of concentration. Hypoglycaemic attacks are usually short lasting but he could be missing a few key items while his blood glucose is low and be unable to catch up.

At a psychological level, the double handicap of deafness and diabetes could be affecting his morale and self-confidence. Perhaps he would be helped by meeting other boys of his age who also have diabetes. This often helps children to realize that diabetes is compatible with normal life and activities.

My son was recently awarded a scholarship to a well-known public school but when they found he had diabetes, he was refused admission on medical grounds. They can give no positive reason for this and our consultant has tried very hard to make them change their minds. Why should he be so penalized?

This was a disgraceful decision based on old-fashioned prejudice. It looks as if nothing will make the school change its mind but, if Diabetes UK were told, they might have brought more pressure to bear. The Disability Discrimination Act will also cover access to education. You could also consider seeking legal advice.

Should my son tell his school friends about his diabetes?

It is very important that your son tells his close friends that he has diabetes. He should explain about hypos and tell them that if he does behave in an odd way they should make him take sugar and he should show them where he keeps his supplies. If your son shows his friends how he measures his blood glucose they will almost certainly be interested in diabetes and be keen to help him with it. We know several young people who bring their closest friend to the hospital diabetes clinic with them. As he becomes older and spends more time away from home he will come to depend more on his friends.

My 10-year-old son moves on to a large comprehensive school in a few months time. Up till now he has been in a small junior school where all the staff know about his diabetes. I worry that he will be swamped in the 'big' school where he will come across lots of different teachers who know nothing about his condition. Have you any advice on this problem?

Moving up to a big comprehensive school is always a daunting experience and is bound to cause the parents of a child with diabetes extra worry. The important thing is to go and talk to your son's form teacher, preferably before the first day of term when he or she will have hundreds of new problems to cope with. Assume that the teacher knows nothing about diabetes and try to get across the following points.

- My child needs daily insulin injections.
- He may need to eat at certain unusual times.
- Describe how your son behaves when hypo and emphasize the importance of giving him sugar. If he is hypo do not send him to the school office or to home alone.
- Staggered lunch hours may be a problem as he may need to eat at a fixed time each day.
- If he needs a lunchtime injection, then you need to arrange with his teachers how he should store and have access to his insulin, syringe or insulin pen, and blood testing equipment.
- Please let us know if he is going to be kept in late (e.g. for detention) as parents tend to worry if their children fail to show up.
- Ask the form teacher to make sure all your son's other teachers know these facts.

Diabetes UK supplies a School Pack which should help explain diabetes to his teachers and it is especially important to speak personally to his sports and swimming instructors. If there are problems with the school over such things as sports, outings or school meals, your diabetes clinic may have a diabetes specialist nurse or health visitor who could go to the school and explain things. You will probably have to repeat this exercise at the beginning of every school year.

What arrangements can I make with school about my 9-year-old daughter's special requirements for school dinners?

It is important to go and see the head teacher and preferably the caterer to explain that your daughter must have her dinner on time. Explain that she needs a certain amount of carbohydrate in a form which she will eat and that she should avoid puddings containing sugar. If your diabetes clinic has a diabetes specialist nurse or health visitor, she may be able to go to the school and give advice.

Most parents of children with diabetes get round the whole problem by providing a packed lunch. This means that you have more control over what your daughter eats and you can supply the sort of food she likes and what is good for her. Point out to your daughter that it would be best for her to eat the contents of her own lunch box, and not to swap them with other children!

When she goes on to secondary school she may be faced with a cafeteria system. This should allow her to choose suitable food but she may also choose unsuitable items (e.g. jam doughnuts).

My son has diabetes. Can I allow him to go on school trips?

In general the answer is yes, but for your own peace of mind you would want to be satisfied that one of the staff on the trip would be prepared to take responsibility for your son. Day trips should be no problem as long as someone can be sure that he eats on time and has his second injection if necessary. At junior school level long trips away from home, especially on the continent, could be more difficult and it really depends on you finding a member of staff that you can trust. They will need to keep an eye on your son and to know how to cope sensibly with problems like a bad hypo.

Once in secondary school most children manage to go away on trips with the school, scouts or a youth group. Of course one of the adults in the party should be responsible, but as your son gets older he will be better able to look after himself. Diabetes UK has the following check list for things to take on school trips and holidays.

- Identification necklace or bracelet
- Glucose
- Insulin, syringe or insulin pen, needles
- Testing equipment for blood/urine
- Food to cover journeys with extra for unexpected delays
- Hypostop Gel.

This is part of the Information for Schools and Youth Organizations Pack which is available from Diabetes UK – the address is in Appendix 3.

My 10-year-old child has heard about Diabetes UK camps from the clinic. I am a bit worried about letting him go off on his own for two weeks. Do you not think that I should wait a few years before sending him to a camp?

No, he's not too young to go. Diabetes UK has been organizing holidays for children since the 1930s and it has become an enormous enterprise. About 600 children take part in these holidays each year, so in one sense your son will not be on his own. Young children love going on group holidays, and the fact of being with other children with diabetes gives them a great sense of confidence – for once they are not the odd ones out. The children learn a great deal from each other and from the staff. Your son will have an exciting holiday and you will have a few weeks off from worrying about his diabetes.

Is it safe to let my little girl go on a Diabetes UK camp?

Perfectly safe. The care interventions team of Diabetes UK has had years of experience in running holidays for children. The average camp consists of 30–35 children who are supervised by the following staff:

Warden, responsible for planning;
Senior Medical Officer, who is experienced in diabetes;
Junior Medical Officer;
2–4 Nurses, usually with a special interest in diabetes and/or children;
3 Dietitians;
1–2 Deputy Wardens;
8 Junior Leaders, young adults with diabetes themselves, who give up two weeks to help.

The staff/child ratio is about 1:2 and there is always close supervision on outings and all sports, especially swimming.

Diabetes and the adolescent

My 16-year-old son is only 5′ 2″ (157 cm) and very immature. I have heard that children with diabetes reach puberty a year or two later than anyone else. Will he grow later?

If your son is sexually underdeveloped then he will certainly have a growth spurt when he goes into puberty. However, 5′ 2″ (157 cm) is undersized for a boy of 16. It could be poor diabetes control that has stunted his growth but there are other possible factors, including the physical stature of his father and yourself. If you are both a normal height, there could be some other medical reason for your son's short size. It would be worth consulting your GP or clinic doctor rather than blaming it automatically on his diabetes.

My daughter and I are getting extremely anxious although our GP tells us there is nothing to worry about. She developed diabetes when she was 14, one year after her periods had started. They stopped completely with the diabetes and have never started again, although we have now waited for two years. Is our GP right to be calm and patient, or are we right to be worried?

A major upset to the system such as diabetes may cause periods to stop in a young girl. It is a little unusual for them not to reappear within two years and we would like to be certain that your daughter's diabetes is well controlled and that she is not underweight. Your doctor will be able to answer these two questions. If her control is good and she is of normal weight, then it would be reasonable to wait another year or two before embarking on further investigations. There is a very good chance that her periods will return spontaneously. If they do not return, nothing will be lost by waiting for another two years.

I am nearly 16 and have not started menstruating yet. Is this because I have diabetes? Since I was diagnosed, I have put on a lot of weight.

On average, girls with diabetes do tend to start their periods at an older age. We assume from your question that you are now overweight and this may be another cause for delay in menstruation. Presumably you have begun to notice other signs of puberty such as breast development and the growth of pubic hair. If so, you should make a determined effort to lose weight and control your diabetes carefully. This will involve a reduction in your food intake and probably an adjustment in your dose of insulin. If, after another year, you have still not seen a period then you should discuss the matter with your doctor.

My son has just heard that he will be going to university next year. While we are all delighted and proud of him, I worry because he will be living away from home for the first time. For the seven years of him having diabetes I have accepted most of the anxiety and practical arrangement of his meals and he has done his best to ignore his diabetes. How is he now going to face it alone?

If your son is bright enough to get into university, he should be quite capable of looking after his diabetes. However, you are right to point out that your son's attitude towards his diabetes is also important. All mothers worry when their children leave home for the first time and it is natural for a child with diabetes to cause extra worry. You can be sure, however, that the training you have given him over the years will bear fruit. Most children like to spread their wings when first leaving home and you can expect a period of adjustment to his new responsibilaities. Provided he realizes why you regard good control of his diabetes as important, he will probably become more responsible in good time. It would also be sensible for your son to contact the diabetes clinic in his university town, so that they can give him support if necessary.

How does diabetes affect my prospects for marriage?

We have never heard a young man or woman complain that diabetes has put off potential marriage partners, although we suppose it could be used as an excuse if someone was looking for a convenient way out of a relationship.

If your diabetes has affected your own self-confidence and made you feel a second-class citizen, then you may sell yourself short and lose out in that way.

I have type 1 diabetes and have recently made friends with a super boy but am frightened that he will be put off if I tell him I have diabetes. What should I do?

The standard answer is that you must tell your new boyfriend at the beginning. However, you have obviously found this a problem or you would not be asking the question. There is no need to broadcast the fact that you have diabetes. It would be possible to conceal diabetes completely from a close companion, although sooner or later he will inevitably discover the truth.

Once you get to know him better, your best plan would be to drop a few hints about diabetes without making a song and dance about it, perhaps during a meal together. If the relationship grows, you will want to share each other's problems – including diabetes. We have never known a serious relationship break up because of diabetes.

My 15-year-old son developed diabetes at the age of 12. Initially he was very sensible about his diabetes but recently he has become resentful saying that he is different from everyone else and blaming us for his disease. What do you suggest?

You must first realize that most people of all ages (and their parents) feel resentful at some stage about this condition which causes so much inconvenience in someone's life. Many 12-year-old children conform with their parent's wishes and generally do as they are told. However, by the age of 15 other important pressures are beginning to bear on a developing young person. In the case of a boy, the most important factors in life are (1) his friends and (2) girls. While you as parents are prepared to make allowances and provide special meals etc, most young lads want to join the gang and do not wish to appear 'different'.

At a Firbush camp (which was restricted to hand-picked, well adjusted young adults with diabetes), the organizers were horrified to discover how angry the young people felt about their condition. Of course this anger will often be directed at the parents. We can only give advice in general terms which apply to most adolescent problems.

- Keep lines of communication open.
- Boost his self-esteem by giving praise where praise is due even if your own self-esteem is taking a hammering.
- Allow your son to make his own decisions about diabetes. If you force him to comply, he will simply avoid confrontation by deceiving you.
- Remember that difficult adolescents usually turn into successful adults.

Our 15-year-old daughter has had diabetes for four years and until recently has always been well controlled. Now it is very difficult to get her to take an interest in her diabetes and she has stopped doing blood tests. At the last clinic visit, the doctor said that her HbA_{1c} was very high and he thought she was probably missing some of her injections. I really do not know what to do.

This is a very upsetting situation for all concerned and unfortunately it is not uncommon. Diabetes is difficult because it places great demands and restrictions on people but in the short term they have nothing to show for their efforts. Non-compliance (not following the prescribed treatment) is very common and the reasons for it are very complex. Like most girls of her age, your daughter probably wants to lose weight and she may have discovered that allowing her glucose levels to float up is a very effective way of quickly losing a few pounds in weight. Thus there may be positive gain to your daughter in missing a few insulin injections.

There is no easy solution to this problem especially as many girls in this situation brightly turn up at the clinic and announce that 'everything is fine'. Simply challenging your daughter and threatening her with the long-term complications of diabetes is unlikely to do much good. It is better to try and get her to realize that you understand that living with diabetes is not easy and allowing her to express her own feelings about it. Of course she may be at a stage of feeling that parents are light-years away from her own experience in which case she is more likely to unburden herself to a close friend, especially someone else with diabetes.

9

Long-term complications

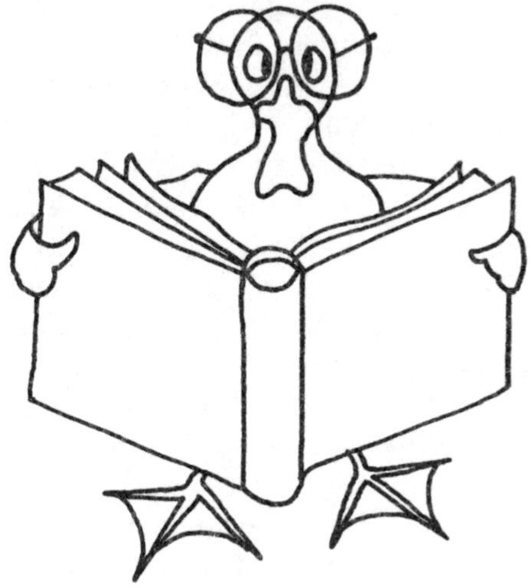

Introduction

Before insulin was discovered, people with diabetes did not survive long enough to develop diabetic complications as we know them today. In the early days after the great discovery, it was commonly believed that insulin cured diabetes. We are now in a better position to realize that although insulin produced nothing short of miraculous recovery in those on the verge of death from diabetic coma and allowed them to return to a full, active and enjoyable life, it is no cure for the condition. However, used properly, insulin results in full health and activity and a long life.

Life expectancy has increased progressively since insulin was first used in 1922 and there are now many hundreds (and probably many thousands) of people who have successfully completed more than 50 years of insulin treatment. Increased longevity has brought with it a number of the so-called 'long-term complications', some of which (such as heart disease and gangrene of the legs) occur not uncommonly in people who do not have diabetes and are generally considered to be inevitable consequences of the ageing process (we all have to die sometime!). Others are not seen in people without diabetes. These conditions are therefore considered the long-term complications specific to diabetes: the three most important are eye damage (*retinopathy*), nerve damage (*neuropathy*) and kidney damage (*nephropathy*).

Diabetic retinopathy can lead to loss of vision and indeed is the commonest cause of blindness registration in people under 65 in the United Kingdom. Fortunately it only leads to visual loss in a small proportion of people. Diabetic neuropathy, by leading to loss of feeling, particularly in the feet, makes affected people very susceptible to infections and occasionally gangrene, with the subsequent need for an amputation. It can also cause impotence. Diabetic nephropathy can cause kidney failure and is now the commonest reason for referral for renal dialysis and transplantation in the United Kingdom and Europe in young people, although again it only occurs in very small numbers.

It is not surprising that people dread the thought of diabetic complications. In the past they worried about them but never enquired about them as they were a taboo subject. This meant that they were only for discussion between doctors and not between doctor and patient.

The world has changed and today people rightly demand to know more about their condition ('whose life is it anyway?') and the majority now find out about the dreaded 'complications' very soon after they are diagnosed. There are so many old wives' tales circulating about diabetic complications and it is perhaps the most important area in diabetic counselling where the facts rather than opinions must be stated.

Although medical science has made impressive progress since the discovery of insulin there is still a long way to go. The scientific evidence from studies of experimental diabetes in animals is very strongly in favour of the specific complications of diabetes being directly related to the degree to which the blood glucose is raised, and their prevention being possible by control of the blood glucose concentration. We believe that the specific diabetic complications in humans are also a direct result of a raised blood glucose level over many years and that they are all preventable by maintenance of normal blood glucose values, HbA_{1c} or fructosamine values. This view has recently been supported by the results of a very large multicentre clinical trial in the USA – the Diabetes Control and Complications Trial (DCCT) which conclusively proved that complications can be avoided by strict blood glucose control. There is more information about the trial in the section on ***Control and monitoring*** in Chapter 4.

Some of the questions in this chapter relating to eyes and feet are not strictly questions about complications, but as they do not easily fit in anywhere else in the book they have been included in this chapter under their specific headings.

General questions

Can someone who is controlled only by diet suffer from diabetic complications?

Complications may occur with any type of diabetes. The cause of diabetic complications is not completely understood although bad control of diabetes is the most important predisposing factor. The duration of diabetes (the length of time for which you have had it, diagnosed or not) is also important – complications are rare in the first few years and occur more commonly after many years.

People treated with diet alone are usually diagnosed in middle or later life. At the time the diagnosis is made, the disease may have been present for a long time, often many years, without the person having any knowledge of it, and therefore without any attempt being made to control it. Thus it is not surprising that complications can occur in some people even when they are treated with diet alone. Good control in these people is clearly just as important as with people who have treatment with tablets or who have type 1 diabetes.

My child has had diabetes for three years and I am trying to find out more about the disease. I recently read a book which said that some people with diabetes may go blind. I don't know if this is true and find it very upsetting. Surely they shouldn't be allowed to write such things in books that young people might read?

You raise a very important matter. Diabetes was almost always fatal within one or two years of diagnosis until the outlook was revolutionized by the discovery of insulin. None the less, it still required a lot of work and experimental development in the manufacture of insulin before someone with diabetes was able to lead an almost normal life, with the aid of one or two insulin injections a day, as they do today.

After several years it became obvious to doctors that some people were developing what we now call 'chronic complications' or 'long-term complications'. It was clear that these took many years to develop. This became the object of a massive research drive, requiring the investment of much effort and entailing many years of work by doctors and other scientists. We now understand how some of these complications occur, and we know how to treat them if they occur. We realize that strict control of diabetes is important in their prevention. For this reason, all doctors and other medical personnel treating people with diabetes spend much of their time and effort trying to help them improve their control and keep their blood glucose as near normal as possible. These complications do not occur in all people by any means, although nowadays, with people living longer than ever before, the complications are becoming more important.

You ask whether facts like these should be made available to people with diabetes. The majority of people like to be correctly informed about their condition, its management and its complications. Modern treatment involves increasing frankness between doctors and patients in discussing all aspects of the condition. A survey among our own patients showed the majority expected to be told the facts about complications.

What are the complications and what should I keep a lookout for to ensure that they are picked up as soon as possible?

The complications specific to diabetes are known as diabetic retinopathy, neuropathy and nephropathy. Retinopathy means damage to the retina at the back of the eye. Neuropathy means damage to the nerves. This can affect nerves supplying any part of the body but is generally referred to as either 'peripheral' when affecting nerves supplying muscles and skin, or as 'autonomic' when affecting nerves supplying organs such as the bladder, the bowel and the heart. Nephropathy is damage affecting the kidney, which in the first instance makes them more leaky, so that albumin appears in the urine. At a later stage it may affect the function of the kidneys and in severe cases lead to kidney failure.

The best way of detecting complications early is to visit your doctor or clinic for regular review. Regular attendance at the diabetes clinic is important so that any complications can be picked up at an early stage and treatment started where appropriate.

Prevention is, however, clearly better than treatment and, if you can control your diabetes properly, you will be less likely to suffer these complications.

Is it possible to avoid complications in later life? If so, how?

Yes. We believe that all people could avoid complications if they were able to control their diabetes perfectly from the day they were diagnosed. There are now many people on record who have gone 50 years or more with type 1 diabetes who are completely free from any signs of complications.

The best advice we can give you on how to avoid complications is to take the control of your blood glucose and diabetes seriously from the outset and to attend regularly for review and supervision by somebody experienced in the management of people with diabetes. Focus on learning how to look after yourself in such a way that you can achieve and maintain a normal HbA_{1c} or fructosamine level (there is a section on these measurements in Chapter 4). If you can do that and keep your HbA_{1c} normal you can look forward to a life free from the risk of diabetic complications.

To what extent are the complications of diabetes genetically determined?

This is a very difficult question. Most specialists believe that there is a hereditary factor which predisposes some people to develop complications and makes others relatively immune from them, but so far scientific evidence to prove this is not very strong.

What is the expected life span of someone with type 1 diabetes and why?

The life span depends to a very great extent on how old the person is when the diagnosis is made. The older the person at the time of diagnosis the closer their expected life span is to that of someone who does not have diabetes.

Looking back to the past we know that, when diabetes was diagnosed in early childhood, then the life span in people with type 1 diabetes was generally reduced, mainly because of premature deaths from heart attacks and kidney failure. We know, however, that the life span has improved with better medical care. We believe that the life expectancy of a child diagnosed with diabetes in the 1990s is longer than ever previously possible and may be nearly as good as an equivalent child who does not have diabetes. We also know that longevity is greatest in people who make regular visits to their clinic and who keep their diabetes under strict control. Those who die prematurely are more likely to be those who do not attend clinic regularly, are not being supervised adequately and do not control themselves well, and who smoke. This is why we have kept emphasizing the importance of good control throughout this book.

My diabetes specialist has said that it does not follow that badly controlled people get all the side effects and ill health in later life; often the reverse is true. Is this really so?

There is an element of truth in this but the word 'often' should be replaced by 'very occasionally'. Well controlled people rarely become ill and develop side effects, whereas people who have unstable and unbalanced diabetes often develop ill health and side effects in later life. This has been confirmed by the results of the Diabetes Control and Complications Trial (DCCT) in the USA –

there is more information about this trial in the section on ***Control and monitoring*** in Chapter 4.

For the last two years my cheeks have become increasingly hollow although my weight is static – is this due to diabetes?

Quite a lot of middle-aged and elderly people become slim up top and pear shaped below, whether or not they have diabetes. However, there is a rare form of diabetes called lipoatrophic diabetes and this could possibly be the explanation for the hollowing of your cheeks. This is not a recognized complication of diabetes but a rare form of the condition. Mention it to your doctor the next time you go to your diabetes clinic.

I have had diabetes for the past 10 years and have recently developed an unsightly skin condition on my shins. I was referred to a skin specialist who told me it was related to my diabetes and would be very difficult to cure. What is it and why does it occur?

Necrobiosis lipoidica diabeticorum (otherwise known as necrobiosis) is a strange non-infective but often unsightly condition that most commonly appears on the shins, although it may occasionally appear elsewhere. It may occur in people years before they develop diabetes or at any time thereafter. Nobody knows much about it and treatment can be very disappointing, but achieving good control of diabetes may help. Local steroid injections and freezing with liquid nitrogen (cryotherapy) have been tried without much success. With time the red raised patches quieten down and usually leave rather transparent scars.

Eyes

I had a tendency towards short-sightedness before being diagnosed as having diabetes. Is this likely to increase my chances of developing eye complications later on?

Short-sightedness makes not the slightest difference to developing diabetic eye complications – it has been said that those with severe short-sightedness may actually be less, rather than more, prone to retinopathy.

Vision may vary with changes in diabetes control. Severe changes in blood glucose levels can alter the shape of the lens in the eye and thus alter its focusing capacity. It is therefore common for those people with high blood glucose levels (i.e. with poor control) to have difficulty with distance vision – a situation which changes completely when their diabetes is controlled and their blood glucose reduced. When this occurs, vision changes again, so that a person experiences difficulty with near vision and therefore with reading. This can be very frightening, at least until it is understood. After two or three weeks, vision always returns to the state it was in before diabetes developed.

I have just been discovered to have diabetes and the glasses that I have had for several years seem no longer suitable, but my doctor tells me not to get them changed until my diabetes has been brought under control – is this right?

Yes. When the glucose concentration in the body rises this affects the focusing ability of the eyes, but it is only a temporary effect, and things go back to normal once the glucose has been brought under control. If you change your glasses now you will be able to see better but as soon as your diabetes is brought under control you will need to change them yet again. It is better to follow your doctor's advice and wait until your diabetes has been controlled for at least a month before going to the optician again.

As someone with diabetes how often should I have my eyes checked?

If your diabetes is well controlled and your vision is normal and you have no signs of complications, then once a year is generally sufficient. It is important that you do have your eyes checked once a year by someone trained in this examination, as after many years diabetes can affect the back of the eye (the retina). The routine eye checks are aimed at picking this up at an early stage before it seriously affects your vision and at a stage where it can be effectively treated.

Who is the best person to check my eyes once a year?

This can be done by either the specialist in your diabetes clinic, the specialist in the hospital's eye clinic, your general practitioner or your local ophthalmic optician if they are sufficiently well trained to do this.

You need to undergo two examinations. The first is to test your visual acuity – which is basically your ability to read the letters on the chart down to the correct line. The second is to have the back of your eyes looked at with an ophthalmoscope: this is the more difficult of the two examinations and can only be done by somebody with special training. These days some clinics offer a service to GPs which enables people to have the backs of the eyes photographed: the photographs are then looked at by an eye specialist, and the results are sent to the GP.

Last time I was having my eyes checked from the chart, the nurse made me look through a small pinhole. Why was this?

The pinhole acts as a universal correcting lens. If your vision was improved when looking through the hole it indicates that you may need spectacles for distance vision.

Why do they put drops in my eyes at the clinic?

These drops enlarge the pupil and make it easier for the doctor, who is examining the back of your eye with an ophthalmoscope. It is sometimes not possible to examine the eye properly without dilating the pupil to get a clearer view. As these drops also paralyse the lens, which allows your sight to focus properly, you should not drive immediately after leaving the clinic. The effect of the drops may last as long as 24 hours. It is worthwhile taking sunglasses with you to the clinic if they are likely to put drops in your eyes, as otherwise the bright sunlight can be very uncomfortable until the drops have worn off.

I have had diabetes for 20 years and seem to be quite well. When the doctor looked in my eyes at my last visit he said he could see some mild diabetic changes and referred me to a clinic called the Retinopathy Clinic. Am I about to go blind?

There is no need for alarm. It would be surprising if after 20 years of diabetes there were not some changes in your eyes. He probably considers it appropriate that you should be seen by an eye specialist and maybe have some special photographs taken of your eyes in order to examine them in more detail and to be of use for future reference.

What is retinopathy?

Retinopathy is a condition affecting the back of the eye (the retina) which may occur in people with long-standing diabetes, particularly those in whom control has not been very good. There is a gradual development of abnormalities of the blood flow to the back of the eye that can lead to deterioration of vision, as a result either of disturbance of the function of the eye itself or of bleeding into the eye from the abnormal blood vessels.

Retinopathy is usually diagnosed by examination of the eye with an ophthalmoscope, and it can usually be picked up a long time before it leads to any disturbance in vision. Treatment at this stage with a laser usually arrests the process and slows or stops further deterioration.

On a recent TV programme it was stated that people with diabetes over 40 years of age were likely to become blind. This has horrified me because my 9-year-old son has diabetes and unfortunately some of his school friends have told him about the programme. What can I say to reassure him?

Some damage to the eyes (retinopathy) occurs quite commonly after more than 20 years of diabetes. Retinopathy is, however, usually slight and does not affect vision. Only a very small proportion of people actually go blind, probably no more than 7% of those who have had diabetes for 30 years or more. Because of the tremendous advances that have occurred in diabetes over the last 20 or 30 years, this proportion will be much less when your son has had diabetes for 30 years. The figure is likely to be smaller in people with well controlled diabetes and larger in those who are always badly controlled.

Can I wear contact lenses and if so would you recommend hard or soft ones?

The fact that you have diabetes should not interfere with your use of contact lenses or influence the sort of lens you are given. Of greater importance in the choice of type would be local factors affecting your eyes and vision, and the correct person to advise you would be an ophthalmologist or qualified optician specializing in prescribing and fitting contact lenses. It would be sensible to let him or her know that you have diabetes and you must follow the advice you are given, particularly to prevent infection – but this applies to everyone, whether or not they have diabetes.

Are flashes of light and specks across one's vision symptoms of serious eye trouble?

Although people with diabetes do get eye trouble, flashing lights and specks are not usually symptoms of this particular problem. You should discuss it with your own doctor who will want to examine your eyes in case there is any problem.

Why does diabetes affect the eyes?

A simple question but difficult to answer. Current research indicates strongly that it is the excess glucose in the blood stream that directly damages the eyes, mainly by affecting the lining of the small blood vessels that carry blood to the retina. The damage to these vessels seems to be directly proportional to how high the blood glucose is and how long it has been increased. This is the reason why we all believe that it can be avoided by bringing the blood glucose down to normal.

What causes cataracts in diabetes?

Cataracts occur in people who do not have diabetes as well as those who do, and as such are not a specific complication of diabetes. There is a very rare form of cataract that can occur in childhood with very badly controlled diabetes, which is known as a 'snowstorm' cataract from its characteristic appearance to the specialist. The normal common variety of cataract which occurs in people with diabetes is exactly the same as that occurring in people without diabetes, although it may occur at a slightly earlier age in people with diabetes. It is really due to the ageing process affecting the substance that makes up the lens of the eye. It begins to develop wrinkles and becomes less clear than it was, until eventually it becomes so opaque that it is not possible to see properly through it.

What are microaneurysms of the eye?

Microaneurysms are little balloon-like dilatations in the very small capillaries of the blood vessels supplying the retina at the back of the eye. They are one of the earliest signs that the high blood glucose has damaged the lining to these capillaries. They do not interfere with vision as such, but give an early warning that retinopathy has begun to develop. There is some evidence to suggest that these can get better with the introduction of perfect control whereas, at later stages of diabetic retinopathy, reversal is not usually possible. Anyone who has microaneurysms must have regular eye checks, so that any serious developments are detected at an early stage.

What is laser treatment?

Laser treatment is a form of treatment with a narrow beam of intense light used to cause very small burns on the back of the eye (retina). It is used in the treatment of many eye conditions including diabetic retinopathy. The laser burns are created in the parts of the retina not used for detailed vision, sparing the important areas required for reading, etc. This form of treatment has been shown to arrest or delay the progress of retinopathy, provided that it is given in adequate amounts at a sufficiently early stage before useful vision is lost. It is sometimes necessary to give small doses of laser treatment intermittently over many years, although occasionally it can all be dealt with over a relatively short period. The eyes need continuous assessment thereafter, as it is possible that further treatment may be needed at any stage.

Can photocoagulation damage the eyes?

The strict answer to this is yes, but uncommonly. Photocoagulation is treatment of retinopathy by light beams, nowadays always lasers. Occasionally the lesion produced by photocoagulation can spread and involve vital parts of the retina so that vision is affected. Normally treatment is confined to the parts of the retina which have no noticeable effect on vision other than perhaps to narrow the field of view slightly. Photocoagulation can also occasionally result in rupturing of a blood vessel and haemorrhage and after a great deal of photocoagulation there is a slight risk of damage to the lens causing a type of cataract.

Is glaucoma related to diabetes?

Yes. Although glaucoma can occur quite commonly in people who do not have diabetes, there is a slightly increased risk in those who do. This is usually confined to those who have advanced diabetic eye problems (*proliferative retinopathy*).

Occasionally the eye drops that are put in your eyes to dilate the pupil to allow a proper view of the retina can precipitate an attack of glaucoma (increased pressure inside the eye). The signs of this would be pain in the affected eye together with blurring of vision coming on some hours after the drops have been put in. Should this occur you should seek urgent medical advice either from your own doctor or from the accident and emergency department of your local hospital, as it is reversible with rapid treatment but can cause serious damage if not treated.

Every time I receive my copy of *Balance*, Diabetes UK's magazine, I have the impression that the print gets smaller. Is this true or is there something wrong with my eyes?

Unfortunately eyesight does tend to deteriorate with age, whether or not someone has diabetes. The first thing to do is to visit your optician and get your eyesight checked to see if it can be improved with glasses, as this may be all that is required. You should mention the fact that you have diabetes to your optician.

For people who are unfortunate and suffer from retinopathy to the degree that reading becomes impossible there are things that can help. *Balance*, for example, is available to members of Diabetes UK as a cassette recording and this service is free of charge although, to satisfy Post Office regulations, you have to have a certificate of blindness before the cassette can be sent to you.

Public libraries can also help – most carry a wide selection of books in large type and most also lend books on cassette. Some larger libraries now have Kurtzweil machines, machines that can translate printed material into speech. So, in effect, they can read to you, although the 'voice' sounds a little mechanical. This can be useful for any material which you feel is confidential, such as letters, where you might not want another person to read them to you. Libraries usually have these machines in rooms of their own, so once you have been shown how to use them you can be quite private.

The Royal National Institute for the Blind also has a talking book service which is excellent. *Diabetes at your fingertips* is available as a talking book from the RNIB.

Feet, chiropody and footwear

I have just developed diabetes and have been warned that I am much more likely to get into trouble with my feet and need to take great care of them – what does this mean?

If you keep your diabetes well controlled, have no loss of sensation and good circulation to your feet, then you are no more at risk than a person without diabetes. In the long term people with diabetes are more likely to develop foot trouble and it pays to get into good habits – inspecting your feet daily, keeping your toenails properly trimmed and avoiding badly fitting shoes right from the outset. When you have diabetes you usually have access to the local NHS chiropodist (nowadays called a podiatrist), who will check your feet and advise you, free of charge, on any questions that you may have.

I have had diabetes for 10 years and as far as I can see it is quite under control and I am told that I am free from complications, but I cannot help worrying about the possibility of developing gangrene in the feet – can you tell me what it is and what causes it?

Gangrene is the death of tissues in any part of the body. It most commonly occurs in the toes and fingers. Gangrene also occurs in people without diabetes, and people with diabetes develop it only if they have a serious lack of blood supply to their feet or reduced sensation. It can also be caused by smoking which is the main cause of clogged-up blood vessels. Generally it occurs only in older people and is related to the progressive hardening of the arteries that is part of the ageing process.

The other form of gangrene that can occur in people with diabetes is caused by the presence of infection. This usually affects the feet of people who have reduced sensation because of diabetic neuropathy (see the ***Introduction*** to this chapter). This can occur even in the presence of a good blood supply. Any infected break in the skin of your feet must be treated promptly and seriously. If you are worried about anything you see on your feet, then you should consult your doctor or chiropodist/podiatrist immediately.

As someone with diabetes do I have to take any special precautions when cutting my toenails?

It is important for everyone to cut their toenails straight across, following the shape of the end of the toe, and not cutting deep into the corners. Your toenails should not be cut too short, and you should not use any sharp instrument to clean down the sides of the nails. All this is to avoid the possibility of ingrowing toenails. If you have problems cutting your toenails consult your NHS chiropodist or podiatrist.

I have a thick callus on the top of one of my toes – can I use a corn plaster on this?

No. Do not use any corn remedies on your feet. They often contain an acid which softens the skin and increases the risk of an infection. Consult a State Registered chiropodist to have it treated – as you have diabetes you should have access to an NHS chiropodist or podiatrist who will treat you free of charge.

My son has picked up athlete's foot. He has diabetes treated with insulin – do I have to take any special precautions about using the powder and cream given to me by my doctor?

No. Athlete's foot is very common and is due to a fungal infection which should respond quickly to the treatment with the appropriate antifungal preparation which can be bought without prescription. Do not forget the usual precautions of making sure he keeps his feet clean, dries them carefully and changes his socks daily.

FEET FACTS

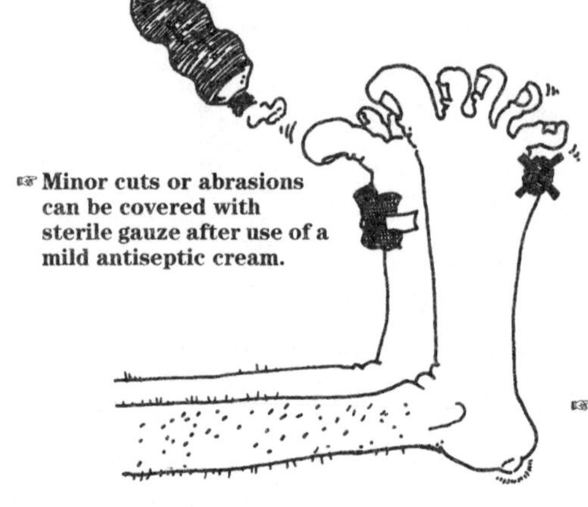

☞ **Minor cuts or abrasions can be covered with sterile gauze after use of a mild antiseptic cream.**

☞ **Avoid using corn plasters – they contain acids which can cause problems.**

☞ **Don't prick blisters, instead treat as for a minor abrasion.**

☞ **Corns, callouses or ingrowing toenails must always be treated by your chiropodist.**

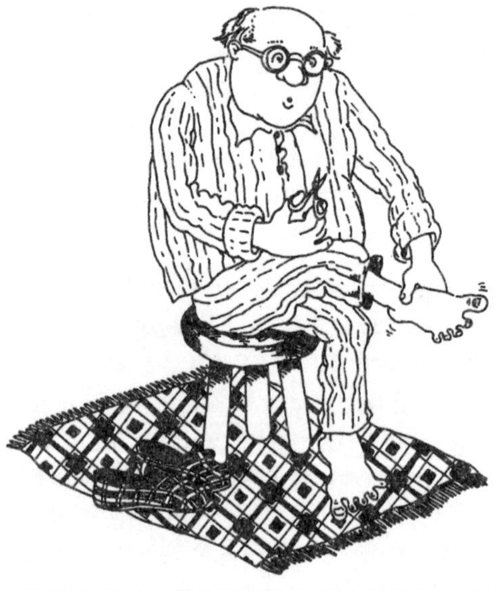

☞ **When your toenails need cutting, always do this after bathing.**

☞ **Cut the nail edge following the shape of the end of the toe.**

☞ **Don't cut the corners of your toenails back into the nail grooves.**

☞ **Avoid using a sharp instrument to clean the free nail edge or the nail grooves.**

Figure 9.1 Foot care information

☞ If your skin is too dry, apply a small amount of emollient cream (e.g. E45).

☞ Check and bathe your feet every day, then pat dry gently, particularly between the toes.

☞ If your skin is moist, dab gently with surgical spirit and then dust lightly with talcum powder.

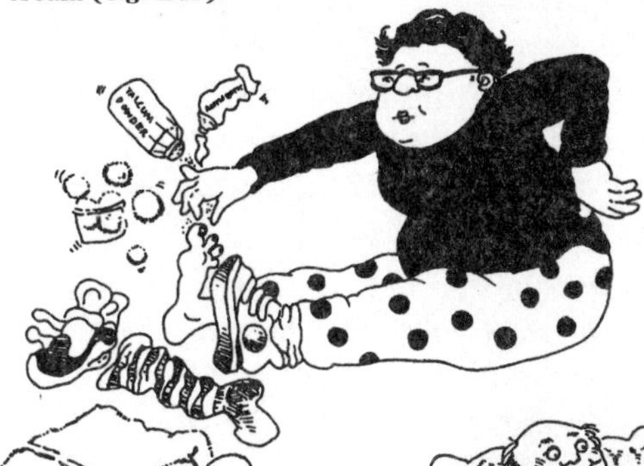

☞ Remove hot water bottles before getting into bed, and switch off your electric blanket.

☞ If thick woollen bed-socks are worn, they must be loose fitting.

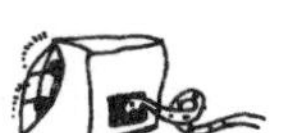

☞ Be careful not to sit too close to heaters or fires.

☞ Choose shoes which provide good support. They must be broad, long and deep enough. Check that you can wriggle all your toes.

☞ Shoes should have a fastening.

☞ Check shoes daily for any small objects, such as hairpins, stones or buttons.

☞ If socks have ridges or seams, wear them inside out. Loose fitting ones are best.

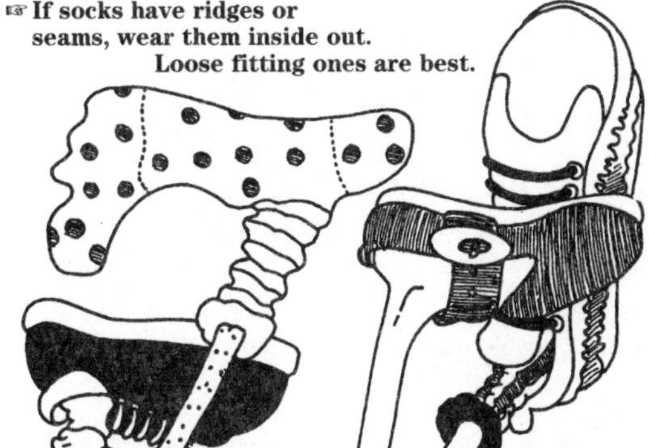

☞ Avoid very hot baths.

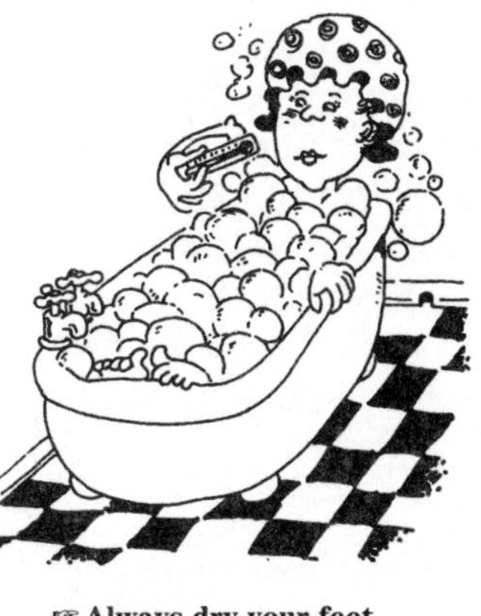

☞ Always dry your feet carefully after bathing.

Does diabetes cause bunions?

No. Bunions are no more common in people who have diabetes than in those who do not.

I have had diabetes for 25 years and I have been warned that the sensation in my feet is not normal. I am troubled with an ingrowing toenail on my big toe which often gets red but does not hurt – what shall I do about it?

You should seek help and advice urgently in case it is infected. If it is, you are at risk of the infection spreading without you being aware of it, because it would hurt less than in someone with normal sensation. This is potentially a serious situation.

I am 67 and have had diabetes for 15 years. As far as I can tell my feet are quite healthy but as my vision is not very good I find it difficult to inspect my feet properly – what can I do about it?

Do you have a friend or relative who could look at your feet regularly and trim your nails? If this is not possible then the sensible thing to do would be to attend a State Registered chiropodist regularly. Ask your GP or diabetes clinic about local arrangements for seeing an NHS chiropodist (nowadays called a podiatrist).

Do I have to pay for chiropody?

Most hospital diabetes departments provide a chiropody service free of charge. Outside the hospital service chiropody under the NHS is limited to pensioners, pregnant women and school children. Although local rules do vary, most districts consider people with diabetes as a priority group and do offer free chiropody. You should check locally before obtaining treatment. If you are seeing a chiropodist or podiatrist privately, make sure that he or she is State Registered (they will have the letters SRCh after their name).

What are the signs that diabetes may be affecting my feet?

There are two major dangers from diabetes that may affect the feet. The first is due to reduced blood supply from arterial thickening. This leads to poor circulation with cold feet, even in warm weather, and cramps in the calf when you are walking (*intermittent claudication*). This is not a specific complication of diabetes and does occur quite commonly in people who do not have diabetes. The major problem here is arterial sclerosis and smoking is a more important cause of this than diabetes. In severe cases this can progress to gangrene.

The second way that diabetes can affect the feet is through damage to the nerves (neuropathy) which reduces the feeling of pain and awareness of extremes of temperature. This can be quite difficult to detect unless the feet are examined by an expert. The danger is that any minor damage to the foot, be it from a cut or abrasion or badly fitting shoe, will not cause the usual painful reaction, so that damage can result from continued injury or infection spreading. It is important that you should know whether the sensation in your feet is normal or reduced. Make sure that you ask your doctor this at your next clinic review.

My daughter has diabetes and often walks barefoot around the house. Should I discourage her from doing this?

It is well known that people with diabetes are prone to problems with their feet which are, for the most part, due to carelessness and can be avoided. The usual reason these problems occur is that, with increasing duration of diabetes, sensation in the feet tends to be reduced. Most people are unaware of this, and so the danger is that damage to the feet maybe the first indication of the problem. By then it could be too late!

The dangers to the feet of children with diabetes, however, are really very slight and there is no reason to discourage your daughter from walking about barefoot at an early age.

What special care should I take of my feet during the winter?

In older people with diabetes, the blood supply to the feet may not be as good as in those who do not have diabetes and this will make their feet more vulnerable to damage by severe cold. As winter is cold and wet we tend to wear warmer thick clothing, and a pair of shoes which, although comfortable in the summer, may be unpleasantly tight when worn with thick woolly socks or stockings. This may damage the feet and also make them more sensitive to the cold. It could numb the sensation completely. All these effects will be made worse if your feet become wet.

Make sure your shoes are comfortable, fit well, and allow room for you to wear an adequately thick pair of socks, preferably made of wool or other absorbent material. Use weather-proof shoes, overshoes or boots if you are going to be out for any length of time in the rain or snow, and dry your feet carefully if they get wet. Do not put your cold – and slightly numb – feet straight onto a hot-water bottle or near a hot fire because you may find that, when the feeling comes back, the heat is excessive, and chilblains may occur. Feet also need protection during the summer as wearing open sandals can cause problems from possible damage by sharp stones, etc.

How can I give continual protection to my feet?

It is extremely difficult. If the sensation in your feet is normal then generally you have very little need to worry but, if there is even slight numbness of your feet, you should check them daily and seek the advice of someone else to look at the areas that you have difficulty in seeing. If your circulation is poor try hard to keep your feet warm and well protected.

I have suffered from foot ulcers for many years and would be grateful if you could suggest a cleaning fluid.

You should not attempt treatment of these yourself and should seek medical advice and expert chiropody. Foot ulcers in people with diabetes are most often associated with reduced sensation in the feet (neuropathy), and you need to have your feet examined by your specialist and find out whether this is the case. If this is so then you need to attend for regular chiropody and to learn all the ways of avoiding trouble once sensation is reduced. It may be necessary to have special shoes made by a shoe fitter (an orthotist) which your hospital consultant can arrange.

Can you give me a simple list of rules for foot care?

The list of foot rules that follows is aimed specifically for those who have abnormalities of either blood supply (*ischaemia*) or nerve damage (*neuropathy*). If you have poor sight then you should get somebody else with good eyesight to help you in your regular inspection and care of your feet. These 'Feet Facts' are shown in a more entertaining form in Figure 9.1!

Foot care rules

Do Wash your feet daily with soap and warm water. Do not use hot water – check the temperature of the water with your elbow.

Do Dry your feet well with a soft towel, especially between your toes.

Do Apply a gentle skin cream, such as E45, if your skin is rough and dry.

Do Change your socks or stockings daily.

Do Wear well-fitting shoes. Make sure they are wider, deeper and longer than your foot with a good fastening that you have to undo to get your foot in and out of the shoe. This will prevent your foot from moving inside the shoe.

Do Run your hand around the inside of your shoes each day before putting them on to check that there is nothing that will rub your feet.

Do Wear new shoes for short periods of time and check your feet afterwards.

Do Cut your toenails straight across following the shape of the end of your toes, not deep into the corners. This is easier after a bath as the toenails soften in the water.

Do Check your feet daily and see your chiropodist/podiatrist or doctor about any problems.

Do See a State Registered chiropodist or podiatrist if in any doubt about foot care.

Do not Put your feet on hot-water bottles or sit too close to a fire or radiator, and avoid extremes of cold and heat.

Do not Use corn paints or plasters or attempt to cut your own corns with knives or razors under any circumstances.

Do not Wear tight garters. Wear a suspender belt or tights instead.

Do not Neglect even slight injuries to your feet.

Do not Walk barefoot.
Do not Let your feet get dry and cracked. Use E45 or hand lotion to keep the skin soft.
Do not Cut your toenails too short or dig down the sides of your nails.
Do not Wear socks with holes in them.
Do not Sit with your legs crossed.
Do not Smoke.

Seek advice immediately if you notice any of the following

- Any colour change in your legs or feet.
- Any discharge from a break or crack in the skin, or from a corn or from beneath a toenail.
- Any swelling, throbbing or signs of inflammation in any part of your foot.

First aid measures

- Minor injuries can be treated at home provided professional help is sought if the injury does not improve quickly.
- Minor cuts and abrasions should be cleaned gently with cotton wool or gauze and warm salt water. A clean dressing should be lightly bandaged in place.
- If blisters occur, do not prick them. If they burst dress as for minor cuts.
- Never use strong medicaments such as iodine.
- Never place adhesive strapping directly over a wound: always apply a dressing first.

Kidneys

Why does diabetes sometimes affect the kidneys and if it does how is it revealed?

There are several ways in which diabetes may affect the kidneys, and they will show up in the routine urine and blood tests that you have at your diabetes clinic.

A lot of glucose in the urine puts you at risk of infection that can spread from the bladder up to the kidneys (*cystitis* and *pyelonephritis*). Occasionally chronic kidney infections may produce very little in the way of symptoms and only be revealed by routine tests.

In people with long-standing and poorly controlled diabetes, high blood glucose can affect the small blood vessels supplying the kidney in the same way as it may affect the small blood vessels supplying the retina of the eye. This does not produce any symptoms but will be picked up on a routine urine test carried out at the diabetes clinic. Many clinics now use a special test for detecting *microalbuminuria*, which as the name implies is a microscopic amount of albumin (protein) in the urine. This is a useful test as it can pick up the very early signs of kidney damage.

With more severe kidney disease, massive amounts of albumin may be lost in the urine, which may make the urine froth and lead to accumulation of fluid in the body and the development of swelling around the ankles (*oedema*). Kidney failure may eventually develop in people who have had long-standing kidney problems. This is usually picked up by blood tests and urine tests many years before the symptoms develop.

Are people with diabetes with kidney failure suitable for dialysis and transplantation?

Yes. The majority of people who are unfortunate enough to end up with kidney failure are suitable for both forms of treatment.

Dialysis (or chronic renal replacement therapy) is of two major types. The older type is haemodialysis where the blood is washed in a special machine twice a week; the more recent is a type of dialysis known as CAPD (chronic ambulatory peritoneal dialysis) where fluid is washed in and out of the abdomen on a daily basis. People with diabetes seem to be rather good at this, and it is in many ways simpler and cheaper than haemodialysis.

Eventual transplantation is the aim of most dialysis programmes but the supply of suitable kidneys is a limiting factor here. The source of kidneys is from either people dying accidentally, who have donated their kidneys, or live related donors, who have agreed to give one of their two normal kidneys, usually to a relative suffering from kidney failure. A normal person can manage perfectly well with one kidney without any shortening of life providing that the kidney does not get damaged. The donor will, of course, have to have an operation and will be slightly more vulnerable as a result because they will have only one kidney to rely on instead of two.

I was found to have protein (albumin) in my urine when I last attended the diabetes clinic – what does this mean?

If it was only a trace of protein, it may mean nothing, but you should get your urine checked again to make sure it remains clear. If it is a consistent finding, it may indicate that you have an infection in the bladder or kidney (*cystitis* or *pyelonephritis*) or it could indicate that you have developed a degree of diabetic kidney damage (*nephropathy*). There are innumerable other causes of protein (albumin) in the urine and it is not necessarily related to the fact that you have diabetes. If it is a consistent finding, it will usually need to be investigated, and you should ask your doctor to keep you informed of the results of the investigation.

At my last clinic visit I was told that I had microalbuminuria. What is this?

The very earliest stages of diabetic kidney disease are associated with a leak of very small amounts of the protein albumin into the urine. If it is a consistent finding, it indicates that your kidneys have been damaged by your diabetes. If this is the case, then attention to control of your blood glucose and treatment of any tendency that you may have towards raised blood pressure is of great importance, as this can stabilize or even reverse the condition.

Nerves

I have been on insulin for three years. Eighteen months ago I started to get pains in both legs and could barely walk. Despite treatment I am still suffering. Can you tell me what can be done to ease this pain?

There are many causes of leg pains, and only one is due specifically to diabetes. This is a particularly vicious form of *neuritis* – in other words, a form of nerve damage which causes singularly unpleasant pain, chiefly in the feet or thighs, or sometimes both. The pain sensation is either one of pins and needles, or of constant burning, and is often worse at night causing lack of sleep. Contact from clothes or bedclothes is often acutely uncomfortable.

Fortunately this form of neuritis is rather uncommon and always disappears, although it may take many months before doing so. Very good control of your diabetes is important as it will help to alleviate the symptoms and speed their recovery. Relief is otherwise obtained by good painkillers, as recommended by your doctor, and sometimes assisted by sleeping tablets. Always remember that eventually recovery occurs, as otherwise you will find that it is easy to get despondent. Also remember that the diagnosis must be made by a doctor who will consider all the various causes of leg pains before coming to a diagnosis of diabetic neuritis.

I have had diabetes for many years but my general health is good and I am very stable. During the last year, however, I have developed an extreme soreness on the soles of my feet whenever pressure has been applied, e.g. when digging with a spade, standing on ladders, walking on hard ground or stones, even when applying the accelerator in the car. If I thump an object with the palm of my hand I suffer the same soreness. The pain is extreme and sometimes lasts for a day or so. Could you tell me if you have heard of this condition in other people and what is the reason for it?

These symptoms may be due to diabetic neuropathy, a condition which occasionally occurs in long-standing diabetes, from damage to the nerves. It affects the feet more often than other parts of the body and often produces painful tingling or burning sensations in the feet, although numbness is perhaps more common. Strict control of your diabetes is important for the prevention and treatment of this complication and it can be made worse by moderate or high alcohol consumption.

I have diabetes controlled on diet alone. I suffer from neuritis in my face. My GP says there is no apparent reason for this but I wondered if it had anything to do with my diabetes.

Not necessarily, as there are a number of types of neuritis affecting the face which have absolutely nothing to do with diabetes. Examples include both shingles (herpes zoster) and Bell's palsy although, of course, both can occur in diabetes.

There are forms of diabetic neuritis that do affect the face: one form occasionally affects the muscles of the eye leading to double vision while another form can cause numbness and tingling. There is also a very rare complication known as 'gustatory sweating' where sweating breaks out across the head and scalp at the start of a meal.

I have recently been told that the tingling sensation in my fingers is due to carpal tunnel syndrome and not neuropathy as was first thought. Can you please explain the difference?

In carpal tunnel syndrome (which commonly occurs in people who do not have diabetes), the nerves supplying the skin over the fingers, the palm of the hand and some of the muscles in the hand get compressed at the wrist. Occasionally injections of hydrocortisone or related steroids into the wrist will relieve it, or it may require a small operation at the wrist to relieve the tension on the nerve. This usually brings about a dramatic relief of any pain associated with it and a recovery of sensation and muscle strength with time.

Diabetic neuropathy more commonly affects the feet than the hands and is usually a painless loss of sensation starting with the tips of the toes or fingers and moving up the legs or arms. It is only very occasionally painful. It is due to some form of generalized damage to the nerves, not to compression of any one nerve, and is much more difficult to treat.

I have had diabetes for 27 years and have developed a complaint called bowel neuropathy. Please can you explain what this is and what the treatment is?

Bowel neuropathy is one of the features of autonomic neuropathy, which may occur in some people with long-standing diabetes, where there is loss of function of the nerves supplying various organs in the body. In your case, the nerves that regulate the activity of your bowels have been affected. The symptoms include indigestion, occasionally vomiting, and episodes of alternating constipation and diarrhoea. Occasionally the episodes of diarrhoea are preceded by rumblings and gurglings in the stomach and not uncommonly this responds quite well to a short course of antibiotics. Otherwise eating a high-fibre diet is encouraged to prevent constipation. Irritable bowel syndrome can cause symptoms not unlike this – it has nothing to do with diabetes although it not uncommonly occurs in people with diabetes. If there is ever passage of blood or mucus within your stools, then you should seek medical advice without delay.

The calf muscle in one leg seems to be shrinking. There is no ache and no pain. Is this anything to do with diabetes? I have been taking insulin for 30 years.

You do not mention whether you have noticed any weakness in this leg. Occasionally diabetic neuropathy can affect the nerves which supply the muscles in such a way that the muscle becomes weak and shrinks in size without any accompanying pain or discomfort. It sounds as if this may be your problem.

Please explain the condition called diabetic amyotrophy.

Diabetic amyotrophy is a rare condition causing pain and weakness of the legs and is due to damage to certain nerves. It usually occurs when diabetes control is very poor, but occasionally affects people with only slight elevation of the blood glucose. Strict control of diabetes leads to its improvement but it may take up to two years or so for it to settle. The nerves affected are those usually supplying the thigh muscles which often become wasted and get weaker.

Heart and blood vessel disease

I have read that poor circulation in the feet is a problem for people with diabetes. Is there any way I can improve my circulation?

Narrowing ('hardening') of the arteries is a normal part of growing older – and the arteries to the feet can be affected by this process, leading to poor circulation in the feet and legs. This occurs in people with diabetes as well as those without, but it is a little more common in those who do have diabetes. The causes of arterial disease are not very well understood, but we do know that smoking and poor diabetes control makes it worse. So if you have diabetes and smoke, the risk of bad circulation really does increase. Stop smoking, control your blood glucose, and keep active – these are the only known recipes for helping the circulation.

Could you tell me if diabetes is likely to affect the heart of an elderly person? Is such a person likely to develop other ailments such as high blood pressure at this stage?

Heart disease is twice as common in people with diabetes and it tends to go hand in hand with high blood pressure, excess body weight and raised cholesterol. There is increasing realization that this grouping of risk factors is an important cause of premature death in diabetes. This highlights the importance of controlling blood pressure and cholesterol in people with diabetes.

My husband died recently from a heart attack. He had had diabetes for 12 years and was controlled on tablets, and at about the same time that he developed diabetes he started having angina attacks. I wondered whether these were related and whether poor control had anything to do with his fatal heart attack?

There is certainly a connection between heart disease and diabetes. At present there is no proven way of reducing the risk and it is not established that tight control of diabetes reduces the risk of heart attacks. However, it has been shown that control of high blood pressure and cholesterol are effective in preventing heart disease.

Is a couple of years of not very good control in a healthy young person with diabetes likely to have much effect upon the arteries?

No. It is unlikely to have much of an effect although any period of poor control is not going to do any good either. Our arteries get more rigid and more clogged up as we get older and this process is aggravated by periods of poor diabetes control and smoking.

My left leg has been amputated due to diabetic gangrene and I get a lot of pain in my right foot and calf. Could too much insulin be the cause of this pain?

No. It sounds very much as if the blood supply to your legs is insufficient and that the pain that you are getting in the foot and calf is a reflection of this poor blood supply, which was the reason why you developed gangrene in your left leg.

My husband had a heart attack last year. Nine months later he had part of his leg amputated. We have been told that he could have further problems but have been given no advice. Please give us some information on what we should do to try and avoid this.

It sounds as though your husband has generalized arterial disease (*arteriosclerosis*) affecting his blood vessels to the heart and to the leg. There are a number of things which you and he can do which may be of help in preventing further trouble. Firstly, if he smokes, he should stop smoking; secondly, he should keep his diabetes as well controlled as possible; thirdly, he should keep his remaining foot and leg warm and make sure that he has expert foot care, either by a chiropodist or by you, under the supervision of a chiropodist or district nurse. If you see any signs of damage to his foot or any discolouration then seek medical advice immediately.

Blood pressure

Are people with diabetes more prone to high blood pressure and strokes?

No, not unless they develop diabetic kidney trouble, when the blood pressure can rise as a complication of kidney problems. Strokes are definitely more common in people with high blood pressure.

I have been told that my blood pressure is raised as a result of diabetic kidney problems and, because of this, that it is very important that I take tablets to lower it – why is this?

There is good evidence to show that lowering the blood pressure to normal in people such as yourself protects the kidneys from further damage and helps delay any further kidney problems.

The mind

My 68-year-old mother has had diabetes for 44 years. In the past few years her mental state has deteriorated considerably and she is now difficult to manage. Is this common for someone who has been on insulin for so long?

Memory loss (most commonly Alzheimer's disease) is mainly a problem of the elderly. People are also more likely to develop diabetes as they get older, so it is likely that both these problems may sometimes affect the same person. There is some disturbing evidence that memory loss may be more common in old people with diabetes than those without. However, the extra risk in diabetes is only small, and we do not know the importance of other factors such as smoking and high blood pressure. So it is possible, but not certain, that your mother's memory problem is related to diabetes.

What illnesses or complications could occur in a man with diabetes who had a brain haemorrhage 18 months ago?

Brain haemorrhages and strokes are no more common in people with diabetes than in those without, unless there is also a history of high blood pressure. The management of somebody who has diabetes and a stroke is really no different than from anyone else with a stroke. The complications that a doctor would be on the lookout for are primarily chest infections and pneumonia, which need to be treated early, and secondarily injuries from accidents if the stroke sufferer had difficulty in getting about.

Are people with diabetes more prone to depression, suicide and other psychiatric illnesses?

There is some evidence to suggest that people with diabetes may be prone to depression, and the suicide rate is higher than in the general population. Recent studies have found that the tendency to depression can be relieved in many people by more involvement in their own management of their diabetes.

I have read that hypos can cause brain damage – is this true?

The strict answer is yes, but only very occasionally. It is only with hypos associated with long periods of unconsciousness that brain damage develops, and then it is extremely unusual. There is no evidence to suggest that the repeated hypos, to which most people who are insulin-treated are exposed, do any permanent damage to the brain at all.

10

Research and the future

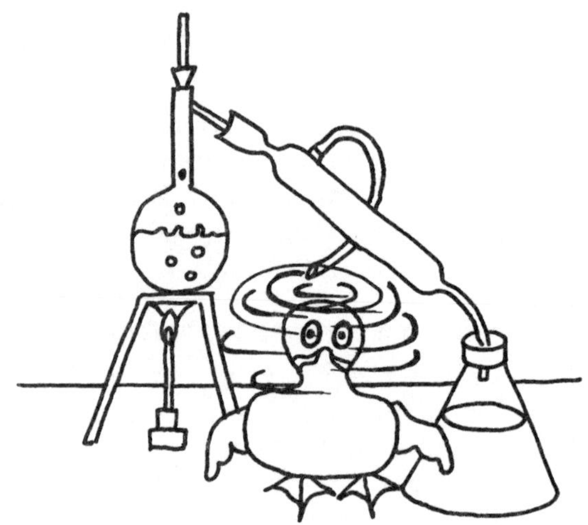

Introduction

New developments and improvements in existing treatments can only occur through research; therefore research is vital to every person with diabetes. In the United Kingdom Diabetes UK spends large sums each year (£4.5 million in 1996) on research into diabetes; similar large amounts of money are contributed by the Medical Research Council, the Wellcome Trust and other grant-giving bodies. The more money that is raised for research into diabetes, the greater the benefits to the population with diabetes. At the time of writing, it costs about £30,000 to support a relatively junior research worker for just one year. The discovery of insulin was made by a doctor and a medical student (Banting and Best) doing research together for just one summer (1921). There have been many important but less dramatic discoveries since then, each in some way contributing to our understanding of diabetes and many improving the available treatment.

Look at Diabetes UK's Website (http://www.diabetes.org.uk) for details of BDA research activities.

Searching for causes and cures

Will diabetes ever be cured?

This question cannot be answered – yet. We must always try to take an optimistic view, however, and if diabetes cannot yet be cured it is not for want of research. Not only does Diabetes UK have meetings to discuss research and progress, but there is also an annual European Association for the Study of Diabetes meeting and an International Diabetes Federation congress which meets every third year. In addition there are also a great many national organizations which meet regularly. More has been discovered during the last 20 years about the cause of diabetes than ever before, and during the same period there have been important advances in treatment. This is therefore a very exciting period in diabetes research and we may continue to look forward to improvements in our understanding of the disease even if, for the moment, a cure is a little too much to hope for.

I have a friend who has been treated with insulin for 12 years. He recently came off insulin altogether after having had an operation on his adrenal gland. He now tells me that his diabetes has been cured. I thought there was no cure for diabetes.

It sounds as if your friend was one of the very few people in whom the diabetes was secondary to some other condition. In his case the other condition was an adrenal tumour. When this was eventually diagnosed and appropriately treated by an operation, it resulted in a cure for his diabetes. This result has been recorded in two forms of adrenal tumour. One is called a *phaeochromo-*

cytoma, where the tumour produces adrenaline and noradrenaline, both of which inhibit insulin secretion by the pancreas. The other adrenal tumour is one producing excess of adrenal steroids and cortisone, which again produces a form of diabetes reversible on removal of the tumour.

There are a number of other rare conditions often associated with disturbances of other hormone-producing glands in the body. In these cases cure of diabetes is possible after appropriate therapy of the hormonal disturbance. Unfortunately, less than 5% of all patients with diabetes, who have such a hormonal imbalance, are suitable for surgery. Specialists are always on the lookout for these causes since the benefits from an operation are so tremendous.

Will it ever be possible to prevent diabetes with a vaccine?

There is some evidence to suggest that certain virus infections can cause diabetes but we are not clear how often this happens: it is probably very infrequently. If a virus were isolated which caused diabetes, then it should be possible to produce a vaccine which could be given to children like polio vaccine, to prevent them from developing diabetes later on in life. At present this possibility seems rather remote.

My son's diabetes has recently gone into remission following three months treatment with insulin. I have been told that this is the 'honeymoon period' and is likely to last only a few weeks or a few months. My question is, is there any way this honeymoon period can be extended and turned into a cure?

That is a very good question and some research work has been done on it using antiviral agents and drugs that interfere with the body's immune responses. The results, so far, don't show any positive benefit from the antiviral preparations but do suggest that the immunosuppressive therapy may prolong the honeymoon period in some patients (there is more information about the honeymoon period in the section on ***Insulin*** in Chapter 3). Unfortunately this form of therapy itself is not without risks and it certainly cannot be recommended at present, although it is an active area of research.

I gather that it is possible to identify people by looking at special blood tests within a family who are at high risk of developing diabetes. This sounds like an exciting development, as presumably children who have inherited an increased risk of diabetes will be those most in need of vaccination should a vaccine become available.

Yes, you are quite right. Studies of the so-called HLA tissue antigens in families, where there appears to be a lot of diabetes, indicates that certain patterns of inherited antigens carry with them the susceptibility to diabetes. Using these tissue markers (discovered by using blood tests) it should be possible to identify the children who are likely to benefit most from a vaccine or an effective form of preventive treatment should one become available in the future. It will be in these susceptible individuals that the first clinical trials will need to be done.

I gather that by studying families who have several members with diabetes, it can help find a cure for the condition. Is this true?

Family studies are very important for helping understand the inheritance of diabetes. In some families there is a clear association between a certain genetic background and the development of diabetes. Some members who have not yet developed diabetes may have the 'markers' described in the answer to the previous question that indicate that they are at increased risk of developing the condition. When new forms of treatment aimed at preventing diabetes are tested for efficacy, then it will be important to see if they can prevent diabetes developing in those most at risk. So far the screening tests are rather crude and inaccurate but they are getting better as research continues, and one day it should be possible to prevent diabetes developing in these high-risk people.

I gather there is evidence to suggest smoked meats could have something to do with the cause of diabetes.

There have been at least two reports indicating that there may be a link between the eating of smoked meats and the development of diabetes. In one it was found that there was a suggestion that children in Iceland conceived around Christmas time had a higher risk of developing diabetes. It was suggested that there was evidence to indicate that this may result from the diet peculiar to that time of year in that country, which traditionally contains much smoked meat. The second report, also from Scandinavia, indicated that the families of children developing diabetes ate more smoked meats than other families.

The common factor here is a substance called nitrosamine which is formed during the meat-smoking process. There is some experimental evidence to show that nitrosamines can cause diabetes in experimental animals and there may well be something important in these observations. We await further research to clarify this but meanwhile we should perhaps cut down on smoked meat particularly if we are about to start a family.

Transplantation

I would like to volunteer to have a pancreas transplant. Is there someone I must apply to? How successful have these operations been?

Pancreatic transplantation is still in the experimental stages and it will be difficult to find anyone who will accept you as a volunteer. Technically, pancreatic transplants are even more difficult than liver, kidney or heart transplants. The pancreas is very delicate and, as the seat of many digestive juices, has a tendency to digest itself if damaged even slightly. The duct or passageway through which these juices pass is narrow, and has to be joined up to the intestines in a very intricate way so that the enzymes do not leak. Even if everything goes well technically, the body will still react against transplant so several immunosuppressant drugs have to be given. Some of these (particularly steroids) given in high doses to suppress rejection of the transplant tend to cause diabetes or make existing diabetes worse!

Some hospitals have carried out this operation successfully. At the moment, these centres in the UK do the operation only if another transplant (usually a kidney) is also necessary, as most doctors believe that the risks are too great to do on otherwise well people. In the USA, one hospital in particular has been transplanting half of a pancreas from a normal volunteer relative into well people with diabetes (not otherwise requiring a transplant). The results show that in the majority of patients operated upon the pancreas grafts do quite well and most people can discontinue insulin injections and resume a normal diet, at least for a while.

Although this is very important and exciting, there are a number of problems which make most of us agree that it is still too early to recommend this treatment in the UK. The problems include, in addition to the significant operative risks, the need to stay on immunosuppressive therapy for ever (see next question for further information on the problems of immunosuppression) and many of us have reservations about the ethical issues involved regarding the requirement of finding a suitable normal volunteer to undergo major surgery which is obviously not free from risk.

Are there any hospitals which carry out transplants of the islets of Langerhans? Would I be able to donate my cells to my insulin-treated daughter?

No, there are no hospitals carrying out such transplants yet, and it would not be possible for you to donate your pancreatic islet cells (islets of Langerhans) to your daughter (the islets are the cells in the pancreas that produce insulin).

The question you raise is, however, an important one because experiments carried out in animals show that it is technically possible to isolate the islets of Langerhans of an animal without diabetes and transplant them into an animal with diabetes and so cure the diabetes. There are two main steps to be overcome before this technique is available for humans. Firstly we have to find a way of culturing and growing the islet cells in a laboratory so that we can produce enough of them to transplant into someone with diabetes to produce enough insulin to cure the condition. Secondly, we have to get over the problems of transplantation of tissues from one individual to another: we have to prevent rejection of the transplant. Traditionally in kidney and other organ transplants this is done by giving large doses of steroids and immunosuppressive drugs. This form of treatment unfortunately has its own risks. These risks may be justifiable when the alternative is death through renal failure or heart failure. However, in the person with diabetes there is an effective form of treatment, insulin, which carries with it in the long-term much less hazard to health than the use of immunosuppressive therapy.

Research into 'microencapsulation' of these islets is making some progress which may one day offer a solution which will avoid lifelong immunosuppressive therapy. By enclosing the islets in a porous membrane and transplanting them into an animal with diabetes, it is possible to show that the insulin can get out of the 'bag of islets' and normalize the blood glucose, at the same time as nutrients from the blood stream can get in to sustain the islets – while this is going on the membrane keeps at bay the cells responsible for tissue rejection. Unfortunately, after a while, the membrane tends to get clogged with scar tissue and the islet graft stops working. There has been excitement in the media recently about an article in the medical journal *The Lancet* reporting a successful transplant of encapsulated islets. The man who received the transplant was still being treated with immunosuppressant drugs as he had received a kidney transplant as well. This result is encouraging, but much more research still has to be done before this could be considered as a form of treatment for diabetes.

Until there has been a major breakthrough in the transplantation of tissues from one individual to another, the hazards of long-term immunosuppressive therapy for someone receiving either a pancreas transplant or an islet transplant are far greater than those of having diabetes treated with insulin. There are no tangible benefits yet for this form of therapy as a primary form of treatment for diabetes. This does not mean that the problems are insuperable but that much research remains to be done before the problems are overcome.

Insulin pumps and artificial pancreas

I recently read about a device called a 'glucose sensor' which can control the insulin administered to animals with

diabetes. Will this ever be used on humans and if so what can we expect from it?

The research into the development of a small electronic device which could be implanted under the skin and which could continuously monitor the level of glucose in the blood has been going on in the United States, the United Kingdom and several other countries for many years. The technical problems of such a device are, however, considerable, and it seems unlikely to be of use in people with diabetes for at least some considerable time. Not only are there technical problems in achieving an accurate reflection of blood glucose level by such a subcutaneous implanted glucose sensor, but the further problem of 'hooking it up' to a supply of insulin to be released according to the demand is formidable. It may be that these problems will one day be resolved and we might then hope that very much better control of diabetes could be achieved than can be achieved by the current methods. There is, however, a very long way to go yet.

I have heard about the artificial pancreas or 'Biostator'. Apparently this machine is capable of maintaining blood glucose at normal levels, irrespective of what is eaten. Is this true? If so, why isn't it widely available?

There are several versions of what you describe, namely an artificial pancreas which measures the glucose concentration in the blood stream continuously and infuses insulin in sufficient quantities to keep the blood glucose normal. Unfortunately these machines are technically very complex, bulky and extremely expensive. The currently available, rather crude machines weigh in excess of 20 kg (44 lb) and cost thousands of pounds. Their major value is for research purposes since they are quite unsuitable at present as devices for long-term control.

Their use has, however, taught us a lot about the needs of such a device in the future, when it can be scaled down to something the same size as a cardiac pacemaker. There is a great deal of research going on amongst several bioengineering groups to achieve this aim but it is still likely to be several years before the first machines become available for research studies, and it will be a long time after that before suitably reliable machines are available for daily treatment. Even when the technical problems have been resolved and it has been miniaturized to an acceptable size for implantation, the costs are likely to be a limiting factor governing availability. There is a long way to go before this becomes a viable form of treatment.

I hear that there are pumps available that can be transplanted like pacemakers – is this true? What are the likely developments with insulin pumps within the next five years?

Yes, it is true that insulin pumps have been transplanted into people as part of research studies and there has been some encouraging progress in this field. Although still experimental and with a long time to go before being a regular form of treatment, some pumps have been developed that are small enough to be transplanted into the muscles forming the wall of the abdomen and have been left there for several years. These pumps do not have a sensor to detect glucose, they simply infuse insulin at a slow rate that can be regulated from the outside using a small radio transmitter. This can be used to command the pump to infuse more insulin just before a meal, or to reduce the rate of infusion if the blood glucose readings are too low. The pumps have a reservoir of insulin that can be refilled with a syringe and needle, through the skin, without too much trouble but changing the batteries requires an operation! Although promising, the major disadvantages are cost and complexity. This is still very much a research procedure and cannot yet be recommended for routine treatment.

New insulin and oral insulin

What advances can we expect in the development of new insulin?

Over the last 20 years we have gone through a stage of producing purer and purer insulins with patterns of absorption varying from the very quick-acting to the very long-acting formulations. In recent times biosynthetic human insulins have replaced the animal insulins for most patients. We go into more detail about human insulins in Chapter 3, but basically they are manufactured by interfering with the genetic codes of bacteria and yeasts and inserting material that 'instructs' the organisms to produce insulin. By inserting the genetic material coding for human insulin, scientists can get the organisms to produce human insulin. They can equally well get them to make any insulin with a known structure, indeed they can even get them to make 'new' insulins with 'invented' structures! We are now in the era of 'designer' insulins! There is virtually unlimited capability to modify the natural insulin and see if we can improve on this: by analogy to other areas we expect to be able to develop a whole new range of insulins with new properties that should be able to make therapy better.

We are already beginning to see the benefits from this remarkable advance in scientific manufacturing. Trials have shown that one of these insulins is absorbed much more quickly than any of the existing fast-acting insulins, is very good for covering meals and can be given immediately before the meal rather that 15–30 minutes before. This insulin has now been released for general use, 'Humalog' from Lilly (see Table 3.1).

We are also looking for variations in the structure of the insulin which will 'target' the insulin more directly onto the liver, the major organ responsible for glucose production in the body. Normally insulin is produced by the pancreas and goes directly to the liver but, unfortunately, in insulin-treated people the insulin which is injected only reaches the liver after it has been through all the other tissues in the body. It should be possible to modify the structure in such a way that it can be targeted at the liver and in that way perhaps it may turn out to be a more effective and easier way of controlling blood glucose levels.

I have heard that it is possible to get away from insulin injections either by using nasal insulin sprays or some form of insulin which is active when taken by mouth. Are these claims true and are we going to be able to get away from insulin injections in the future?

There is no doubt that a small proportion of any insulin put in the nose is absorbed through the membranes into the blood stream and can lower the blood glucose. Unfortunately only a small percentage of that which is put into the nose is ever absorbed and it is therefore an inefficient and expensive way of administering insulin. Because the absorption is erratic the blood glucose is not very stable. Experiments have been done with insulin suppositories showing that they too can lower the blood glucose without the need for injections but again the absorption is only incomplete and the response erratic. It is possible that new methods will be found for increasing the absorption from these sites and making this a possible alternative mode of insulin administration.

Regarding oral insulins, it is possible to prevent the stomach from digesting the insulin by incorporating it into a fat (lipid) droplet (liposome) which enables it to be absorbed from the gut without being broken down by the digestive juices. Unfortunately again, the absorption is erratic, the whole lipid droplet with the insulin is absorbed, and there is no way of knowing when the insulin will be released from the droplet and become active. So far technical problems with this have not been solved despite a lot of research, and at present it seems unlikely that effective oral insulins will be developed in the foreseeable future.

New technology

What benefits to people with diabetes are going to come from the computer and microelectronic revolution?

You will have already seen some of the benefits in the blood glucose monitoring devices currently available, and all the modern insulin pumps rely heavily on microchips to control the rate of infusion.

We have microcomputer programs which help store and analyse home blood glucose monitoring records. It should be possible soon to simulate the blood glucose response to different insulin injections and in this way produce means of exploring the effect of different types and doses of insulin, and simulating the body's response. We are also using computers as a way of teaching people about diabetes and its management, as well as a way of testing people about their knowledge of diabetes. There is now a multimedia interactive CD ROM which contains a great deal of excellent educational material but, as it is very expensive, it is only suitable for Diabetes Clinic or Practice use. Microcomputers are being used to help record and analyse information from the diabetes clinic as well as to help to plan and organize monitoring of diabetes care and to write letters. It is quite likely that this will lead to an improvement in the efficiency of the organization of diabetes clinics, as it has done to the organizing of airline tickets and flights. There are early experiments going on in the use of so-called 'expert systems' to transfer the expert knowledge and reasoning of specialists to general practitioners in order to facilitate their management of people with diabetes within general practice, without the need for them to attend hospital diabetes clinics so often.

It is not unreasonable to expect that the microelectronic revolution will produce a lot of benefits over the next 10 years.

Our local diabetes unit has just run a successful Christmas Fair to raise a lot of money for a mass spectrometer. What good is this going to do for diabetes research?

A mass spectrometer is a very complicated machine which can be used to measure minute amounts of very similar substances present in the blood stream or in other body constituents. It is often used to measure the amounts of naturally occurring stable isotopes which can be administered to people with diabetes to investigate their body's metabolism in great detail. In the past this type of study could only be done by injecting radioactive isotopes which could then be followed in the body as they were metabolized. Radioisotopes produce, as their name indicates, radiation which can have harmful effects on cells in the body. As we know, even the smallest amount of radiation is best avoided: mass spectrometry allows even more detailed research into metabolism than radioisotopes with none of the risk. Your local researchers are very lucky to have this facility.

11

Self-help groups

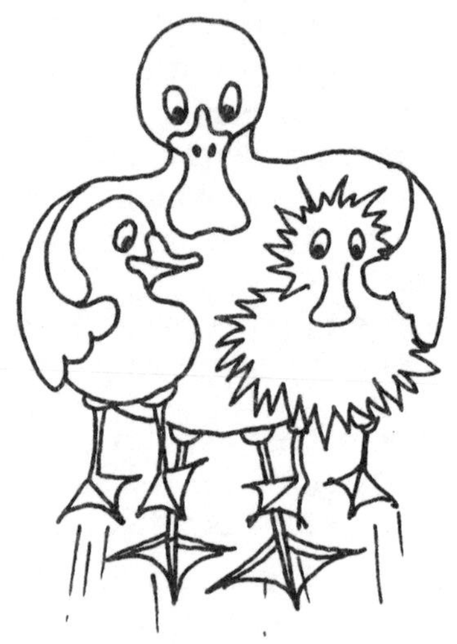

Introduction

This chapter is about the various organizations that have grown up to help their members. It is a straightforward description of what is available and is not written as questions and answers.

People react in different ways to the shock of diabetes: some try to become recluses and hide, while others set out to try to solve all the problems of mankind (including diabetes) in a few weeks. Whatever your reaction, you should make contact with your local Diabetes UK group. You will come across people who are *living* with diabetes and who have learnt to cope with many of the daily problems. These people should provide an extra dimension to the information you have been given by doctors, nurses, dietitians and other professionals.

Diabetes UK

This was founded in 1934, under the name of the British Diabetic Association, by two people with diabetes, H. G. Wells the author and R. D. Lawrence, a doctor based at the diabetes clinic of King's College Hospital, London. In a letter to *The Times* dated January 1933, they announced their intention to set up an 'Association open to all diabetics, rich or poor, for mutual aid and assistance, and to promote the study, the diffusion of knowledge, and the proper treatment of diabetes in this country'. They proposed that people with diabetes, members of the general public interested in diabetes, and doctors and nurses should be persuaded to join the projected association. More than 60 years later Diabetes UK is a credit to its founders. It has more than 170,000 members, and an annual budget in excess of £12 million. In many countries there are separate organizations for patients and for professionals, but Diabetes UK draws its strength from the fact that both interest groups are united in the same society. In the UK it is the biggest provider of funds for research into diabetes.

Diabetes UK also provides help and advice on all aspects of diabetes. The Diabetes Care and Information Services welcome general questions on living with diabetes, either by post or telephone on their Careline on 0171 636 6112. Many people with diabetes experience discrimination in terms of increased premiums, restricted terms or even can have policies refused when taking out insurance. Faced with the general lack of understanding within the insurance market, Diabetes UK has negotiated its own exclusive schemes to provide policies suited to the needs of people with diabetes and those living with them. Diabetes UK Services offers competitively priced home and motor, travel and personal finance products. For home and motor insurance ring 0800 731 7432; for travel insurance ring 0800 731 7431 and for personal finance ring 0800 731 7433. Up to date information and news is published in *Balance*, a magazine which appears every other month. *Diabetes for Beginners* is provided for newly diagnosed people, both type 1 and type 2 (insulin dependent and non-insulin dependent). Diabetes UK produces its own handbooks, leaflets and videotapes for teaching purposes, and also sells those produced by other publishers. It constantly lobbies for high standards of care for those with diabetes. Diabetic UK's address is given in Appendix 3.

Diabetes UK holidays

The first Diabetes UK holidays for children took place in 1935 and these have grown into a large enterprise. There are approximately 17 holidays each year throughout the UK and abroad, catering for up to 600 children with diabetes aged 6–18 years. These educational holidays are organized by the care interventions team and they give the opportunity for children to meet others with diabetes and to become more independent of their parents. They aim to give the children a good time, to teach them more about their diabetes and to provide a well-earned break for their parents.

Diabetes UK family weekends

The care interventions team also organizes family weekends for parents of children with diabetes. These cater for about 180 families each year. While parents have talks and discussions from specialist doctors, nurses and dietitians, there are activities for children throughout the weekend supervised by skilled and experienced helpers.

Local Diabetes UK branches

There are over 480 branches and parents' groups throughout the country. These are run entirely by volunteers and, because of their commitment, large sums of money are raised for research into diabetes. Diabetes UK branches also aim to increase public awareness of diabetes, and arrange meetings for local people with diabetes and their families for support and information.

Parent support groups

Parents of young children with diabetes often feel they have special needs – and that they can offer particular help to other parents in the same boat. Over 80 parent support groups exist throughout the UK and they have added a sense of urgency to the main aim of Diabetes UK: the defeat of diabetes. In addition to self-help, the parents' groups also raise money for research.

The care interventions team now runs a 'Parent-link' which is a network support system for parents of children with diabetes that aims to put parents in touch from a gradually expanding database. Parent-link sends out a newsletter called *Link-Up* four times a year.

Joining Diabetes UK

Diabetes UK works to influence the decisions made about living with diabetes, and the more members it has, the greater its influence. Diabetes UK cannot continue to provide its services and activities to all people with diabetes without your support. If you would like more information about joining Diabetes UK, contact the Supporter Development department on (020) 7323 1531 or write to Diabetes UK at the address shown in Appendix 3.

Tadpole Club

This is a club for younger children with diabetes, their families and friends, which sends out a regular fun newsletter. More information (including current membership fee) can be obtained from the Diabetes UK (address in Appendix 3).

Youth Diabetes (YD) project

The YD project was founded in 1983 under the inspiration of Professor Jim Farquhar of Edinburgh University. It aims to bring together young people with diabetes to share friendship, ideas, feelings and solutions to problems. The YD project is now membership based and is strongly supported by Diabetes UK and Novo Nordisk. At a national level the YD project organizes two separate events.

YD Holiday Course

Since 1983 this has been held at Firbush, a custom-built activity centre on the banks of Loch Tay. As well as canoeing, sailing, cycling and climbing, the young people share their experiences of living with diabetes and examine some of the problems in a constructive way. For further information contact Dr Ray Newton, Ninewells Hospital, Dundee DD2 1UB.

YD Weekend

This annual weekend forum has been held at a number of university campuses since 1987. It provides a forum for the views of young people with diabetes, and also includes plenty of recreation, socializing and breaking-down of barriers. This is an opportunity to develop a consensus of young people's views with direct feedback to medical services, Diabetes UK and manufacturers. If you want to attend, contact the care interventions team of Diabetes UK (address in Appendix 3).

12

Emergencies

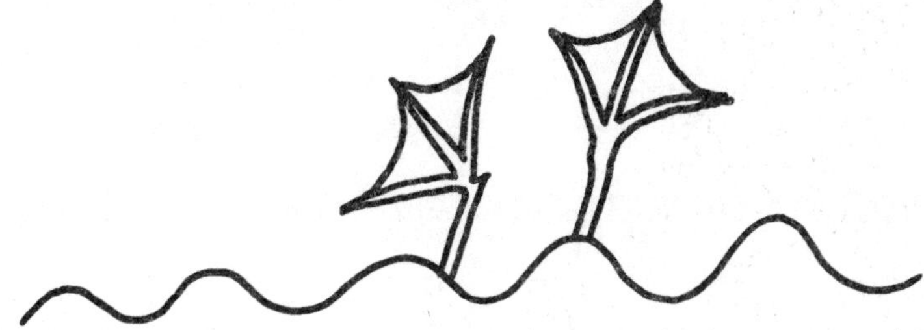

Introduction

This chapter is for quick reference if things are going badly wrong. It includes vital information for people with diabetes themselves, as well as some simple rules for relatives and friends. They are designed to be consulted in an emergency although it would be well worth your checking through them *before* you reach crisis point. It seems a pity to end this book in such a negative way by telling you what to do in a crisis. We hope that by keeping your diabetes well controlled you will avoid these serious situations.

What every person on insulin must know

- NEVER stop insulin if you feel ill or sick. Check your blood sugar – you may need extra insulin even if you are not eating very much.
- If you are being sick, try to keep up a good fluid intake (at least 2½ litres (4 pints) a day). If you are vomiting and unable to keep down fluids, you probably need to go to hospital for an intravenous drip.
- ALWAYS CARRY SUGAR or some similar quick-acting carbohydrate on your person.
- NEVER risk driving if your blood sugar could be low. People with diabetes DO lose their driving licences if found at the wheel when hypo.
- REMEMBER physical exercise and alcohol are both likely to bring on a hypo.

What other people must know about diabetes

- NEVER stop insulin in case of sickness (no apologies for repeating this).
- Repeated vomiting, drowsiness and laboured breathing are bad signs in someone with diabetes. They suggest impending coma and can be treated ONLY in hospital.
- A person who is hypo may not be in full command of his or her senses and may take a lot of persuasion to have some sugar. Jam or a sugary drink (e.g. Lucozade) may be easier to get down than Dextro-energy tablets. Hypostop, a glucose gel, may be useful.
- NEVER let someone drive if you suspect they are hypo. It could be fatal.

Foods to eat in an emergency or when feeling unwell

Each of the following contains 10 g carbohydrate:

100 ml pure fruit juice
100 ml Coca-Cola (*not* Diet Coke)
60 ml Lucozade
Small scoop ice-cream
2 sugar cubes or 2 teaspoons of sugar
1 ordinary jelly cube or 2 heaped tablespoons of made up jelly
$\frac{1}{3}$ pint (approx. 200 ml) of milk
Small bowl of thickened soup
2 cream crackers
1 natural yogurt
1 diet fruit yogurt
1 apple or pear or orange
1 small banana
3 Dextro-energy tablets

If you are feeling unwell, eating solid foods may not be possible and you may need to rely on sweet fluids to provide the necessary carbohydrate. Liquids such as cold, defizzed (i.e. allowed to stand and go flat) Coca-Cola or Lucozade are useful if you feel sick. Do not worry about eating the exact amount of carbohydrate at the correct time but take small amounts often.

If you continue to vomit, SEEK MEDICAL ADVICE.

Signs and symptoms of hypoglycaemia and hyperglycaemia

Hypoglycaemia

This is LOW blood sugar. Also called a hypo, a reaction or an insulin reaction. Signs and symptoms include:

- FAST onset

- Tingling of the lips and tongue
- Weakness
- Tiredness
- Sleepiness
- Trembling
- Hunger
- Blurred vision
- Palpitation
- Nausea
- Headache
- Sweating
- Mental confusion
- Stumbling
- Pallor
- Slurred speech
- Bad temper
- Change in behaviour
- Lack of concentration
- Unconsciousness (hypoglycaemic or insulin coma).

Hyperglycaemia

This is HIGH blood sugar. Signs and symptoms include:

- SLOW onset (usually more than 24 hours)
- Thirst
- Excess urine
- Nausea
- Abdominal pain
- Vomiting
- Drowsiness
- Rapid breathing
- Flushed, dry skin
- Unconsciousness (hyperglycaemic or diabetic coma).

Glossary

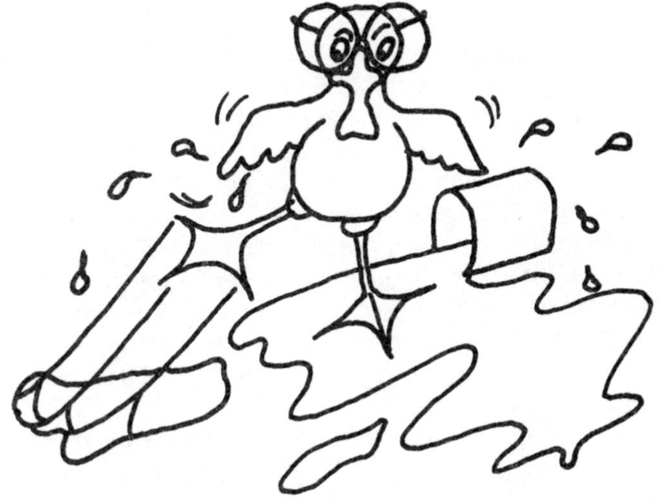

Terms in *italics* in these definitions refer to other terms in the glossary.

acarbose A drug which slows the digestion and absorption of complex *carbohydrates*.
Acesulfane-K A low-calorie intense sweetener.
acetone One of the chemicals called *ketones* formed when the body uses up fat for energy. The presence of acetone in the urine usually means that more insulin is needed.
adrenaline A hormone produced by the adrenal glands which prepares the body for action (the 'flight or fight' reaction) and also causes an increase in blood glucose levels. Produced by the body when the blood glucose falls too low.
albumin A protein present in most animal tissues. The presence of albumin in the urine may denote a kidney or bladder infection or early kidney damage.

alpha cell The cell that produces glucagon – found in the *islets of Langerhans* in the *pancreas*.
antigens Protein substances which the body recognizes as 'foreign' and which trigger an immune response.
arteriosclerosis or **arterial sclerosis** or **arterial disease** Hardening of the arteries. Loss of elasticity in the walls of the arteries from thickening and calcification. Occurs with advancing years in those with or without diabetes. May affect the heart, causing thrombosis, or affect the circulation, particularly in the legs and feet.
aspartame A low-calorie intense sweetener. Brand name NutraSweet.
autonomic neuropathy Damage to the system of nerves which regulate many autonomic functions of the body such as stomach emptying, sexual function (potency) and blood pressure control.
bacteria Germs.
balanitis Inflammation of the end of the penis, usually caused by the presence of sugar in the urine.
beef insulin Insulin extracted from the *pancreas* of cattle.
beta-blockers Drugs which block the effect of stress hormones on the cardiovascular system. Often used to treat angina and to lower blood pressure. Change the warning signs of *hypoglycaemia*.
beta cell The cell which produces insulin – found in the *islets of Langerhans* in the *pancreas*.
biguanides A group of antidiabetes tablets which lower blood glucose levels. They work by increasing the uptake of glucose by muscle, by reducing the absorption of glucose by the intestine and by reducing the amount of glucose produced by the liver. The only used preparation is metformin.
blood glucose monitoring System of measuring blood glucose levels at home using special reagent sticks or a special meter.
bran Indigestible husk of the wheat grain. A type of *dietary fibre*.
brittle diabetes Term used to refer to diabetes that is very unstable with swings from very low to very high blood glucose levels.
calories Units in which energy or heat are measured. The energy value of food is measured in calories.
carbohydrates A class of food which comprises starches and sugars and is most readily available by the body for energy. Found mainly in plant foods. Examples are rice, bread, potatoes, pasta, dried beans.
cataract Opacity of the lens of the eye which obscures vision. It may be removed surgically.
clear insulin Soluble or regular insulin.
cloudy insulin Longer-acting insulin with fine particles of protamine or zinc.

coma A form of unconsiousness from which people can only be roused with difficulty. If caused by diabetes, may be a *diabetic coma* or an *insulin coma*.
complications Long-term consequences of imperfectly controlled diabetes.
control Usually refers to blood glucose control. The aim of good control is to achieve normal blood glucose levels (4–7 mmol/l).
coronary heart disease Disease of the blood vessels supplying the heart.
cystitis Inflammation of the bladder causing frequency of passing urine and a burning sensation when passing urine.
Dextro-Energy Glucose tablets.
diabetes insipidus A disorder of the pituitary gland accompanied by excessive urination and thirst.
diabetes mellitus A disorder of the *pancreas* characterized by a high blood glucose level. This book is about diabetes mellitus.
diabetic amyotrophy Rare condition causing pain and/or weakness of the legs from the damage to certain nerves.
diabetic coma Extreme form of *hyperglycaemia*, usually with *keto-acidosis*, causing unconsciousness.
diabetic foods Food products targeted at people with diabetes, in which ordinary sugar (*sucrose*) is replaced with substitutes such as *fructose* or *sorbitol*. These foods are not recommended as part of your food plan.
diabetic nephropathy Type of *nephropathy* which may occur in diabetes.
diabetic neuropathy Type of *neuropathy* which may occur in diabetes.
diabetic retinopathy Type of *retinopathy* which may occur in diabetes.
dietary fibre Part of plant material which resists digestion and gives bulk to the diet. Also called fibre or roughage.
diuretics Agents which increase the flow of urine, usually called water tablets.
epidural Usually referring to the type of anaesthetic that is commonly used in obstetrics. Anaesthetic solution is injected through the spinal canal to numb the lower part of the body.
exchanges Portions of *carbohydrate* foods in the diabetes diet which can be exchanged for one another. 1 exchange = 10 g carbohydrate.
fibre Another name for *dietary fibre*.
free foods Foods which contain so little *carbohydrate* that people with diabetes may have liberal helpings of them without counting them in their diet. Examples include cabbage, rhubarb, lettuce, cauliflower, tea or coffee without milk.

fructosamine Measurement of diabetes *control* which reflects the average blood glucose level over the previous 2–3 weeks. Similar to *haemoglobin A_{1c}* which averages the blood glucose over the longer period of 2–3 months.

fructose Type of sugar found naturally in fruit and honey. Since it does not require insulin for its *metabolism*, it is often used as a sweetener in *diabetic foods*.

gangrene Death of a part of the body due to a very poor blood supply. A combination of *neuropathy* and *arteriosclerosis* may result in infection of unrecognized injuries to the feet. If neglected this infection may spread, causing further destruction.

gene Unit of heredity controlling a particular inherited characteristic of an individual.

gestational diabetes Diabetes occurring during pregnancy.

glaucoma Disease of the eye causing increased pressure inside the eyeball.

glucagon A *hormone* produced by the *alpha cells* in the *pancreas* which causes a rise in blood glucose by freeing *glycogen* from the liver. Available in injection form and can be used to treat a severe *hypo*.

glucose Form of sugar made by digestion of *carbohydrates*. Absorbed into the blood stream where it circulates and is used for energy.

glucose tolerance test Test used in the diagnosis of *diabetes mellitus*. The glucose in the blood is measured at intervals before and after the person has drunk a large amount of glucose whilst fasting.

glycogen The form in which *carbohydrate* is stored in the liver. It is often known as animal starch.

glycosuria Presence of *glucose* in the urine.

glycosylated haemoglobin Another name for *haemoglobin A_{1c}*.

haemoglobin A_{1c} The part of the haemoglobin or colouring matter of the red blood cell which has glucose attached to it. A test of diabetes *control*. The amount of haemoglobin A_{1c} in the blood depends on the average blood glucose level over the previous 2–3 months.

honeymoon period Time when the dose of insulin drops shortly after starting insulin treatment. It is the result of partial recovery of insulin secretion by the *pancreas*. Usually the honeymoon period only lasts for a few months.

hormone Substance generated in one gland or organ which is carried by the blood to another part of the body to stimulate another organ into activity. *Insulin* and *glucagon* are both hormones.

human insulin Insulin which has been manufactured to be identical to that produced in the human *pancreas*. Differs slightly from older insulins which were extracted from cows or pigs.
hydramnios An excessive amount of amniotic fluid, i.e. the fluid surrounding the fetus.
hyperglycaemia High blood glucose (above 10 mmol/l).
hypo Abbreviation for *hypoglycaemia*.
hypoglycaemia (also known as a hypo or an insulin reaction) Low blood glucose (below 3 mmol/l).
impotence Failure of erection of the penis.
injector Device to aid injections.
insulin A *hormone* produced by the *beta cells* of the *pancreas* and responsible for control of blood glucose. Insulin can only be given by injection because digestive juices destroy its action if taken by mouth.
insulin coma Extreme form of *hypoglycaemia* associated with unconsciousness and sometimes convulsions.
insulin dependent diabetes (abbreviation IDD) Former name for *type 1 diabetes*.
insulin pen Device that resembles a large fountain pen that takes a cartridge of insulin. The injection of insulin is given after dialling the dose and pressing a button that releases the insulin.
insulin reaction Another name for *hypoglycaemia* or a hypo. In America it is called an insulin shock or shock.
intermediate-acting insulin Insulin preparations with action lasting 12–18 hours.
intradermal Meaning 'into the skin'. Usually refers to an injection given into the most superficial layer of the skin. Insulin must not be given in this way as it is painful and will not be absorbed properly.
intramuscular A deep injection into the muscle.
islets of Langerhans Specialized cells within the *pancreas* that produce *insulin* and *glucagon*.
isophane A form of *intermediate-acting insulin* which has protamine added to slow its absorption.
joule Unit of work or energy used in the metric system. About 4.18 joules in each *calorie*. Some dietitians calculate food energy in joules.
juvenile-onset diabetes Outdated name for *type 1 diabetes*, so called because most patients receiving insulin develop diabetes under the age of 40. The term is no longer used because type 1 diabetes can occur at any age.
ketoacidosis A serious condition due to lack of insulin which results in

body fat being used up to form *ketones* and acids. Characterized by high blood glucose levels, ketones in the urine, vomiting, drowsiness, heavy laboured breathing and a smell of *acetone* on the breath.

ketones Acid substances formed when body fat is used up to provide energy.

ketonuria The presence of *acetone* and other *ketones* in the urine. Detected by testing with a special testing stick (Ketostix, Ketur Test) or tablet (Acetest). Presence of ketones in the urine is due to lack of insulin or periods of starvation.

laser treatment Process in which laser beams are used to treat a damaged *retina* (back of the eye). Used in *photocoagulation.*

lente insulin A form of *intermediate-acting insulin* which has zinc added to slow its absorption.

lipoatrophy Loss of fat from injection sites. It used to occur before the use of highly purified insulins.

lipohypertrophy Fatty swelling usually caused by repeated injections of insulin into the same site.

maturity-onset diabetes Another term for *type 2 diabetes* most commonly occurring in people who are middle-aged and overweight.

metabolic rate Rate of oxygen consumption by the body, rate at which you 'burn up' the food you eat.

metabolism Process by which the body turns food into energy.

microaneurysms Small red dots on the *retina* at the back of the eye which are one of the earliest signs of diabetic *retinopathy.* Represent areas of weakness of the very small blood vessels in the eye. Microaneurysms do not affect the eyesight in any way.

micromole One thousandth ($^{1}/_{1000}$) of a *millimole.*

millimole Unit for measuring the concentration of glucose and other substances in the blood. Blood glucose is measured in millimoles per litre (mmol/l). It has replaced milligrammes per decilitre (mg/dl or mg%) as a unit of measurement although this is still used in some other countries. 1 mmol/l = 18 mg/dl.

nephropathy Kidney damage. In the first instance this makes the kidney more leaky so that *albumin* appears in the urine. At a later stage it may affect the function of the kidney and in severe cases lead to kidney failure.

neuropathy Damage to the nerves, which may be *peripheral neuropathy* or *autonomic neuropathy.* It can occur with diabetes especially when poorly controlled, but also has other causes.

non-insulin dependent diabetes (abbreviation NIDD) Former name for *type 2 diabetes.*

pancreas Gland lying behind the stomach which as well as secreting a digestive fluid (pancreatic juice) also produces the hormone *insulin*. Contains *islets of Langerhans*.
peripheral neuropathy Damage to the nerves supplying the muscles and skin. This can result in diminished sensation, particularly in the feet and legs, and in muscle weakness.
phimosis Inflammation and narrowing of the foreskin of the penis.
photocoagulation Process of treating diabetic *retinopathy* with light beams, either laser beams or xenon arc. This technique focuses a beam of light on a very tiny area of the *retina*. This beam is so intense that it causes a very small burn, which may close off a leaking blood vessel or destroy weak blood vessels which are likely to bleed.
polydipsia Being excessively thirsty and drinking too much. It is a symptom of untreated diabetes.
polyuria The passing of large quantities of urine due to excess glucose from the blood stream. It is a symptom of untreated diabetes.
pork insulin Insulin extracted from the *pancreas* of pigs.
protein One of the classes of food that is necessary for growth and repair of tissues. Found in fish, meat, eggs, milk and *pulses*. Can also refer to *albumin* when found in the urine.
proteinuria Protein or *albumin* in the urine.
pruritus vulvae Irritation of the vulva (the genital area in women). Caused by an infection that occurs because of an excess of sugar in the urine and is often an early sign of diabetes in the older person. It clears up when the blood glucose levels return to normal and the sugar disappears from the urine.
pulses Peas, beans and lentils.
pyelonephritis Inflammation and infection of the kidney.
renal threshold The level of glucose in the blood above which it will begin to spill into the urine. The usual renal threshold for glucose in the blood is about 10 mmol/l, i.e. when the blood glucose rises above 10 mmol/l, glucose appears in the urine.
retina Light sensitive coat at the back of the eye.
retinopathy Damage to the *retina*.
roughage Another name for *dietary fibre*.
saccharin A synthetic sweetener which is calorie free.
short-acting insulin Insulin preparations with action lasting 6–12 hours.
Snellen chart Chart showing rows of letters in decreasing sizes. Used for measuring *visual acuity*.
sorbitol A chemical related to sugar and alcohol which is used as a

sweetening agent in foods as a substitute for ordinary sugar. It has no significant effect upon the blood glucose level but has the same number of calories as ordinary sugar so should not be used by those who need to lose weight. Poorly absorbed and may have a laxative effect.

steroids Hormones produced by the adrenal glands, testes and ovaries. Also available in synthetic form.

subcutaneous injection An injection beneath the skin into the layer of fat which lies between the skin and muscle.

sucrose A sugar (containing *glucose* and *fructose* in combination) derived from sugar cane or sugar beet (i.e. ordinary table sugar). It has a high carbohydrate and calorie content.

sulphonylureas Antidiabetes tablets which lower the blood glucose by stimulating the *pancreas* to produce more insulin. Commonly used sulphonylureas are glibenclamide and chlorpropamide.

thrombosis Clot forming in a blood vessel.

tissue markers Proteins on the outside of cells in the body which are genetically determined.

toxaemia Poisoning of the blood by the absorption of toxins. Usually refers to the toxaemia of pregnancy which is characterized by high blood pressure, *proteinuria* and ankle swelling.

type 1 diabetes Name for *insulin dependent diabetes* which cannot be treated by diet and tablets alone. Outdated name is juvenile-onset diabetes. Age of onset is usually below the age of 40 years.

type 2 diabetes Name for *non-insulin dependent diabetes*. Age of onset is usually above the age of 40 years, often in people who are overweight. These people do not always need insulin treatment and usually can be successfully controlled with diet alone or diet and tablets. Also known as maturity-onset diabetes.

U40 insulin The old weaker strength of insulin, no longer available in the UK. It is still the standard insulin in many European countries.

U100 insulin The standard strength of insulin in the UK, USA, Canada, Australia, New Zealand, South Africa, the Middle East and the Far East.

urine testing The detection of abnormal amounts of *glucose*, *ketones*, *protein* or blood in the urine, usually by means of urine testing sticks.

virus A very small organism capable of causing disease.

viscous fibre A type of *dietary fibre* found in *pulses* (peas, beans and lentils) and some fruit and vegetables.

visual acuity Acuteness of vision. Measured by reading letters on a sight testing chart (a *Snellen chart*).

water tablets The common name for *diuretics*.

Appendix 1
Blood glucose meters

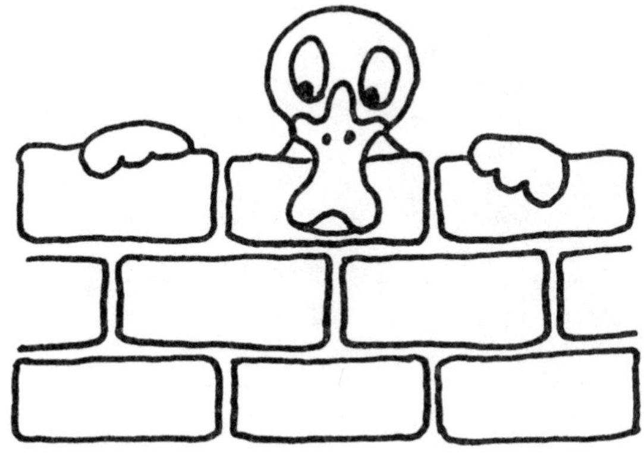

As far as we know, all the information in the table overleaf was correct when this book was printed. However, research and changes in technology mean that manufacturers are constantly updating their meters, and the prices also change at frequent intervals. *Balance*, the BDA's magazine, usually carries advertisements for the latest meters. You can check current prices by contacting the manufacturers – their addresses are given in Appendix 3.

Meter	Manufacturer	Type of strip	Time (seconds)	System technology
One Touch Profile	LifeScan	One Touch test strips	45	No wipe system
One Touch Basic	LifeScan	One Touch test strips	45	No wipe system
Accutrend	Roche Diagnostics	BM-Accutest	12	No wipe system Limited colour chart
Accutrend Alpha	Roche Diagnostics	BM-Accutest	12	No wipe system Limited colour chart
Glucotrend	Roche Diagnostics	Glucotrend strips	30	No wipe system Limited colour chart
Glucometer 4	Bayer	Glucotide test strips	30–40	No wipe system Limited colour chart
Glucometer Esprit	Bayer	Test sensor disc	30	No wipe system Limited colour chart
ExacTech	MediSense	ExacTech test strips	30	No wipe system
Precision Q.I.D.	MediSense	G2 Sensor electrodes	20	No wipe system
MediSense G2 (card)	MediSense	G2 Sensor electrodes (test strips)	20	No wipe system
MediSense G2 (pen)	MediSense		20	No wipe system
Hypocount Supreme	Hypoguard	Hypoguard Supreme	60	No wipe system Colour chart
Hypoguard GA	Hypoguard	Hypoguard GA	90	Wipe system Colour chart

Calibration	Blood glucose range mmol/l	Memory (number of results recalled)
Programme number for each pot of strips	0 – 33.3	250 with date and time
Programme number for each pot of strips	0 – 33.3	Last test result No date and time
Bar code in each vial of strips	1.1 – 33.3	50 with date and time
Bar code in each vial of strips	1.1 – 33.3	9, no date and time
Coding chip	0.6 – 33.0	10, no date and time
Programme number for each pack of strips	0.6 – 33.3	10, no date and time
Programme number for each sensor disc	0.6 – 33.3	100 with date and time
Calibration strip with each pack of strips	2.2 – 25	Last test result No date and time
One step calibration	1.1 – 33.3	10, no date and time
One step calibration	1.1 – 33.3	10, no date and time
One step calibration	1.1 – 33.3	10, no date and time
Factory confidence strip	2.2 – 22.2	14, no date and time
Factory confidence strip	0 – 22	10, no date and time

Appendix 2

Useful publications

At the time of writing, all the publications listed here were available. Those available from Diabetes UK (address in Appendix 3) are marked with an asterisk. Check with your local bookshop or the BDA for current prices.

About diabetes

Books

* *Living with diabetes*, by Jenny Bryan, published by Hodder Wayland
* *Diabetes and your teenager*, by Bonnie Estridge, published by Thorsens
* *Late onset diabetes*, by Rowan Hillson, published by Vermilion

Magazines and booklets

These titles are all published by the BDA.

* *Balance* – the BDA's own magazine which appears every other month.
* *Diabetes for beginners: Type 1*
* *Diabetes for beginners: Type 2*
* *What diabetes care to expect*

Nutrition

Apart from the books listed here, you will also be able to find other titles in your local library. Do check their suitability with your own diabetes clinic before using them, as they may well be out-of-date and include

* titles available from Diabetes UK

information that is not in line with current dietary recommendations for people with diabetes. The Health Development Agency has useful leaflets for people with diabetes and on healthy eating.

Books and leaflets

* *Festive food and easy entertaining* by Jill Myers and Azmina Govindji, published by Thorsons in collaboration with Diabetes UK
* *The Essential diabetic cookbook* by Azmina Govindji and Jill Myers, published by Thorsons in collaboration with Diabetes UK
* *The Diabetes cookbook* by Azmina Govindji and Stella Bowling, published by Sainsbury's in collaboration with Diabetes UK, and available in Sainsbury's supermarkets
* *The Everyday diabetic cookbook* by Stella Bowling, published by Grub Street in collaboration with Diabetes UK
* *Food and diabetes: Food choices*, available from Diabetes UK

Recipe books

These titles are all published by Diabetes UK.

* *Home preserves*
* *Everyday cookery – Healthy recipes for the older person*
* *Home baking*
* *Microwave cookery*
* *Managing your weight*

* titles available from the BDA

Appendix 3

Useful addresses

Bayer plc
Diagnostic Division
Bayer House
Strawberry Hill
Newbury
Berkshire RG14 1JA
Tel: 01635 563000
Fax: 01635 563393

Becton Dickinson (UK) Ltd
Diabetes Health Care Division
Between Towns Road
Cowley
Oxford OX4 3LY
Tel: 01865 781510
Fax: 01865 781551

Bio Diagnostics Ltd
Upton Industrial Estate
Rectory Road
Upton upon Severn
Worcestershire WR8 0XL
Tel: 01684 592262
Fax: 01684 592501

British Parachute Association
5 Wharf Way
Glen Parva
Leicester LE2 9TF
Tel: 0116 2785271
Fax: 0116 247 7662

British Sub-Aqua Club
Telfords Quay
Ellesmere Port
Wirral L65 4FY
Tel: 01513 506200
Fax: 01513 350 6215

D.E.P.T.H.
(Diabetes Education Prevention Treatment Health)
Diabetic Care Centre
7 Spurway Parade
Woodford Avenue
Ilford
Essex IG2 6UU
Tel: (020) 8551 6263

Diabetes UK
10 Queen Anne Street
London W1G 9LH
Tel: (020) 7323 1531
Fax: (020) 3637 3644

Disability Alliance
Universal House
88 Wentworth Street
London E1 7SA
Tel: (020) 7247 8776
Fax: (020) 7247 8765

Eli Lilly Diabetes Care Division
Dextra Court
Chapel Hill
Basingstoke
Hants RG21 5SY
Tel: 01256 315000
Fax: 01256 315858

Golden Key Co Ltd
1 Hare Street
Sheerness
Kent ME12 1AH
Tel: 01795 663403
Fax: 01795 661356

Health Development Agency
(for visits 9.00–5.00)
Trevelyan House
30 Great Peter Street
London SW1P 2HW
Tel: (020) 7222 5300
Fax: (020) 7413 0339 (for catalogue)

Hypoguard (UK) Ltd
Dock Lane
Melton
Woodbridge
Suffolk IP12 1PE
Tel: 01394 387333
Fax: 01394 380152

Insulin Dependent Diabetes Trust
PO Box 294
Northampton NN3 2BN
Tel/Fax: 01604 721325

John Bell & Croyden
50–54 Wigmore Street
London W1H 0AU
Tel: (020) 7935 5555
Fax: (020) 7935 9605

Lifescan
Enterprise House
Station Road
Loudwater
High Wycombe
Bucks HP10 9UF
Tel: 01494 450423
Customer Care Freephone: 0800 121 200
Fax: 01494 463299

Medic-Alert Foundation
1 Bridge Wharf
156 Caledonian Road
London N1 9UU
Tel: (020) 7833 3034
Fax: (020) 7713 5653

MediSense Britain Ltd
Mallory House
Vanwall Business Park
Maidenhead
Berkshire SL6 4UD
Tel: 0845 6073247
Fax: 01628 678805

Novo Nordisk Pharmaceuticals Ltd
Novo Nordisk House
Broadfield Park
Brighton Road
Pease Pottage
Crawley
West Sussex RH11 9RT
Tel: 01293 613555
Fax: 01293 613535

Owen Mumford Ltd
(Medical Shop)
Brook Hill
Woodstock
Oxford OX20 1TU
Tel: 01993 812021
Fax: 01993 813466

Roche Diagnostics UK Ltd
Diabetes and Point of Care
Rapid Diagnostics
Bell Lane
Lewes
East Sussex BN7 1LG
Tel: 01273 480444
Fax: 01273 480266

The Royal National Institute for the Blind
224 Great Portland Street
London W1N 6AA
Tel: (020) 7388 1266
Fax: (020) 7388 2034

Index

Note: the index is in word-by-word order, covering pages 4 to 264. Page references are printed **in bold** for Plates; in *italic* for figures and tables; with letter g added for glossary items.

abdomen, bloating sensation 42
abdomen as injection site 72, *73*, 75
abnormalities, congenital 175
abortion 173
abroad, visiting and living 131–4
acarbose 37, 41, 256g
accidents 10, 130, 146
accommodation for dependent older people 160
Accutrend 266–7
Accutrend Alpha 266–7
Acesulfane-K 256g
acetone 256g
acromegaly 12–13
Actrapid 52, 54, *58*, 76, 102, *103*
Actrapid Penfill/Pen *58*
acupuncture 45–6
acupuncture wrist bands 128
adhesive strapping 226
adjustment of insulin, general guidelines 102, *103*
adolescence 200–4
  puberty delayed 200
  refusing to follow treatment 203–4
  relationships 202
  resentment about diabetes 202–3
adrenal gland 237–8
adrenal steroids 238
adrenaline 84, *85*, 87, 136, 141, 152, 237–8, 256g
advertisements for diabetic products 106
advice
  access to sources 119–21
advice *(continued)*
  Diabetes UK family weekends 250
  see also dietician; doctor; nurse
age factor in starting a family 176–7
AIDS 54
air bubbles in injection syringe 69
air travel 129, 132–4
albumin (protein) 227, 228, 256g
alcohol 26–7, 68, 137, 147–9
  breathalyzers 147
  choice of suitable drink 26–7, 67
  for cleaning skin 68
  diabetic neuropathy made worse by alcohol 229
  drinking and insulin 148–9
  during pregnancy 177
  ideal limit 149
  liver reaction to alcohol 19
  reaction with tablets 38–9, 149
  teenage drinking and diabetes 148–9
  when on antihistamines 140
allergy to bee stings 140
allergy to insulin 55
allowances *see* Social Security benefits
alopecia areata 158
alpha cell 257g
alpha glucosidase inhibitor 37
alternative medicine 46
Alzheimer's disease 234
amino acids 18
amputation owing to gangrene 206, 233
amyotrophy 231, 258g

anaemia 172
anaesthetics 142, 143, 179, 185
anaphylactic shock 140
anger 141
angina 232–3
angle of injection 70
animal insulin 50–4
animals in research 241–2, 242–3
ankles, swelling 151, 227
anti-insulin effect of some drugs 11
anti-yeast cream 6
antibiotics 231
antibodies and insulin 51, 157
anticoagulants 165–6
antifungal preparation for feet 219
antigens 256g
antihistamines 139–40
antiviral preparations 238
anxiety 84, *85*
appetite 36, 39, 65, 153, 154
appointments for check-up 118
arm as injection site 72, *73*
arterial disease 29, 223
arteries, narrowing ('hardening') 153, 165, 219, 223, 232–3
arteriosclerosis 223, 233, 257g
arthritis 11, 12
artificial sweeteners 25, 31
aspartame 25, 257g
aspirin 151, 153
asthma 11
athlete's foot 219
athletics 126
  see also sports
attendance allowance 156
Autolet Lite/Autolet Mini finger prickers 105, 190
automatic injector 76–7
autonomic neuropathy 231, 257g
Autopen 76

B-D Automatic Injector (Inject-Ease) 79
B-D Lancer finger pricker 105, 190
B-D pens **10**, 76
B-D Safe-Clip 80–1
B-D syringe 82
babies
  breathing difficulty in newly born 185–6
  caesarian section 178–9, 183, 185
  care during pregnancy and birth 175
  congenital defects 175, 182–4
  diabetes in babies 188–90
  father's diabetes 176, 181
  feeding 180–1, 188
  food refusal 190
  growth related to control 183, 186
  jaundice at birth 183–4
  risk of hypoglycaemia 179, 180
  urine testing 189–90
  weight at birth 178–80, 183
  see also children; pregnancy
back problems 45–6
bacteria 257g
bad temper 255
Balance magazine (Diabetes UK) 106, 217, 249
balancing blood glucose level 19, 56–7
balancing food, insulin and exercise 62, 93, 102
balanitis (soreness at end of penis) 6, 257g
baldness 158
banana 254
Banting, Frederick 48, 236
'basal + bolus' regimen 55, 77, 134, 135
Bayer Esprit **3**
BCG vaccination 150–1
beans 29, 30
Becotide inhaler 152
bedsocks 158, *221*
bee stings 140
beef insulin 52–3, 257g
beer 5, 27, 147, 149
behaviour change 255
Bell's palsy 230
benefits *see* Social Security benefits
Benefits Agency 156
bereavement 10
Best, Charles 48, 236
beta cell 257g
beta-blockers 152, 153, 257g

Betnovate cream/ointment 150, 152
biguanide 37, 126, 257g
bioengineering 243–4
Biostator (artificial pancreas) 243–4
biscuits 25, 35, 36, 61, 67, 85, 124, 135, 144, 190
bitter gourd (karela) 46–7
blackouts 87
blankets, electric 157–8
blindness 206, 213, 214
  gadgets to help with procedures 82–3, 108, 217–18
blisters on feet *220*, 226
bloating sensation in abdomen 42
blood
  being a blood donor 157
  best finger pricker 105
  blood in stools 231
  haemoglobin 113
  oestrogen levels in the blood 171
  problems with samples 107
  sites for withdrawing blood 104–5
blood glucose 98–108
  feeling hypo when glucose level normal 100–1
  monitoring **1–6**, 99, 257g
  normal range in non-diabetic person 98
  see also glucose level
blood glucose/sugar level *see* glucose level
blood pressure 23, 94, 117, 234
  check at annual review 121
  contraceptive pill 167
  high BP 152, 233, 235
  low BP and impotence 165
blood test
  babies 189
  during infections 195
  during travel 128
  routine testing 4, 96, 110, 114–15, 121
blood vessels 218
  disease 232–3
  eye 215–16
  heart 233
blood vessels *(continued)*
  kidney 227
  legs 233
  photocoagulation 216–17
  see also arteries
blurred vision 7, 84, 255
  see also eyesight
BM Ketur-Test strips 109
BM-Test strips 106–7
boiling of syringes to be avoided 81, 83
bone abnormality (congenital) 175
books, talking books for the blind 218
bottle-feeding babies 180
Bovine Neutral/Isophane/Lente/PZ1, 52
bowel neuropathy 230–1
bowels, loose (diarrhoea) 25
bracelets for identification 160
brain
  and blood glucose levels 84, *85*, 86, 100
  damage through hypos 235
  damage through insulin reactions 88
  damage to baby before birth 182–3
  haemorrhage 235
  see also mind; strokes
bran 28, 257g
bread 27, 30, 61, 190
breast-feeding 180
breathalyzing 147
breathing problems 151, 185–6, 253, 255
British Parachute Association 126
British Sub-Aqua Club 125
brittle diabetes 121–2, 138–9, 257g
bronchodilators 153
BSE (bovine spongiform encephalopathy) 53
bunions 222
burning sensation in feet 229
bus driving 146–7
butter 29, 62, 68
buttocks as injection site 72, *73*

caesarian section 178–9, 183, 185
cakes 25, 62

Calabren *41*
calf
  muscle shrinkage 231
  pain 223, 233
calories 23, 25–6, 29–30, 66, 257g
  in alcoholic drinks 26–7
  ice-cream 36
  importance of total number 62, 68
camps for children (BDA) 199–200
cancer 13, 153, 159
Canderel 31
CAPD (chronic ambulatory peritoneal dialysis 227
car *see* driving
carbohydrates 17, 25–6, 28, 41, 61, 257g
  in alcoholic drinks 26–7, 148
  exchanges 62
  fibre-richness 30, 62–3, 68
  foods for emergency 254
  increasing intake 60, 86–7, 124, 126
  rapidly absorbed type 85
  reducing intake to avoid insulin 44, 60
  school food 198
care
  antenatal 175
  dependent older people 160
  education in self-care 119
  extra care allowance for children 194
  inability to obtain services 121
  newly diagnosed people 119–21
Careline (Diabetes UK) 155, 249
carpal tunnel syndrome 230
cartridges for insulin pen 52, 55, *58*, *59*, 76
cases for carrying syringes 83
cataracts 7, 215, 257g
'catching' diabetes impossible 10
CD ROM about diabetes 247
Centre Point Needle Guide 83
cereals 28, 30
chance discovery of diabetes 7
Channel Tunnel travel 128
charges
  chiropody 222
charges *(continued)*
  prescriptions *see* prescription charges
check-up appointments 118
cheese 29–6, 62, 68
chemical messengers *see* hormones
chemist's supplies 80, 155
  see also OTT (over the counter)
chewing-gum 25, 154
chilblains on feet 224
children 191–200
  accurate information on diabetes 208
  BCG immunization 150–1
  blackouts 87
  blood glucose rise after glucagon 89
  changing schools 197
  checklist for school trips 199
  control difficulties 191
  deafness 196
  dehydration 139, 196
  Diabetes UK holidays 187, 199–200, 249–50
  disability living allowance 155
  dislike of injecting themselves 193
  eating too much sugar 194
  exchanges in foods 62
  'fatty liver' 19
  feelings during hypos 84
  food refusal 190
  giving their own injections 193
  hair loss 158
  hearing impairment 196
  height related to diabetes 191, 192
  human insulin 53
  identification items 199
  improvements in care 119
  incidence of diabetes 9
  intelligence 182–3
  ketones in urine 109, 195
  learning ability 196
  parents' diet when conceiving child 240
  parents' worry about diabetes 187–9, 190
  permanence of diabetes 47
  possibility of future vaccine 238

children *(continued)*
raised glucose level during infections 195–6
refused admission to secondary school 196
risk of weight gain when they stop growing 67
school sports and hypos 65–6
self-confidence 196, 199
site for blood sample 105
Social Security benefits 194
surgical operations 142–3
symptoms of hypo 84
Tadpole Club 251
telling their friends about diabetes 196–7
tiredness after hypos 86
travel precautions 151
vomiting 139, 195–6
see also babies; school
chiropodist 118, 121, 218, 219, 222, 233
chlorpropamide 37–8, 39, *41*, 90, 149
chocolate 36
cholesterol increase 232–3
Christmas, increasing insulin dosage 64
chronic ambulatory peritoneal dialysis (CAPD) 227
chronic renal replacement therapy 155, 206, 227
cider 27
cigarettes *see* smoking
circulation
annual check-up 121
feet 218, 223
problems 7, 153
cleaning
injection site 68
needles and syringes 81
clear insulin (soluble, regular) *see* short-acting insulin
clinics 28, 56–7, 76, 116–21, 118, 201
eye testing at diabetes clinic 212–13
family planning 169
regular attendance essential 209
waiting a long time 117–18
cloudy insulin *see* long-acting insulin
Coca-Cola 85, 120, 253
cold, feeling 158
colds 55, 137, 138, 195
collection service for equipment disposal 81
colour blindness 100, 112
coma 89, 92, 93, 182–3, 194, 253, 255, 258g
companions helping to prevent hypos 125
complementary therapy 46
complications 94, 95, 141, 258g
avoiding them in later life 209
general questions 207–11
long-term problems 205–7
people on diet only 207
pregnancy 182–6
prevention 209
computers and diabetes 246–7
concentration ability 100, 196, 255
conception, good control of diabetes beforehand 177
confectionery *see* sweets
confusion, mental 84, *85*, 87, 253, 255
congenital abnormalities 175
constipation 39, 231
contact lenses 214–15
contraception 162–3
contraceptive pill 11, 104, 152, 167–8
control
advice and discussion 120–1, 358g
affected by changing insulin source 131
assessments of your control 120
babies' growth related to control 182
criteria for good control 57, 92–4, 99, 101
difficulty keeping control 95
difficulty since birth of baby 180–1
during and after operations 142
during shift work 134–5
father's diabetes affecting unborn child 176, 181
good only 1 week per month 103–4
haemoglobinU1cu 95

control *(continued)*
improving by multiple injections 97
ketones in urine 109–10
misleading yourself about ability to cope 115
and monitoring 94–7
necessity for strictness 94
pregnancy 174–5, 177–80
preventing/avoiding complications 208, 209
reducing awareness of hypos 87
relying on how you feel 93
trying to achieve perfection 99, 191
use of HRT 172
using contraceptive pill 168
using insulin pump 78
variation in vision 212
weight gain with good control 67–8
weight gain with poor control 66–7
young children 191
your own role 121
convulsions 84
cooking methods 29
corn remedies 219
coronary heart disease *see* heart disease
costs
food 31–2
mass spectrometer 247
research 236–7
coughs 137, 151–2, 195
cows' insulin 50
Coxsackie virus 10, 14
crackers (biscuits) 61, 254
cramps in the calf 223
cream 29, 62
antifungal 219
E45 cream 225, 226
steroid 150
cricket 124
crispbreads 61
crisps 32, 67
cryotherapy for necrobiosis 211
Cushing's disease/syndrome 12, 13
customs' confiscation of porcine insulin 131
cystic fibrosis 13–14
cystitis 227, 228, 258g

daily living with diabetes 123
danger of increased sugar in blood 5
Daonil 40, *41*, 90
DCCT (Diabetes Control and Complications Trial) 78, 94, 95
deaf children and diabetes 196
death, factors leading to premature death 210
defects, congenital 175, 182–4
dehydration 128, 139, 196
dental treatment 143
Department of Health 81, 119
Department of Social Security 156
depression 141, 235
treatment by drugs 150
Dextro-energy tablets 181, 253, 254
dextrose 181
Dextrosol 85, 258g
Diabenese 149
Diabetamide *41*
diabetes
affecting the eyes 6–7
brittle diabetes 121–2, 138–9, 257g
causes 9–14, 13, 237–40
cure 237
diabetes insipidus/mellitus 8, 258g
discovered by chance 7
first signs 5
history 17, 205, 208, 236
instability 122
insulin-dependent type *see* type 1
maturity onset in diabetes of the young 176
non-insulin dependent type *see* type 2
other diseases 13–14
poor control 19–20
smoking 153–5
so-called 'mild' diabetes 7
temporary diabetes 13
type 1 *see under* type 1
type 2 *see under* type 2
types 8, 121, 125
undetected 4
untreated 6

diabetes *(continued)*
see also adolescence; babies; children; control; glucose level; injections; insulin; pregnancy; young people
Diabetes for beginners magazine (Diabetes UK) 249
Diabetes Care Department of Diabetes UK 132, 249
Diabetes Control and Complications Trial (DCCT) 207, 210–11
Diabetes Federation congress 237
Diabetes Liaison Nurse 118
Diabetes UK 22, 28, 48, 53, 113, 119, 132, 249
family weekends 250
holidays 187, 199, 249–50
information on services 120, 146, 188, 194, 197, 237
research 236–7, 249
Website 237
Youth and Family Service 155, 194, 250
Diabetes UK holidays for children 194, 199–200
diabetic amyotrophy *see* amyotrophy
Diabetic Community Nurse 118
diabetic foods 24–5, 35–6
diabetic gangrene *see* gangrene
Diabetic Health Visitor 118
diabetic nephropathy *see* nephropathy
diabetic neuropathy *see* neuropathy
diabetic retinopathy *see* retinopathy
Diabinese 38, 39, *41*, 90
Diabur test (5000) 110, 189
diagnosis, care immediately following 119–21
dialysis, kidney/renal 227–8
Diamicron *41*
Diapen 1 and 2 (insulin pens) 76–7
diarrhoea 25, 39, 42, 231
Diastix 110, 189
diazepam 150
diet 7, 22–33
changing diet when starting insulin 60
control by diet alone 23–4, 90, 115, 120, 207, 230
diet *(continued)*
drastic dieting not recommended 67
healthy eating 28
high-fibre 231
inability to stick to diet 115
and insulin 60–8
ketones in urine when dieting strictly 109–10
losing weight 10, 34–5, 67
main recommendations 29–30
metformin tablets 101
monitoring yourself 99
parents' diet at conception of child 240
responding well to diet 5, 24
seeking advice 27–8
'special diabetic' food 25, 156
tablets and diet treatment 26, 151
for thin people taking insulin 60
dietician 2, 26, 28, 35, 66
for the newly-diagnosed person 119
digestion 16, 17, 41, 54–5
Disability Alliance 155–6
disability living allowance for child care 194
discrimination against people with diabetes 137
discussion with diabetes team 120
diseases that increase chance of getting diabetes 13–14
disposal of syringes and needles 80–1
diuretics 12, 151, 258g, 264g
dizziness 38, 84, 159
doctor
advice to employer 136, 137
asking doctors' advice 68, 104, 121, 153
conflicting advice 191
contraceptive advice 169
diabetic clinic in local practice 116–17
diagnosis of leg pains 229
fee for signing insurance form 145
frankness in discussion 208
prescriptions for equipment 80
smoking advice 153–4
specialists in diabetes 116

doctor *(continued)*
  see also prescriptions
dosage *see* injections; insulin
dreaming 89
drinks
  in emergency 254
  see also alcohol; *individually named drinks*
drips 128, 138–9, 142, 179
driving 91, 123, 143–7, 253
  buses 145, 146
  carrying food in the car 135
  high mileage in certain jobs 135, 143–4
  implications of diabetes on driving 119, 135, 143–4
  influence of alcohol 149
  influence of drugs 146
  licence application 144–5
  motor accidents and hypos 146
  rules for those with diabetes 146, 253
Driving and Vehicle Licensing Agency *see* DVLA
drops for eyes 213, 217
drowsiness 38, *85*, 89–90, 139, 194, 253
drugs 150–3
  affecting or precipitating diabetes 11–12
  driving under influence 146
  immunosuppressive drugs 240–2
  low blood pressure and impotence 165–6
  tablets 37–44
dry mouth 94
DVLA and implications of diabetes 119, 144–5

E111 form for travelling within EU 128, 132
ears 104–5, 159, 189
eating between meals *see* snacks
eating out 127
economic conditions 119
education on diabetes 120, 246–7, 249
eggs 62
ejaculation and impotence 164–5
elderly people *see* older people
electric blankets 157–8, *221*
  see also heating pads
electrolysis for excess hair 158–9
electronics and diabetes 246–7
emergencies 252–5
  alarming rise in blood glucose 128, 138
  babies with diabetes 188
  drinks 254
  food needed while driving 144
  foods to eat in emergency or when feeling unwell 254
  glaucoma 217
  hypoglycaemia and hyperglycaemia 254–5
  identification items 160
  insulin pump breakdown 78
  ketoacidosis 109
  operations 142–3
  sudden severe hypo when driving 145
  vomiting in emergency situation 254
  what every person on insulin must know 253
  what other people must know 253
emotional upsets *see* stress
employers' attitudes to diabetes 136–7
employment *see* work
energy 124
  see also calories
England, incidence of diabetes 9
enlargement of liver *see* 'fatty liver'
entertaining 127
enzymes that react to glucose 100
epidural anaesthetic 185, 258g
epileptic fits 88
equipment
  advice on supplies 120
  availability abroad 131–2
  spares 132
erection and impotence 164–5
Esprit **3**, 266–7
EU (European Union) 128, 132
Euglucon 40, *41*, 90
European Association for the Study of Diabetes 237
ExacTech 266–7

examination worries 141
exchanges and carbohydrates 62
exercise 23, 35, 57, 62, 126
  beneficial effects 120
  blood glucose level 19, 68, 97, 124
  countering depression 141
  eating snacks 64, 66, 124
  see also sports
expiry date of insulin supply 131
eyesight 6–7, 206, 211–18
  affected by hypos 100
  B-D Pen Magniguides for insulin pens 76
  blindness 206, 213–14, 214
  blurred vision 7, 84, 255
  cataracts 7, 215
  colour blindness 100, 112
  contact lenses 214–15
  damage to the lens 7
  damage to the retina 6–7, 206, 209
  double vision 230
  drops used at clinic 213
  flashing lights and specks 215
  foot care problem 222, 225
  laser treatment 145, 216
  measuring blood glucose levels 108
  microaneurysms 216
  pain and blurring of vision 217
  photocoagulation 216–17
  regular checks 94, 117, 121, 212
  short sight 7, 211–12
  test for driving licence 145
  type of testing required 213
  using syringes 82–3
  variation with control changes 212
  visual acuity 264g
  why it is affected by diabetes 215

fabric softeners 189
facial neuritis 230
faith healing 46
families, diabetes running in *see* inheritance
family
  Diabetes UK weekends 250
  starting a family 176–7
  see also inheritance
family planning clinic 169
Family Practitioner Committee 155
family studies and diabetes 238
Farquhar, Professor Jim 251
fast-acting insulin 54–5
fasting, sponsored fasts 157
fat
  breakdown in the body 18
  injection into deep layers below skin 72, *73*, 74
  level in blood 19
  non-milk 36
  too much in food 25, 29, 62–3, 67, 68
fatness *see* weight
fatty acids 18
'fatty liver' 19–20
feeling *see* sensation
feet 218–26, *220*, *221*
  athlete's foot 219
  bedsocks 158, *221*
  blisters *220*, 226
  bunions 222
  burning by hot-water bottles 157–8
  burning or tingling feeling 229
  care and monitoring 94, 121
  chilblains 224
  chiropodist 118, 121, 218, 219, 222, 225, 233
  cold weather care 223–4
  corn remedies 219, *220*, 225
  discolouration 226, 233
  dry skin *221*
  drying carefully *221*, 225
  first aid measures 226
  foot spa 161
  footwear 218, *221*, 223–4, 225
  gangrene 206
  hot-water bottles 157–8, *221*, 224, 225
  infections 219, *220*, 222, 223, 225, 226
  injuries 223, 225, 226
  loss of feeling 206
  need for special care 218
  nerve damage 223, 230
  neuropathy 230
  numbness 224, 229

pain 229, 233
poor circulation 223, 232
rules for care 224–6
signs of trouble 222–3
socks/stockings 219, *221*, 223–4, 225, 226
soreness on the soles 229
toenails 219, *220*, 222, 226
ulcers 224
unaware of extremes of temperature 223
walking barefoot 223, 226
ferry, sickness during travel 128
fertility 162, 168
fetus 175, 184
fibre content in food 25, 28–9, 62, 258g
films about diabetes 118
finger prickers *see* prickers
fingertips as site for blood sample 104–6, 189
Firbush activity centre, Scotland 203, 251
first aid for feet 226
fish 20, 32, 62, 67
flatulence 42
flour 28, 30
fluid
accumulation of fluid in body 227
emergency drinks 254
importance of intake during breast-feeding 180
retention of fluid 151
flushing sensation 149, 171
foetus *see* fetus
food
and blood glucose level 19
carrying supply in car 135, 146
cost and budgeting 31–2, 156
diabetic foods 24–5, 35–6, 258g
emergency 253
extra food and extra insulin 64
feeding babies 180–1, 188
finding out about the content 25–6
free foods 259g
labels 23, 25–6
plant foods 29
production of insulin 18, *18*
food *(continued)*
recording meals and snacks in dieting 68
right type and amount 22
school trips and holidays 199
shift work 134–5
'special' 25, 156
standard airline meals 134
weighing food 27
when to stop solids 195
see also diet; meals *and individual foods*
football 124
footwear 218, *221*, 223–4
forceps delivery of baby 179
foreskin soreness (*phimosis*) 6
free prescriptions *see* prescription charges
freezing with liquid nitrogen *see* cryotherapy
frequency
passing urine 94
routine appointments 118
fried foods 68
friends 120, 125, 196–7, 202–3, 204
frigidity 163
fructosamine 93, 114, 207, 209, 259g
fructose 25, 36, 259g
fruit 28, 29, 30, 61, 67, 85, 144, 254
fruit juice 32–3, 85, 190, 253
fungicides 160, 170, 219

gadgets to help visual impairment 76, 82–3
gallstones 171
games *see* sports
gangrene 206, 218–19, 223, 233, 259g
gauges for use with syringes 83
genes 14–15, 50, 210, 259g
German measles 14
gestational diabetes 9, 259g
ginseng 47
glandular disorders 13
glasses (spectacles) 7
glaucoma 217, 259g
glibenclamide 12, 37–8, 39, *41*, 90, 116, 149

Glibenese *41*
gliclazide 37, 39–40, *41*
gliptizide 37, *41*
gliquidone *41*
glitazones 42–3
glucagon 12, 17, 88–9, 90, 128, 129, 259g
Glucobay 37, 41–2
Glucolet finger pricker 105, 190
Glucometer 266–7
Glucophage 37, 39, 40
glucose 259g
  as fuel for the body 6, 17–18
  glucose sensor 242–3
  inability to take it by mouth 89
  production in the body 17
  spilling into urine 108–9, 112, 170
  tablets 85, 124, 125, 126, 128
  taken for hypos 85, 86, 181, 253
  tolerance test 259g
glucose level
  above 10 mmol/l, 39, 42, 56, 65, 86, 99, 110
  above 13 mmol/l, 109
  alcohol effect 27
  artificial pancreas 243–4
  associated with ketones and vomiting 139
  babies 9, 188
  below 4 mmol/l, 38, 86, 87, 129
  below 7 mmol/l, 56, 64
  children 191, 199
  criteria for good control 101
  dangers of long-term high level 100–1
  diet to reduce level 10
  dizziness 38
  driving 146
  drowsiness 38
  early morning high in children 191
  estimating alcohol effect 148–9
  extra Actrapid insulin 102
  eyesight problems 215
  fluctuations 104
  fructosamine tests 114
  giving up testing 96
  haemoglobin test 113–16
  high concentration 6, 92, 170, 180, 255
glucose level *(continued)*
  increase 5, 11, 13, 128
  instant measurement available 135
  with intercurrent illness 43
  kidney problems 227
  lack of sleep 136
  low concentration in babies 9
  lowest time 89
  lumps at injection site 72
  maintaining normality 19
  measuring 56, 57, 85, 96, 98, 135
  medicines that might increase level 152–3
  monitoring 93
  pregnancy 175, 179, 181, 182, 183, 186
  pure fruit juice effect 32
  reasons for rise 97
  related to weight loss 33–4
  renal threshold 99, 108–9
  research into complications 206–7
  retina of eye affected 212, 214, 215, 216–17
  swings over 24 hours 122
  symptoms of high level 255
  symptoms of low level 254–5
    see also hypos
  see also blood glucose; control
Glucotrend **6**, 266–7
Glurenorm *41*
glycogen 259g
glycosuria, renal 108, 112, 259g
glycosylated haemoglobin *see* haemoglobin A
GP (general practitioner) *see* doctor
growth
  adolescents 200
  babies 182, 186
  children 191, 192
growth hormone treatment 153
gum infection 143
gustatory sweating 230

haemochromatosis (iron overload) 13
haemodialysis 227
haemoglobin A_{1c} 93, 95, 111, 113–16, 139, 207, 209, 259g

haemoglobin *(continued)*
 in pregnancy 175, 184
 too high 115, 116, 203
 too low 115
hair 158–9
hand 229, 230
handbooks on diabetes 249
hardening of arteries 153
hare-lip 175
Harmogen 153
hay fever 139–40
headaches from hypos 84, *85*, 86, 90, 256
healing crusade claims 47
Health, Department of 81, 119
health centres, dieticians 26
hearing impairment and diabetes 196
heart attack 10, 14, 232
heart disease 23, 29, 63, 206, 232–3, 258g
heart failure 151
heartbeat, rapid 84, *85*, 255
heating pads, electric 158
heel as site for blood sample 189
height related to diabetes *see* growth
herbal remedies 46–7
hereditary factor *see* inheritance
Hermesetas 31
herpes zoster (shingles) 230
HLA tissue antigens 239
holes in the heart 175
holidays 128–34, 155, 198–9
 checklist of things to take 128, 132, 199
 Diabetes UK holidays for children 187, 199, 249–50
 school trips 198–9
 Youth Diabetes holiday course/ weekends 251
homes for the elderly 160
'honeymoon period' of diabetes 55, 56, 192, 238, 259–60g
hormones 11–12, 238, 260g
 disturbances of glands 238
 during menstrual periods 103–4
 excessive amounts 12
 exess growth hormone 13
hormones *(continued)*
 female hormone and menopause 171
 glucagon 12, 88–9
 growth hormone treatment 153
 impotence problem 164
 production by pancreas 16–17
 production during pregnancy 180
 steroid 11
 thyroid 12, 158
 see also adrenaline
hospital, needless trips 136
hospital care for diabetes 28
hospital operations 142–3
hot flush, facial 39
hot-water bottles 157–8, *221*, 224, 225
HRT (hormone replacement therapy) 153, 171–2
Humaject I *58*, 76
Humaject (M1, M2, M3, M4) *59*, 76
Humaject S *58*, 76
Humalog 54, 56, *58*, 245
Human Actrapid 76
Human Insulatard *58*, 76
human insulin 50–4, 87, 260g
Human Mixtard (10, 20, 30, 40, 50 Pen) *59*, 76
Human Mixtard (30), (50) *59*, 76
Human Velosulin *58*
Humapen Ergo **12**
Humulin I *58*, *103*
Humulin Lente *58*
Humulin (M1, M2, M3, M4) *59*
Humulin S *58*, *103*
Humulin ZN *58*
hunger *85*, 89, 190, 255
hydramnios in pregnancy 184, 260g
hydrocortisone injections 230
hyperglycaemia 122, 163, 255, 260g
hypnosis 47
Hypocourt Supreme 266–7
hypoglycaemia 9, 68, 84, 122, 260g
 danger while driving 135, 145
 newly born babies 175, 177, 183, 184
 prolonged attack 88
 risk to baby during labour 179, 180
 stress effect 97
 symptoms 254–5

hypoglycaemia *(continued)*
  see also hypos
Hypoguard GA 266–7
Hypolet finger pricker 105
hypos 17, 24, 49, 63, 84–91
  adjusting insulin 102, *103*
  advice on what to do 120
  after sexual intercourse 167
  alcohol effects 148–9
  at the dentist's surgery 143
  bad attacks 90, 156
  best thing to take 85
  beta-blockers 152
  blackouts 87
  breast-feeding 180
  caused by insulin 55–6
  change in character 51–2
  children with negative testing 191
  comas 89, 92, 93, 182–3
  confusion with hay fever treatment 139–40
  denying the occurrences 86
  dilemma of control and risk 95
  dizziness 38
  driving 145
  epileptic fits 88
  eyesight problem 100
  feeling hypo with normal blood glucose 100–1
  food refusal in young children 190
  frequent occurrence 86, 102, 137
  insulin analogues 54
  motor accidents 146
  night-time 64
  people on diet alone 90
  people taking tablets 90
  pregnancy 181
  prevention during exercise 124, 125
  proof of hypo 84–5
  reducing unexpected hypos 29
  related to mealtimes 65
  result of vomiting 128
  sports 65–6, 124–7
  stress effect 141
  symptoms 84–5, *85*
  telling friends and workmates 135–6, 196
hypos *(continued)*
  vomiting 255
  warning of onset 51–2, 53, 87–8
  young people living alone 90–1
Hypostop jelly 89–90, 128, 253
Hypurin Bovine Isophane/Lente *59*
Hypurin Bovine Neutral 52, *58*
Hypurin Bovine PZI *59*
Hypurin Porcine 30/70 mix *59*
Hypurin Porcine Isophane *58*
Hypurin Porcine Neutral 52, *58*
hysterectomy 172

ice-cream 36, 61, 190, 254
ice-cube technique for injections 70
Iceland 240
IDD (insulin-dependent diabetes) *see* type 1 diabetes
identification items 128, 143, 160, 199
illness
  affecting diabetes 137–43
  and blood glucose levels 87
  intercurrent illness while on tablets 43, 140
  rules for those with diabetes 138
  severe 13
immune responses of the body 238
immunosuppressive therapy after transplant 241–2
impotence 162–7, 206, 260g
  treatment 166–7
inadequacy feelings 141
Income Support 143
Inderal 153
indigestion 151, 231
industrial tribunals 137
infants *see* babies
infection
  after finger pricking 106
  causing gangrene in feet 219, 226
  ear-piercing 159
  gums 143
  needing increased insulin 195
  possibility of infection when using pump 79
  'triggers' 10, 139
  using IUDs 170

infection *(continued)*
viruses 238
infertility 162, 173
information
Diabetes UK Website 237
computers and software 246–7
foot care *220*, *221*
local Diabetic Associations 248
need for accuracy 208
pregnancy pack 175
schools and youth organizations 193
state benefits 155–6
inhalers, steroid type 152
inheritance 12, 14–16, 169, 176, 210, 239
injections
air bubbles in syringe 69
angle of injection into site 70
arrangements at secondary school 197
automatic injector 76–7
away from home 127, 199
babies 189
bleeding at site 71
bulges caused at top of thighs 74
change from diet and tablets 116
children giving their own 193–4
difficulty with injecting 74, 79
fear of injecting yourself 44, 49, 116, 141
frequency 19
future change to sprays or oral droplets 246
holidays 127, 199
importance of timing 56, 63, 64–5
increase in number 54
increasing dose at different sites 74–5
injection sites 72–5
leaking of insulin at site 71–2
length of time before food 63
lump under the skin 71
lumps at injection sites 72
missing injections in adolescence 203–4
mixing two types in one syringe **2**, 69, 80
injections *(continued)*
multiple injections 67–8, 77, 80, 97
painful injections 70
peak effects during day 63
practical aspects 80–4
reasons for this method 49
sites 72–5, *73*
'sucking-back' of insulin into bottle 69
synthetic insulin analogues 54–5
taking a long time to complete 70
technical problems 97
technique **9**, 68–72, 120
used as excuse for missing school 192–3
visual impairment problems 82–3
what to do if you miss one 56
when needed 8, 10, 18, 33, 43–4
see also injectors; insulin; pens; pumps
Injectomatic injector 79
injectors 79–80, 260g
instability of diabetes 122
Insulatard 52, *58*, 76, *103*
insulin 260g
alcohol when on insulin 148–9
allergy 55
animal insulin 50, 51, 52–3, 131
anti-insulin effect of some drugs 11–12
anti-insulin effect of some hormones 141
availability abroad 131–2
care for those taking insulin 120
changing from one source to another 51–4
changing from tablets 44, 89, 116
changing to diet alone 192
controlling body's fuel supply 17–18
coughs and colds in children 195
diet whe non insulin 60–8
different types on market 57, *58–9*
dosage 38, 40, *41*, 42, 51, 57, *61*, 64, 156
dosage during air travel 132–4
dosage for frequent hypos 86

insulin *(continued)*
- dosage increase 11, 54, 74–5, 97, 102, *103*, 141, 150, 195
- dosage reduction 88, 124, 126
- drawing up **7**
- driving licence 144–5
- effect of hospital operations 142
- emergency checklist 253
- extra insulin 102
- five common regimens *61*
- gradual decrease to none 192
- guidelines for adjustment 102, *103*
- history 48–50, 236–7
- holiday supply 128, 129, 199
- 'honeymoon period' 55, 56, 192
- human insulin 50–4, 87, 245
- 'insulin resistance' 22
- isophane 86
- lack of insulin 17
- lente 156, 261g
- long-acting *58*, 69, *103*, 144
- losing insulin while travelling 129
- the making of long-acting insulin 50
- maximum dose of tablets before insulin needed 43
- medium-acting 60, 63, 89, *103*, 134
- menstrual periods effect 103–4
- mixed *59*
- mixing **8**
- new type 244–5
- oral insulin 245
- parachuting 126
- pens for giving insulin **11**, **12**, 45, 49, 53, 54, 63, 75–7, 127, 260g
- problems and self-help 52
- production *18*, 19
- requirement decreasing over years 57
- severe reaction 12
- shelf life and expiry date 131
- shift work 134
- short-acting 54–5, 60, 69, *103*, 124, 128, 134, 144, 195
- sliding scale of insulin 142
- soluble *58*, 86
- sources 50
- stopping altogether 138, 192

insulin *(continued)*
- storage and release in body 18
- storage of supplies 84, 120, 129, 131
- taking abroad 128, 129, 131
- times *58*, *59*, 60
- trying to avoid 44
- two types in one syringe 69
- U40 supplies 131
- U100 availability 131
- weight gain 66–7
- when to increase dosage 11
- why the body needs insulin 17

insulin-dependent diabetes *see* type 1 diabetes

Insulin-dependent Diabetes Trust 52

insurance 128, 130, 136–7
- doctor's fee for signing form 145
- implications of diabetes on 119
- motor 145

insurance examinations 7

intercurrent illness while on tablets 43, 140

intermediate-acting insulin *see* medium-acting insulin

intermittent claudication *see* cramps in the calf

intestine and pancreas 16–17

iodine 226

iron overload (haemochromatosis) 13

iron shortage in body 158

irregular hours and diabetes control 135, 136

irritable bowel syndrome 231

ischaemia 224

islets of Langerhans (in pancreas) 17, 241–2, 260g

Isophane 52, 86, 260g

itching around the genitals 6, 7, 38, 160

IUD (intrauterine contraceptive device) 170

jam 25, 253

jaundice in newly born babies 183–4

jelly (sugar-free) 25, 32

jet injector 80

jet lag *see* time zones, schedules for air travel

jewellery for identification purposes 160
job *see* work
jogging 126
joules 23, 260g
jumping, parachute 126
juvenile-onset diabetes 8

karela or bitter gourd 46–7
keep fit classes 126
Kenwright, Dawn 126
ketoacidosis 79, 102, 109, 158, 261g
KetoDiastix strips 109, 110
ketones 6, 109, 138, 139, 146, 157, 189, 195, 261g
  glucose and ketones in urine 109–10
Ketostix 109, 189
Ketur Test 189
kidneys 108, 111, 206, 209, 226–8
  CAPD 227
  dialysis 155, 206, 227
  failure 227–8
  haemodialysis 227
  high blood pressure 234
  how diabetes affects kidneys 226–7
  transplantation 206, 227–8
kilocalories *see* calories
kilojoules *see* joules
King's College Hospital, London 249

labels on foods 23, 25–6
laboratory testing 99–100
labour, control during 175, 179, 184–5
lack of sleep 89, 136
lactic acidosis 39–40
lager 27, 147, 149
Lancet, The 242
lancet used in finger pricking 105
laser treatment in eyes 145, 261g
Lawrence, R. D. 48, 249
leaflets on diabetes 249
leakage of insulin at injection 71–2
learning ability 196
leaving home *see* living alone
legs 84, 121, 206, 226, 228–9, 231
lemonade 85, 148
lens of the eye 7
Lentard MC *58*
lentils 29
Lentizol 150
LGV driving licences 145, 146–7
Libanil *41*
life span *see* longevity
light-headedness 90
Lion Alcolmeter 147
lipoatrophic diabetes 74, 211, 261g
lipohypertrophy 72, 74, 261g
liver 17–18, 19–20, 42, 88, 149, 171
living alone 90–1
local Diabetic Associations 248, 250
location tray 83
Loch Tay, Scotland 251
London to Los Angeles flying time schedule 133
London to New York flying time schedule 132
long-acting insulin 50, *103*, 258g
longevity 205–6, 210
Los Angeles to London flying time schedule 133–4
losing warning symptoms of hypos 87–8
losing weight *see* weight, diet to lose
loss of consciousness *see* unconsciousness
low renal threshold to glucose 108, 112
Lucozade 85, 86, 128, 195, 253, 254
luggage, where to keep insulin 129
lumps at injection sites 72, 74, 261g
lungs 153, 183, 185

magnifiers for syringes 83
malaria 130
Malix *41*
management of diabetes during pregnancy 178–81
marathon running 126
margarine 29, 62, 68
marriage prospects 169–70, 176, 181, 202
Mars bars 181
mass spectrometer 247
maturity onset diabetes of the young (MODY) 8, 176, 261g

meals
  delayed or missed 24, 29, 127, 128, 144
  during air travel 132–4
  eating out 127
  food refusal in young children 190
  irregular hours of work 135, 144
  planning on a budget 32
  related to hypos 85, 86, 135
  related to timing of injections 56, 65, 77
  school dinners 193, 198
  shift work 134–5
  standard airline food 134
mealtimes
  arrangements at secondary school 197
  flexibility with insulin pen 97, 144
  regularity 23–4, 54, 77
  urine testing 111
measurement of blood glucose 57, 93, 96–100, 110
  doing more than normal 134
  instant result available 135
meat 29, 62, 67, 239
medallion for identification 160
medical attention abroad 132
Medical Research Council 236
medication *see* drugs; medicine; tablets
medicine 11–12, 137, 152–3
  see also drugs; tablets
MediSense sensors **4**, **5**, 266–7
medium-acting insulin 60, 63, 89, *103*, 134, 260g
meetings with diabetes team 120
memory loss 234
menopause 168, 171
menstruation *see* periods (menstrual)
mental confusion 255
mental slowing 158
  see also mind
mental states *see* mind
metabolic rate and weight loss 34–5, 261g
metallic burning taste in mouth 40
meters **1–7**, 105, 106, 108, 265–7
meters *(continued)*
  accuracy 107
  correct technique 107
  taking on holiday 128
metformin 37, 38, 39–40, 90, 101
microalbuminuria 111, 227, 228
microaneurysms of the eye 216, 261g
microelectronics and diabetes 246–7
microencapsulation of islets of Langerhans 242
micromole/millimole 261g
Middle East, living in 131
middle-aged people 10, 16, 97
migraine 86
mileage driven in certain jobs 135
milk 29, 32, 68, 188, 195
millimole (mmol) 98, 261g
mind 158, 234–5, 255
minibus driving 145
Minodiab *41*
'miracle cures' 46
miscarriages 177
Mixtard 52
  see also Human Mixtard
Mixtard (10, 20, 30, 40, 50 Penfill) *59*
mixtures of insulin 69
MODY (maturity onset diabetes of the young) 176
mole *see* millimole
monitoring
  blood glucose **1–6**, 99, 257g
  your own role in care 92–4, 99, 121
Monoject syringes 79
Monojector finger pricker 105, 190
Monotard 52, *58*, 69, *103*, 191
moody behaviour 86
motor insurance 145–6
motor racing 125
mountaineering 124
mouth, continuous metallic burning taste in 40
mucus in stools 231
muesli 32
mumps 14
muscle wasting 231
Muslim attitude to porcine insulin 131
myopia (short sight) *see* eyesight

myxoedema 158

nappies in urine testing 189
nasal sprays for insulin 245–6
nausea 39, *85*, 92, 109, 255
Navidrex 151, 152
necklets for identification purposes 160
necrobiosis 211
needles
  best types 81–2, *82*
  Centre Point Needle Guide 83
  disposable 80–1
  with insulin pens 75–6, 79
  with insulin pumps 78, 79
  re-use 81
  with syringes 49, 70, 72
negative urine tests for glucose 101
Neo-Naclex 152
nephropathy 111, 206, 209, 228, 258g 261g
nerve supply to legs and feet 121
nerves 228–31
  see also neuropathy, diabetic
neuritis 229, 230
neuropathy, 159, 161, 206, 209, 229, 258g 262g
  of bowel 230–1
  feet 219, 223, 224, 229
New York to London flying time schedule 133
Newton, Dr Ray 251
NHS Prescriptions – How to get them free form 155
nicotine gum/patches 154
NIDD (non-insulin dependent diabetes) *see* type 2 diabetes
night tests for blood glucose level 115
nightmares 89
non-compliance with prescribed treatment 203
non-insulin dependent diabetes *see* type 2 diabetes
noradrenaline 238
nose, hay fever 140
Novo Nordisk 251
Novopens **11**, 76
numbness 230
numbness of feet 224, 229
nurse
  asking advice 66, 68, 88, 104
  specialist 118–19, 198
NutraSweet 25
nuts 62
Nystatin cream 160

obesity 10
obstetric complications 175
oedema of ankles 227
oestrogens 171
oil, cooking 62
older people
  Alzheimer's disease 234
  cataracts 215
  chlorpropamide problem 38
  complications 207
  damage to eyesight 6–7
  dependence on others 160
  diabetes discovered by chance 7
  diet 21
  eyesight deterioration 217–18
  heart disease and diabetes 232
  homes for the elderly 160
  indications for going on insulin 44–5
  insulin pens 45
  memory loss 234
  mental deterioration 234–5
  narrowing of arteries 232
  not feeling particularly unwell 5, 21
  obesity as common cause of diabetes 10
  reduction in insulin dosage 57
  retinopathy 214
  warning of hypos 87
One Touch Basic **2**, 266–7
One Touch Profile **1**, 266–7
operations 14, 142–3
ophthalmologist 215
ophthalmoscope 121, 213
optician 213
oral insulin 246
orienteering 124
osteoporosis 172
OTT (over the counter) items 80, 105, 128

ovaries 172
overweight people *see* weight
oxygen in blood 113

packed lunch for schoolchildren 198
pain
  abdomen 255
  eye 217
  legs 228–9, 233
  sole of foot and palm of hand 229
painkillers 151, 229
pallor 255
palpitation 255
palpitations *85*
pancreas
  artificial 243–4
  cancer 13
  description 16–17, *1.1*, 262g
  diseases 13–14
  effect of certain drugs 150
  effect of tablets in pregnancy 177
  function before baby's birth 180, 183
  insulin failure 9, 10–11, 43
  islets of Langerhans 241, 260g
  normal functioning 63
  pancreatitis 13
  producing extra insulin 77
  starting again to produce insulin 57
  surgical removal 14
  transplant 240–1
pancreatitis 13
panic 84
papaverine for impotence 164
parachuting 126
Parentlink support system 250
parents
  resentful adolescents 203
  support groups 250
  worry about children with diabetes 187–9, 190
Parents Group, Diabetes UK 53
Parstelin 150
pasta 27, 30, 61
pastilles, (sugar-free) 25
pastries 62
patches
  HRT 172
patches *(continued)*
  nicotine/gum 154
  red patches on shins *see* necrobiosis
PCV driving licences 145
peas 29
penis 6, 164
pens (insulin) 44, 49, 52, 54, *58*, *59*, 63, 71, 75–7, 260g
  advantages 77, 79–80, 97, 127
  children at school 193
  how to use **10**, **11**, **12**
  looking after equipment 120
  preloaded *58*, *59*, 76
  taking on holiday 128
people with diabetes, two main types 4–5
periods (menstrual) 103–4, 168, 172, 200–1
phaechromocytoma (type of adrenal tumour) 238
phimosis (soreness of foreskin) 6, 262g
photocoagulation treatment of retinopathy 216, 262g
physiology of diabetes 16–20
pierced ears 159
pigs'/pork insulin 50, 51, 262g
pill
  contraceptive *see* contraceptive pill
  for travel sickness 129
pinhole device in eye testing 213
pioglitazone 42
pituitary gland abnormality 8
plants said to reduce high level of blood glucose 46
plasma, blood 114
plunger, drawing back after inserting needle 71
pneumonia 14
podiatrist *see* chiropodist
polydipsia *see* thirst
polyuria *see* urine, excess
popcorn, home-made 32
porage *see* porridge
Porcine Neutral/Isophane/30/70 Mix insulin 52
Pork Insulatard *58*
pork insulin *see* pigs' (pork) insulin

Pork Mixtard (30) *59*
Pork Velosulin *58*
porridge 30, 32, 126
post, insulin by 131–2
potatoes 27, 61, 190
poultry 29, 67
pounding heart *85*
powder, glucagon 88
practical aspects of insulin injections 80–4
Precision Q.I.D. **7**, 266–7
predisposition to diabetes 10
prednisolone 11, 12, 152
pregnancy 174–5
  antenatal clinic attendance 179–80
  caesarian section 178–9, 183
  complications 182–6
  contrasting treatment in hospital 178–9
  diabetes developed in pregnancy 8–9, 11, 35, 178, 259g
  fructosamine tests 114
  haemoglobin tests 114
  hydramnios 184
  improvements in outcome 119
  ketones in urine 109
  management 178–81
  need for good control 174–5, 182
  pre-pregnancy 176
  termination 173
  toxaemia 184
  unwanted 168–9
prejudice against people with diabetes 137, 196
Prempac 153
prepregnancy 176
prescription
  blood lancets 105
  charges 119, 155–6
  click-count syringe 83
  free 155
  Hypostop 90
  strips for testing 100, 106, 109, 110
  syringes and needles 80
preserves *see* jam
prevention of complications 209
prevention of diabetes not possible 11
prickers for obtaining blood sample 105, 107, 190
progesterone 171
progesterone-only pill 168
Progynova 153
protamine 50, 55
protein 18, 29, 61–2, 68, 111, 227, 262g
pruritis vulvae (itching around vagina) 6, 7, 160, 262g
psychiatric illnesses 235
puberty, delayed 200
public libraries and help with eyesight 217–29
publicans with diabetes 136–7
pulmonary embolism 167
pulses 62, 262g
pulses, *see also* beans; peas
pumps (insulin) 77–9
  in control experiment 95
  during labour 179, 184–5
  how they work 77–8
  main difficulties 79
  research 242–4
  slow infusion pumps during operations 142
  transplanted into people 244
pyelonephritis 227, 228, 262g
PZ1 insulin 52

quick-acting insulin *see* short-acting insulin

radioisotopes 247
Rastinon *41*
re-stabilization 122
re-using needles and syringes 81
reading
  difficulty with vision 212
  problems with print size 217–18
recipe books 22
recording, meals and snacks when dieting 68
refrigerator, storing insulin 84, 129, 131
refusal to follow treatment in adolescence 203–4

regimens for insulin treatment *61*
relationships 202
relatives 120
relaxation 45
remission of diabetes 238
renal dialysis 155, 206
renal glycosuria 109
renal threshold 99, 108–9, 110, 112, 262g
renal transplantation 206
research 236–7
- artificial pancreas 243–4
- blood tests in high risk families 239
- close control of blood glucose 95
- complications of diabetes 206–7, 208
- Diabetes UK Website 237
- eyesight and diabetes 215
- inheritance 210
- injecting air into bottle of insulin 69
- insulin pumps 78, 242–4
- mass spectrometry 247
- new and oral insulin 244–6
- new technology 246–7
- pancreas transplant 240–2
- parents' diet at conception of child 240
- production of human insulin 50
- unexpected deaths *perhaps* due to hypoglycaemia 54, 91
- vaccines 238
- warning of hypos 87
- *see also* DCCT

resentment against diabetes in adolescence 202–3
resistance to insulin 22
Respiratory Distress Syndrome (RDS) 183, 185
restaurants 127
results and discussion with doctor 117–18
retina 212, 214, 216, 262g
retinopathy, 6–7, 112, 206, 209, 211, 216, 258g 262g
- photocoagulation treatment 216–17
- proliferative type 217
- what it is 214

Retinopathy Clinic 213–14
review, formal annual review by doctor 120–1
rheumatoid arthritis 11
rice 27, 30, 31, 61
risk, to unborn babies 177–8
rosiglitazone 42–3
roughage *see* fibre
routine, getting used to it permanently 96
Royal National Institute for the Blind 218
rubella 14
rugby 124
running 65–6

saccharin *see* sweeteners
sailing 124
St Vincent Declaration on diabetes 119
sales reprsentatives' special problems 135
sandals and foot care 224
sandwiches 32, 85, 124, 148
Saudi Arabia, living in 131
saunas 159
scales for weighing food 27
Scandinavia 240
school
- cafeteria system problems 198
- changing to comprehensive school 197–8
- dinners 193, 198
- drowsiness in clas 194
- prejudice against children with diabetes 196
- resisting attendance 192–3
- special schools for childen with diabetes 192
- sports 65–6, 124, 198
- teacher and swimming 125, 198
- telling friends about diabetes 196–7
- trips 198–9, 200
- *see also* adolescence; children; teachers; young people

Schools and Youth Organizations Pack (Diabetes UK) 193, 197, 199
scouts organization 199

screening tests 239
scuba diving 125
sea travel 128
Sea-Legs anti-sickness tablets 128
seasickness 128, 129
self-care 119
self-confidence 196, 199, 202, 203
self-help groups 52, 248–51
sensation, loss of feeling in feet 206, 218
sensors **6–7**
severe illness and diabetes 13
sex and diabetes 162–3
  delayed puberty 200
  erection and ejaculation 164, 165
  impotence 163–167
  marriage 169–70, 176, 181, 202
shaking *85*, 152
shelf life of insulin 131
sherry 27, 149
shift work 134–5, 136
shingles 230
shins, skin condition (necrobiosis) 211
shock 10–11, 141
  insulin shock 260g
shoes *see* footwear
short sight *see* eyesight
short stature in children 191
short-acting insulin, 50, 56, 60, 63, *103*, 124, 128, 257g 263g
  during infections 195
  on shift work 134–5
shortness of breath 151
SI units 98
sickness 89, 128–9
side-effects
  and bad control 210–11
  Glucobay 42
  metformin 39–40
  steroid cream 150
  steroids 12
  vasectomy 169
sites for injection 57, 72–5, *73*
skating 130
skiing 125, 130
skin
skin *(continued)*
  conditions treated with steroid cream 150
  flushed and dry skin 255
  infection in feet 219
  injecting quickly 70–1
  irritation 160
  necrobiosis on shins 211
  sunbathing 130
sleep, lack of it 89, 136
sleepiness 38, 255
sliding scale for insulin 142
slimline tonic 148
slimming magazines 25
slurred speech 255
smoked meats 239–40
smoking 153–4, 177, 218, 226
snacks
  between meals 24, 63–4, 130, 134, 144
  extra energy for sports 66, 124
  treatment for hypo 85
  when drinking alcohol 148, 149
social conditions 54, 119
Social Security benefits 122, 155–6, 194
socks/stockings 219, *221*, 225
soft drinks 25
Soft Touch finger pricker 105, 190
Softclix finger pricker 105
sorbitol 25, 36, 263g
soreness around the genitals 6
soup 254
Spain, living in 132
Special Care Unit (babies) 185–6
spectacles 7
speech difficulty *85*, 255
speed of food absorption 85
spirit
  (alcoholic drinks) 27, 148, 149
  for cleaning finger before pricking 105
  for cleaning skin before injection 68, 74
  for storing syringes 81, 83
  for use on feet *221*
  for wiping top of insulin bottle 84

sports 65–6, 124–7, 141, 198, 200
  Firbush activity centre 251
  food before and after 124
  see also individual sports
sprays, insulin 245–6
squash, fruit 195
stability
  of diabetes 122
  emotional 122
stabilization of insulin dosage 19
staff at Diabetes UK camps for children 200
starch, and glucose 17, 28
statistics
  gestational pregnancy 178
  incidence of diabetes in England 9
  inheriting diabetes 14–16, 176
  insulin injections 8
  life expectancy 205–6
  loss of glucose in urine 6
sterilization 169
steroids 11, 12, 150, 152, 263g
  excess of adrenal steroids 238
  excess steroid hormone 13
  excessive amounts 12–13
  given in transplants 241–2
  injections for necrobiosis of shins 211
  side-effects 12, 158
sticks for blood glucose monitoring 99, 106
stomach, irritation of the lining 151
stools, blood or mucus 231
stopping insulin altogether 138
stopping tablets 38
storage of insulin 84
stress, and blood glucose level 14, 19, 46, 55, 97, 141
strips
  for blood testing 100, 106, 106–7
  correct technique for testing 107
  taking strips on holiday 128
  for urine testing 33, 110
stroke 165, 171, 234
studying and stress 141
stumbling 255
sucrose (sugar) 42
sugar 68, 85, 254
  added in food and drinks 20–30, 195
  in alcoholic drink 137
  in the blood *see* glucose
  in cough mixtures 151–2
  in wines 27
sugar level *see* glucose level
sugar substitutes 24–5
suicide 235
sulphonylureas 37, 40–1, *41*, 126, 263g
sun cream 130
sunbathing 130
sunbeds 159
sunglasses after eye test 213
Supreme Test Strips 107
surgery, major 14
susceptibility to diabetes *see* tendency to diabetes
sweating 84, *85*, 152, 159, 230, 255
Sweet 'n' Lite 31
Sweet 'n' Low 31
sweetened foods 25
sweeteners (artificial) 25, 31
Sweetex 31
sweets 25, 35, 85, 143, 181, 194
swelling around ankles 227
swimming 91, 124–5, 198, 200
symptoms of diabetes 5–7
syringes
  air bubbles in 69
  availability abroad 131
  best types 81–2
  care of syringes 81, 120
  carrying-cases 83
  disposable 80–1
  drawing back plunger 71
  gauges for visual problems 83
  for giving glucagon 88
  for injection 49
  location tray 83
  Monoject 79
  re-using 81
  sizes 81–2, *82*
  taking on holiday 128, 199
  use with pumps 78
  use with U40 insulin 131

tablets 7, 21–2, 37–44
  advice and care 120
  affecting diabetes 152–3
  against malaria 130
  anti-sickness 128, 129
  appetite suppresssants 36
  causing or worsening diabetes 11–12, 152–3
  changing to insulin 44, 89
  dextrose 181
  'diabetic' types 37
  diet and tablets treatment 26, 151
  dosage 38, *41*, 42–3
  driving licence 144
  duration of action 37–8, 40–1
  glucose 85, 124, 125, 126, 128
  inadvisable during pregnancy 177
  intercurrent illness while on tablets 43, 140
  making people fat 37
  monitoring yourself 99
  reaction to alcohol 38–9, 149
  responding well to tablets 5
  stopping tablets 38
  thyroid 158
  'water tablets' 12, 151, 264g
  weight loss when taking tablets 39
  see also drugs
Tadpole Club for children with diabetes 251
takeaway meals 127
talking book service 218
targets in diabetes care 119
taste, continuous metallic burning taste in mouth 40
teachers
  arrangements for school dinners 193, 198
  concern over pupils with diabetes 194, 197
  overprotective attitude 193
  school trips 198–9
  see also school
technology, new 246–7
teenagers *see* adolescence; young people
teeth 31, 143
telling friends about diabetes 196–7, 202
temperature
  feet unaware of extremes 223
  of skin during sunbathing 130
  for storing insulin 129
tendency to diabetes 10, 14
tennis 124
Tenormin 153
termination of pregnancy 173
testing book 96
testosterone 165
tests
  blood testing techniques 100
  blood tests 4, 96, 99, 115, 128
  blood and urine tests on babies 189–90
  eyesight 212–13
  fructosamine 114
  giving up testing 96
  glucose tolerance 99, 112, 259g
  HbA_{1c} 113
  instruction on testing 120
  for ketones in urine 109–10
  night tests for blood glucose level 115
  reliability of blood test 190
  screening 239
  sticks and strips 106–8
  testing arrangements on holiday 199
  see also urine testing
thiazide 151, 152
thighs
  as injection site 72, *73*, 74, 75
  pain in 229
thinking ability 152, 158
thirst 5, 38, 92, 94, 109, 255
Thompson, Leonard (first person to receive insulin) 49–50
thrombosis 167, 171, 263g
thrush, vaginal 170–1
thyrotoxicosis 12, 13
time
  importance of timing injections 56, 63, 64–5
  long time taken in injecting 70

time zones, schedules for air travel 132–4
Times, The 249
tingling sensation *85*, 229, 230, 255
tiredness 7, 84, *85*, 86, 94, 141, 190, 255
tissue markers indicating susceptibility 239, 263g
tissue transplant *see* transplantations
tobacco *see* smoking
tobogganing 130
toenails 218, 219
Tolanase *41*
tolazamide *41*
tolbutamide 37, *41*
Toronto 48, 49
toxaemia of pregnancy 184, 263g
training in diabetes for doctors 117
transfusions, being a blood donor 157
transplantation 206, 240–2
travel 128–34
  checklist of things to take 128, 132
  rules to be kept 134
treatment
  advances 237–40
  advice on individual treatment 119
  complementary therapy 45–6
  diet and tablets 26
  different methods 21–2
  indefinite length of time 12
  laser treatment for eye conditions 216
  non-compliance in adolescence 203–4
  non-medical treatment 45–7
  starting treatment 4
  unorthodox methods 22, 45
trembling *85*, 255
'trigger' infections 10
trips, school 198–9
Trisequens 153
troglitazone 43
tropical climate and insulin storage 129
tumour, adrenal gland 237–8
twins, identical 16
type 1 diabetes 8, 260g, 263g
type 2 diabetes 8, 262g, 263g
types of people with diabetes 4–5

U40 insulin 131, 263g
U100 insulin availability 131, 263g
ulcers of foot 224
ultrasound in pregnancy 175
Ultratard *58*, 69
ultraviolet radiation 159
unconsciousness 84, 87, 89, 93, 255
underblankets, electric 157
unfair dismissal 137
United States of America 132, 241, 243
university, going for first time 201–2
urine 108–13
  albumin in 227, 228
  excess 5, 8, 12, 92, 109, 255
  formation 108
  frequency in passing 92, 94
  frothing of urine 227
  ketones 109, 111
  losing glucose in urine 6, 112
  microalbuminuria 111, 227, 228
  normal amount passed 5
urine testing 263g
  for albumin (protein) 111
  annual only 114–15, 117
  at annual review 121
  at home or clinic 111
  best time of day 111
  consistently negative 101
  failure to get true blood glucose 110
  general 4, 7, 33, 99
  ignoring test results 108
  for micro-albuminuria 111
  negative to glucose in test 40
  result sometimes misleading 40, 93
  strips for testing 33
  type of laboratory tests 111
  young children 189–90
Uruguay, living in 131–2

vaccination 130, 150
  against diabetes 238
vacuum in bottle of insulin **1**, **2**, 69
vagina, itching around the 6
vasectomy 169

vegetables 28, 29, 30, 32
Velosulin 52, *58*, *103*
Ventolin bronchodilator 153
vertigo 159
vials of insulin for injection 55, *58*, *59*
videotapes on diabetes 118, 249
viruses 10, 14, 238, 264g
vision *see* eyesight
visual fields test for driving licence 145
visual handicap and state benefits 155
vitamins 139
vodka 148
vomiting 89, 92, 128, 129, 139, 194, 195–6, 231
  emergency situation 253, 254

waiting a long time at clinics 117
warning
  beta-blockers 152
  breakdown of insulin pump 79
  informing airlines of diabetes requirements 134
  of onset of hypos 51, 53, 87–8
  telling others about your own hypos 135–6
  see also emergencies
washing powders 189
water, needing to drink during night 5
'water tablets' (diuretics) 12, 151, 264g
wax for removing excess hair 158–9
weakness, feeling of 84, 92, 255
weather and insulin requirement 57
weekends, Diabetes UK holidays 250
weight
  in adolescence 201
  diet for thin people 60
  diet to lose 10, 22–3, 29–30, 67–8
  difficulty in losing 34–5, 36, 68
  effect of smoking 154
  heavy babies 8–9, 178–80, 182, 183
  how much to lose 34
  increase after long-term insulin 66
  increase since diabetes diagnosis 66
  loss in babies with diabetes 189
  loss as first sign of diabetes 5
  loss with nausea and diarrhoea 39
  loss in untreated diabetes 6
weight *(continued)*
  need for insulin 33–4
  overweight problems 33–7, 97
  recording at annual review 121
  restricting alcohol 148
  scales for weighing food 27
  why people gain weight 23
welfare benefits *see* Social Security benefits
Wellcome Trust 236
Wells, H. G. 48, 249
What diabetes care to expect 26, 94, 119
wind (flatulence) 42
wine 26–7
winter sports 130
withdrawal symptoms 38
womb removal (hysterectomy) 172
work 134–7
  abroad 131–2
  absence from work 140
  discrimination 137
  implications of diabetes 119
  irregular hours 135, 136
  shift work 134–5, 136
  stopping because of brittle diabetes 122
  warning fellow employees of hypos 135–6
workouts at home 126
worry *see* stress
wrist bands for seasickness 128
wrist operation (carpal tunnel syndrome) 230

X-ray of luggage containing insulin 129

yeast infection 6, 170
yoghurt 25, 32, 67, 195, 254
young people
  alcohol and diabetes 148–9
  arterial disease 233
  becoming well without insulin 4–5
  depression 141
  diabetes discovered by chance 7
  diabetes in the young 187–8
  diabetic nephropathy 206

young people *(continued)*
difficulty in keeping control of diabetes 95
difficulty in losing weight 68
examination stress 141
eyesight affected 6–7
'fatty liver' 19
hypos 86–7
impotence and diabetes 166
insulin essential 21, 49
living alone/away from home 90–1, 201–2
maturity onset diabetes 176, 261g
smoking 153
socializing 251
special clinics 118
twins 16
type of diabetes 8
Youth Diabetes (YD) project 251
see also adolescents
Youth Department of Diabetes UK 155, 194, 250
Youth Diabetes (YD) project 251
youth organizations 193, 199

zinc 50, 55
ZN insulin 69

Epilepsy at your fingertips
£14.99
Brian Chappell and Dr Pamela Crawford

The authors answer over 220 real questions from people with epilepsy – giving you the knowledge to lead an active and fulfilled life!

Kidney failure explained
£14.99
Dr Andy Stein and Janet Wild

Everything you always wanted to know about dialysis and transplants but were afraid to ask.

> 'I would recommend this book to all kidney patients, new or old, as standard reading.'
> *Professor John Walls, Leicester General Hospital*

Eczema and your child
£11.99
Dr Tim Mitchell, Dr David Paige and Karen Spowart

This practical and medically accurate handbook will guide you through the maze of old wives' tales, unscientific advice and outdated treatments.

> 'The tone of the book is very sensible and considered. It addresses the questions we are asked all the time.'
> *Mercy Jeyasingham, Director of Education and Information, National Eczema Society*

Your child's epilepsy £11.99
Dr Richard Appleton, Brian Chappell and Margaret Beirne

If your child has epilepsy, you will find this practical guide invaluable.

Of related interest:

Vital diabetes
NEW SECOND EDITION! £14.99
Dr Charles Fox and Mary MacKinnon

If you are a busy healthcare professional involved in primary care diabetes, this brief and practical book is a must for you. It presents all the vital facts and figures of diabetes care in an easy-to-use format. This handy reference book gives you the confidence of knowing that you are up to date with the facts and can advise your patients with confidence.

Providing diabetes care in general practice
£21.95
Mary MacKinnon

This practical handbook contains everything you need to know to manage people with diabetes in primary care.

Mary MacKinnon's 'bible' gives you all the back-up and information you need to run a high-quality, effective diabetes service within your practice – in just 320 pages.

Diabetes in the real world
£19.95
Dr Charles Fox and Dr Tony Pickering

This is the real world, inhabited by real people, and by GPs with limited resources and a desperate shortage of time – rather than the artificially ordered environment of the textbook.

Charles Fox and Tony Pickering confront the issues and problems of diabetes care in general practice, from the perspective of the GP at the coal face.

PRIORITY ORDER FORM

Cut out or photocopy this form and send it (post free in the UK) to:

Class Publishing Customer Service
FREEPOST (no stamp needed)
LONDON W6 7BR

Tel: 01752 202301

Fax: 01752 202333

Please send me urgently
(tick boxes below)

Post included price per copy (UK only)

☐	**Diabetes at your fingertips** (Ref: 62 79 6)	£17.99
☐	**Heart health at your fingertips** (Ref: 90 09 8)	£17.99
☐	**Stroke at your fingertips** (Ref: 62 98 2)	£17.99
☐	**Multiple sclerosis at your fingertips** (Ref: 62 94 X)	£17.99
☐	**Asthma at your fingertips** (Ref: 90 06 3)	£17.99
☐	**High blood pressure at your fingertips** (Ref: 62 81 8)	£17.99
☐	**Stop that heart attack!** (Ref: 62 85 0)	£17.99
☐	**Psoriasis at your fingertips** (Ref: 62 99 0)	£17.99
☐	**Cancer at your fingertips** (Ref: 62 56 7)	£17.99
☐	**Epilepsy at your fingertips** (Ref: 62 51 6)	£17.99
☐	**Kidney failure explained** (Ref: 62 90 7)	£17.99
☐	**Eczema and your child** (Ref: 62 86 97)	£14.99
☐	**Your child's epilepsy** (Ref: 62 61 3)	£14.99
☐	**Vital diabetes** (Ref: 62 93 1)	£17.99
☐	**Providing diabetes care in general practice** (Ref: 62 74 5)	£24.95
☐	**Diabetes in the real world** (Ref: 62 53 2)	£22.95

TOTAL: _____

Easy ways to pay

Cheque: I enclose a cheque payable to Class Publishing for £__________

Credit card: please debit my ☐ Access ☐ Visa ☐ Amex ☐ Switch

Number: Expiry date:

Name

My address for delivery is

Town County Postcode

Telephone number (in case of query)

Credit card billing address if different from above

Town County Postcode

Class Publishing's guarantee: remember that if, for any reason, you are not satisfied with these books, we will refund all your money, without any questions asked. Prices and VAT rates may be altered for reasons beyond our control.

REF: DAYF4